Health and Disease
in Old Age

Health and Disease in Old Age

Edited by

John W. Rowe, M.D.

Associate Professor of Medicine and Director, Division on Aging, Harvard Medical School; Chief, Gerontology Division, Beth Israel and Brigham and Women's Hospitals; Director, Geriatric Research Education Clinical Center, Veterans Administration Outpatient Clinic, Boston

Richard W. Besdine, M.D.

Assistant Professor of Medicine and Director, Geriatric Fellowship Training Program, Division on Aging, Harvard Medical School; Director, Geriatric Medical Education, Hebrew Rehabilitation Center for Aged; Gerontology Division, Beth Israel and Brigham and Women's Hospitals, Boston

Little, Brown and Company, Boston

Contents

Contributing Authors

Burt Alan Adelman, M.D.
Instructor in Medicine, Harvard Medical School; Director, Geriatric
Rehabilitation Unit, Brigham and Women's Hospitals, Boston

Jerry Avorn, M.D.
Assistant Professor, Social Medicine and Health Policy, Harvard Medical School;
Staff Internist and Member, Gerontology Division, Beth Israel Hospital, Boston

Richard W. Besdine, M.D.
Assistant Professor of Medicine and Director, Geriatric Fellowship Training
Program, Division on Aging, Harvard Medical School; Director, Geriatric
Medical Education, Hebrew Rehabilitation Center for Aged; Gerontology
Division, Beth Israel and Brigham and Women's Hospitals, Boston

Louis R. Caplan, M.D.
Professor of Neurology, University of Chicago, Pritzker School of Medicine;
Chairman, Department of Neurology, Michael Reese Hospital, Chicago

Gary Gerstenblith, M.D.
Assistant Professor of Medicine, The Johns Hopkins University School of
Medicine; Physician, Department of Medicine, Cardiology Division, The Johns
Hopkins Hospital, Baltimore

David F. Giansiracusa, M.D.
Assistant Professor of Medicine, University of Massachusetts Medical School,
Rheumatology Unit, University of Massachusetts Medical Center, Worcester

Barbara A. Gilchrest, M.D.
Assistant Professor of Dermatology, Harvard Medical School; Assistant
Dermatologist, Dermatology Department, Beth Israel Hospital, Boston

Fred G. Kantrowitz, M.D.
Assistant Professor of Medicine, Harvard Medical School; Chief, Rheumatology
Unit, Beth Israel Hospital, Boston

Edward G. Lakatta, M.D.
Chief, Cardiovascular Section, National Institute on Aging, National Institutes
of Health; Assistant Professor of Medicine, Department of Medicine,
Cardiology Division, The Johns Hopkins Hospital, Baltimore

Benjamin Liptzin, M.D.
Assistant Professor of Psychiatry, Harvard Medical School, Boston; Geriatric
Psychiatry Unit, McLean Hospital, Belmont, Massachusetts

Kenneth L. Minaker, M.D.
Instructor in Medicine, Harvard Medical School; Gerontology Division, Beth Israel and Brigham and Women's Hospitals, Boston

Neil M. Resnick, M.D.
Instructor in Medicine, Harvard Medical School, Gerontology Division, Beth Israel and Brigham and Women's Hospitals, Boston

Richard M. Rose, M.D.
Instructor in Medicine, Harvard Medical School; Assistant in Medicine, New England Deaconess Hospital, Boston

John W. Rowe, M.D.
Associate Professor of Medicine and Director, Division on Aging, Harvard Medical School; Chief, Gerontology Division, Beth Israel and Brigham and Women's Hospitals; Director, Geriatric Research Education Clinical Center, Veterans Administration Outpatient Clinic, Boston

Carl Salzman, M.D.
Associate Professor, Department of Psychiatry, Harvard Medical School; Director, Psychopharmacology Research, Massachusetts Mental Health Center, Boston

Scott T. Weiss, M.D.
Assistant in Medicine and Associate Chief, Pulmonary Unit, Beth Israel Hospital; Assistant Professor of Medicine, Harvard Medical School, Boston

Terrie T. Wetle, Ph.D.
Macy Fellow and Assistant Professor of Medicine, Division of Health Policy and Education and Division on Aging, Harvard Medical School, Boston

Vernon R. Young, Ph.D.
Professor of Nutritional Biochemistry, Department of Nutrition and Food Science, Massachusetts Institute of Technology, Cambridge

Preface

The past 10 years have seen American geriatrics advance from obscurity to visibility through numerous programs in medical schools and teaching hospitals. This increasing interest has been accompanied by an increased demand for educational materials and curriculum offerings in geriatric medicine at the undergraduate levels. We offer this textbook in the hope that it will be of value to medical students, physicians-in-training, and practitioners. In its development, we have attempted to strike a balance between the desire for completeness and the recognition that much of what is generally considered to be geriatric medicine is discussed very adequately in textbooks of primary care or general internal medicine.

This book has several characteristics that we hope will make it useful. We have included substantial information about the normal physiologic and psychosocial changes that occur with age, both in introductory chapters and in the initial portions of each individual chapter. This reflects our belief that much of the influence of age on disease presentation, response to treatment, and ensuing complications results from the interaction of a disease process with an age-altered physiologic substrate. The juxtaposition of normal age-related changes and disease characteristics should help the physician to identify the separate clinical consequences of aging and disease. This book generally contains information only on diseases that occur late in life or that present special characteristics in the elderly as compared to younger individuals. Since our aim was to write a book that could appropriately serve as a supplement to a more general text rather than to reproduce a textbook of internal medicine, we have chosen not to include information regarding many diseases and, in the case of hematology, an entire organ system. We have included subjects not usually found in general texts, such as the biology and physiology of aging, the social context of geriatric medicine, long-term care, nutrition, ethical issues in geriatrics, and a consideration of the research methodologies appropriate for clinical gerontologic investigations.

We hope that this book will provide physicians with a gerontologic data base and with principles of geriatric medical practice so that they can better arm themselves to care for the disproportionate burden of illness borne by our increasingly large elderly population.

J. W. R.
R. W. B.

1. The Data Base of Geriatric Medicine

Richard W. Besdine

For a generation in many western European countries, medical education and health care have had a special focus on the elderly; Britain has even developed a specialty with freestanding academic and service departments. In the United States, however, little special attention has been given to old people, either in terms of medical education or in health care systems design [1,2]. Congress in 1976 identified gaps in physician education and expressed concern about the capability of American practitioners to meet successfully the medical care needs of an increasing number of old people in the population [3]. In 1974, only one program was offering postgraduate training in geriatrics [4].

Recently, an extensive report by the Institute of Medicine of the National Academy of Sciences [5] recommended substantial specific innovation in American medical education, both predoctoral and postdoctoral, in order to provide information about aging. The goal in America should not be the creation of another clinical specialty, since there already exist adequate numbers of physicians who could provide care for elderly patients [6]; rather, establishment of an academic specialty was recommended to equip the educational mainstream with information enabling students, house staff, and practicing physicians to manage sickness and disability in the American elderly population. The data base needing to be taught is both broad in perspective and disease-specific. Its major components include demography, health care delivery, gerontology (study of normal aging), and geriatric medicine (disease in old age). *Geriatrics* is a general term that covers relevant information in all four areas. This chapter will outline the components of the data base required in the health care of elderly individuals, emphasizing the interrelationships among the multiple disciplines needed for successful treatment of elderly Americans.

Demography

Like Europe before us and developing nations in the future, the United States population is becoming top-heavy with elders. Many factors have collaborated over the past century to "age" our society. Understanding the greying of America provides the clinician with an important perspective. The longest-lived Americans are no older today than during the Revolutionary War, the aged survivors still living approximately 100 years. Maximum human life span has not changed [7], but a dramatic increase in average life expectancy has allowed many more people to survive into old age, creating a new medical care need in Western countries that Bernard Isaacs has called "the survival of the unfittest." Previously unimagined numbers of people are surviving into extreme old age with burdens of disease,

1

social disadvantage, emotional vulnerability, and the inevitable poverty such burdens create [8]. Average life expectancy in America has increased by more than 25 years for an individual during the twentieth century—from 47 years in 1900 to 73 years in 1980 [9]. In the next 50 years the elderly population will double, reaching more than 50 million individuals, while the total United States population growth is projected at only 40 percent, resulting in more than one in five citizens being over 65 years of age. The "old-old" subset of elderly will increase even faster. Americans older than 75 years of age will increase from 35 percent to 45 percent of the elderly population, and those 85 years of age and older will increase threefold, from two million to six million individuals [10]. The American demographic shift toward old age demands adequate preparation, both attitudinal and educational, by health care providers.

Normal Aging

Gerontology, the study of normal aging, draws from all of the biobehavioral sciences that contribute to our understanding of changing human function (see Chap. 2). Gerontologic investigation attempts to distinguish effects of normal healthy aging from disease effects. As people age and disease becomes more prevalent, healthy subjects for study are harder to find. Many studies have included impaired elderly subjects; these erroneously attribute observed differences between young and old to aging when the differences actually arise from disease. Furthermore, cross-sectional studies, which are relatively easy to do, may be less useful than longitudinal studies, which are difficult because of subject dropout and the long life span of humans [11]. Although generalizations are dangerous, especially since variability increases with age, most age-related biologic changes show growth and development peaking at or before age 30 with subsequent linear decline until death, even into the ninth decade. Biologic functions declining with age include: renal blood flow and creatinine clearance, cardiac output, glucose tolerance, vital capacity of the lung, lean body mass, and cellular immunity [12]; but, synthetic and metabolic liver functions and total lung capacity remain the same across the age spectrum, and secretion of antidiuretic hormone in response to osmolar stimuli actually increases with age [13]. Although there is certainly need for more good human aging research, a body of gerontologic data does now exist and knowledge is accumulating rapidly. These relevant data are the intellectual frontier of geriatric care and must be assimilated into the specifics of diagnosis and treatment for the elderly. Most physicians have not been taught fundamental data about normal human aging and thus do not know what to expect in terms of cardiac output, kidney function, blood pressure, ventilatory capacity, or glucose removal in a healthy old person. When illness is superimposed on normal age-related changes, the classic parallel lines of normal human biology and disease converge at the elderly patient, causing a dilemma for the clinician unschooled in gerontology. The need for detailed elucidation of normal biologic aging is obvious when we consider the potential for confusion in the practitioner encountering a sick old person. This patient has biobehavioral and functional abnormalities not found in younger healthy individuals, but whether the observed differences are attributable to normal aging or disease cannot be ascertained without a detailed understanding of the multifarious changes resulting from normal human aging. Only with a clear view of normative age-related changes can a sick old person be properly evaluated and treated. Ignorance of these data have two equally dangerous consequences. First, normal, age-related changes may be attributed to disease, initiating treatment that will certainly be ineffective and will likely do harm. Alternatively, disease effects are mistakenly attributed to normal aging and neglected, allowing unchecked progression of a potentially treatable underlying disease. A third outcome, and perhaps the most destructive, is the avoidance of elderly patients altogether by clinicians frustrated and discouraged by unsuccessful interactions with aged individuals whose multiple problems have disease and age-related components.

Health Care Delivery
USE OF HEALTH SERVICES BY THE ELDERLY

Disability, doctor visits, and disease are more prevalent in the elderly and generate increased use of health care services. The prevalence of disease and disability rises sharply with age and is highest in the very segment of the elderly population increasing the most rapidly of all, the old-old. The rapidly growing group of increasingly old and infirm citizens is making demands on the traditional health care delivery system that are qualitatively different from any experienced before. These demands will continue to escalate, and the strain on the health care system will increase disproportionately since the elderly, having more illness, use more services. Although only 11 percent of our population, Americans over 65 account for 40 percent of our "acute" hospital bed days, buy one-quarter of all prescription drugs, spend 30 percent of our over 160-billion-dollar health budget, and account for more than 50 percent of the 40-billion-dollar federal health budget [14]. Nursing home care cost 10 billion dollars in 1976, rose to 21.6 billion in 1980, and in 1990 is expected to reach 75 billion dollars [15]! As early as 1972, institutional beds used for long-term care were more numerous than acute-care hospital beds. Currently the 1.3 million nursing home beds (1.1 million occupants over age 65) outnumber the 850,000 hospital beds used for short-term care by a ratio of more than 3 : 2. With only 5 percent of Americans over 65 years old in nursing homes, it seems reasonable to regard the nursing home experience as largely irrelevant to American elderly in spite of the high cost. Individuals currently 65 years of age and older, however, have a 20 percent chance of being admitted to a nursing home in their remaining lifetime. People over age 80 are much more likely to die in nursing homes than in their own homes.

IMPORTANCE OF EARLY DETECTION OF DISEASE

As disease progresses undetected in elders, prolonged disability and permanent functional losses become increasingly likely. Since illness and loss are predictable, at least statistically, identification of the high-risk elderly and periodic checking for a decline in health is a sensible approach to improving care of older Americans. As informal support networks in communities become less available to provide home-delivered services for dependent elderly (because nuclear families are replacing extended ones, and care-giving daughters and daughters-in-law are entering the work force), the demand for expensive, formal community and institutional services will continue to rise. Early detection of illness and prevention of disability in older people will therefore likely save money on total service consumption and improve life quality by maximizing independence. It is likely that an early detection program will result in higher aggregate costs early on because of the increased demand generated by case-finding and referrals. In the long run, however, overall costs should be lower because of early, less costly interventions that will delay costlier interventions and long-term institutionalization.

The concept of risk is crucial in developing better health services for elderly Americans. One definition of high risk is heavy health service consumption, including long-term institutional care. Although only 5 percent of older Americans live in long-term care institutions at any one time, for each aged nursing home resident there are at least two home-dwelling elderly who qualify for institutional care and differ from the nursing home group primarily in having a capable family network providing the informal supports that allow continued community-dwelling [16]. The most impaired, high service–consuming elderly comprise 15 to 20 percent of the population over 65 years old and are at highest risk for health-related decline.

The frail elderly are those at highest risk for decline based on health-related problems. Careful surveillance of their condition is crucial to detecting early decline based on illness and preventing functional losses that reduce life quality and increase cost. The high-risk, community-dwelling elderly are identifiable by five markers [17]. Those over 75 years of age are three to five times more likely to require assistance due to health impairment than are 65- to 74-year-olds, making advanced age a first reasonable marker. Elderly persons living alone are at greater risk, if only because decline is less likely to be noticed. Persons recently bereaved are at greatly increased risk to become ill and even die in the grieving period and post-bereavement year. Elderly individuals recently discharged from hospitals have a one in four chance of rehospitalization in the following year, marking increased risk. Others who would appear to have increased risk but for whom the risk has not been documented include aged persons with cognitive loss (demented), mobility problems, or incontinence.

The most frail Americans generally reside in nursing homes where round-the-clock "surveillance" already exists. Unfortunately, high-quality surveillance in most long-term care facilities is sadly lacking for a variety of reasons. Most nursing homes are understaffed, particularly with well-trained professionals who are best qualified to assess and monitor the health status and function of patients. Physicians, when they appear in the facility, tend to be oriented toward acute illness crises and are likely to see only those patients identified as "having a problem." Registered nurses have become so administratively burdened that their patient contact is primarily limited to that care that, by law, only they can provide. They therefore are unlikely to monitor patient function in a systematic way and may only become aware of decline if it is called to their attention by aides or other staff. Finally, the nursing home, both by its structure and in societal attitudes toward it, presents multiple incentives to dependency. Decline in independent function may be viewed by family and staff as a "natural adjustment" to the nursing home setting. New initiatives are needed in nursing homes to alert staff to a surveillance role and to prevent unrecognized decline.

ILLNESS BEHAVIOR IN THE ELDERLY
Underreporting of Illness
The first, and a pervasive, phenomenon partly responsible for advanced disease states engendering major disability in frail elderly is the failure of the elderly themselves to report illness. Legitimate symptoms heralding serious but often treatable disease are concealed, or at least not reported, by elderly patients. The first suggestion that older persons did not seek medical attention when suffering health-related functional decline came from Scotland. In the 1950s and 1960s, several pioneer geriatricians screened elderly individuals, seeking information about illness behavior, suspecting that verifiable differences might underlie the clinical impression that old people did not seek medical care promptly when ill [18,19]. The findings in these and subsequent corroborating studies were surprising, even to the investigators. An iceberg of concealed disease was discovered among Scottish elderly enrolled in the British National Health Service, which appeared to have the necessary features to provide adequate service to the elderly: doctors responsible for each older person's outpatient care, free care, and numerous, accessible doctors' offices. Yet startling numbers of problems hitherto unknown to and untreated by the patient's responsible physician were discovered. Nor were the problems esoteric, requiring sophisticated diagnostic methodology. Frequently encountered disorders included congestive heart failure, correctable hearing and vision deficits, tuberculosis, urinary dys-

function, anemia, chronic bronchitis, claudication, cancers, nutritional deficiencies, uncontrolled diabetes, foot disease hampering mobility, dental disease impeding nutrition, dementia, and depression.

Further questioning of subjects and review of primary data led to some clear explanations for this apparently self-destructive illness behavior of elderly Scots. Older people perceive pain, malaise, and disability adequately but choose to conceal their distress or at least not seek treatment. The most common explanation for symptom tolerance and nonreporting was the pervasive belief that old age is inextricably associated with illness, functional decline, and feeling sick. Old and young, lay and professional, men and women, all believe that to be old is to be ill. Obviously this "ageist" view of health and disease guarantees that older individuals, even when afflicted with the same symptoms that impel the middle-aged sick into the mainstream of the health care system, will not seek care, will suffer in silence the progression of many diseases, and endure the functional losses engendered by untreated illness. That old age in the absence of disease is a time of good health and persisting function has been documented by numerous studies of normal aging [12], but while our society labors in ignorance of gerontologic information, elders will continue expecting decline and dysfunction. A useful geriatric maxim to be remembered is that sick old people are sick because they are sick, not because they are old. Although certainly decline in numerous physiologic functions characterize normal human aging, these declines are gradual, and their functional impact is ameliorated by the decades over which they occur and by the remaining, if diminishing, reserve capacities of the individual. Thus, major functional decline, especially if abrupt in an individual already old, is usually attributable to disease, not age.

A second explanation for old people not reporting illness was that the high prevalence of depression, coupled with the many losses common in late life, interfered with the desire to regain vigor. A third block to reporting illness was found to be intellectual loss. Though never normal, the increasing prevalence of cognitive loss with age is doubly dangerous to the detection of disease. Cognitively impaired individuals have a diminished ability to complain and are also evaluated less enthusiastically for associated medical disease or even reversible disease producing the intellectual losses themselves [20]. A fourth explanation for symptom concealment by elderly patients was fear that something would be found and generate diagnostic or therapeutic interventions that in themselves would produce functional loss and jeopardize independent living. Finally, today's octogenarians, having grown up when health care systems produced less salubrious interventions, may be reluctant to seek care even in the present.

The abundant documentation that disease is not being reported by the elderly appears to contradict a clinical rule of thumb that identifies hypochondriasis as common among aged patients. Many clinicians caring for elderly patients cite an individual or two who tries their patience and good-will with endless complaints rooted in trivial or nonexistent illness. Yet when studied, the hypochondriacal, doctor-shopping, old person appears to be one more unverifiable mythical figure in people's ideas about aging [21]. Not only is hypochondriasis less common among older people, but when elders do complain, important disease is found underlying their complaints substantially more often than in younger, nonhypochondriacal individuals [22].

Nonreporting of symptoms of underlying disease in elderly persons is an especially dangerous phenomenon when coupled with the American organizational structure of health care delivery. Our health care system is passive, especially for elderly people, and lacks prevention-oriented or early detection efforts. American medical care of the critically ill, elderly hospitalized patient is the best in the world. Science and technology are most expertly blended to help the sick. But American hospital beds, HMOs, physicians' offices, emergency rooms, and neighborhood health centers all wait passively for the symptomatic patient to activate the system. For the most part, this passive system of health care provision is adequate for children, who have parental advocates, and for young and middle-aged adults who have the need to work and earn impelling them to seek medical relief of function-impairing symptoms. But aged persons, without advocates and usually without jobs, burdened by society's and their own ageist views of functional loss in the elderly, cannot be relied upon to initiate appropriate health care for themselves, especially early in the course of an illness when intervention is most likely to have a favorable outcome. In summary, our health care system relies on the patient to enter the system and initiate care; and that is precisely the one illness behavior most often missing in aged individuals. These factors make undetected decline especially likely and suggest that adding a more active case-finding facet to the system for the elderly would be beneficial.

"Predeath" Among Hospitalized Elderly
A second phenomenon endangering older Americans in our health care system was again identified in Scotland. A year-long study of 4,000 hospital deaths in individuals over 65 years of age revealed a recurring pattern of preadmission debility and surprisingly long stays for those patients destined to die [23]. The older the patients were, the longer they survived before dying in the hospital. A high proportion—nearly three-quarters—of the deaths were preceded by a period of increasing dependency prior to hospitalization. A high correlation of dependency with advancing age and death following hospitalization led to naming the dependent period "predeath." The most common causes of the predeath dependency were immobility, incontinence, and mental impairment, often in combination. The durations of predeath and attendant hospitalization were strikingly age-

related, as was the likelihood of hospital death. Although deaths of the very old occurred more often in beds allotted to geriatric or psychiatric patients (in which average hospital stays were substantially longer than for patients in American beds used for acute or short-term care) than in those used for patients undergoing medical or surgical care, it was astonishing to find that the average hospital stay before death was three months for patients 65 to 74 years of age, six months for those 75 to 84 years of age, seven months for men 85 years and older, and 13 months for women over 85 years old! Retrospective analysis of a small subject sample revealed a high proportion having potentially reversible or at least improvable causes for the predeath dependency if appropriate evaluation and treatment were undertaken early. Immobility, incontinence, and dementia are clarions of serious underlying disease in old people and demand prompt evaluation. Once again it appears that long, costly, discouraging dependency among old people might be avoided by a more active case-finding component of the health care system.

Multiple Pathology
A third factor predisposing elderly individuals to functional decline based on late detection of potentially treatable disease is the common occurrence of illness-clustering in aged patients. Usually called multiple pathology, the existence of several concurrent diseases in an old person who either is not obviously ill or is under treatment for a different problem has a profound negative influence on health and functional independence in old age. A random sample of community-dwelling subjects over 65 years of age found nearly 3.5 important disabilities per person [19]. An earlier study of elderly patients being admitted to hospitals documented six pathological conditions per person [24]. A recent American clinical experience tabulated common problems often coexisting in elderly individuals [25]; these were congestive heart failure, depression, dementia syndrome, chronic renal failure, angina pectoris, osteoarthritis/osteoporosis, gait disorder, urinary difficulty, constipation, arterial or venous insufficiency in the legs, diabetes mellitus, chronic pain, sleep disturbance, multiple drug regimens, and anemia.

The number of pathologic conditions in an individual is strongly related to age, often rising to more than a dozen in the very old. If the entire spectrum of multiple pathologic conditions is not identified and carefully considered, virtually any diagnostic or therapeutic initiative is as likely to produce harm as benefit. In the absence of obvious flare-up of one problem, major danger still exists for the patient with multiple pathology. Korenchevsky [26] first pointed out the destructive, insidious virulence of unattended multiple pathologies in the uncomplaining elderly patient. The undetected, untreated diseases create ricochetting stress in several organ systems or tissues, producing deterioration of a previously diseased but compensated physiologic function. As each overburdened organ fails, there is created "what rapidly becomes an irreversible concatenation of deteriorations, passing multiple points of no return, leading to infirmity, dependence, and, if uninterrupted, death" [25]. The retrospective identification of previously unidentified disorders that have led to fixed functional losses in a once independent elder is a truly depressing but improvable aspect of geriatrics.

In summary, considering the preceding observations about illness behavior and disease patterns in old people, our health care system seems especially vulnerable when it attempts to meet the health needs of an aging population and to prevent institutionalization of members of this population. Inadequate reporting of illness by the elderly coupled with the passivity of our medical apparatus make it highly probable that disease will be far advanced before the aged patient gets into the health care system. During the delay between onset and detection, it is possible for multiple pathologies to interact, harming the patient and producing irrevocable disability in spite of eventual excellent care. For some elderly patients, delay is lengthened because of neglect of a number of nonspecific but serious problems, including immobility, incontinence, and cognitive loss, any or all of which can herald eventual death. These risks, which delay treatment and allow irretrievable losses for elderly sick people, might be avoided by adding an active case-finding surveillance mechanism for the elderly to our current passive health care system.

Approach to the Elderly Patient
GENERAL
Successfully approaching the elderly patient requires the use of special strategies during the history and physical examination. The setting should take into account problems likely to be encountered. Because the prevalence of hearing and vision deficits approaches two-thirds in the frail elderly, an interview/examining room should be quiet, and speech should be clear, slow, and uttered while facing the old person directly in order for him or her to lipread or pick up other visual clues. If voice volume is increased, it should be at a low pitch in recognition of the greater high-tone hearing loss in the elderly. The examiner should ask questions periodically to be sure the subject understands what has been said. When there is uncertainty concerning comprehension, the question or statement should be rephrased in different words.

Light should be adequate, but it should be remembered that too-bright light can be painful for those who have had cataract surgery. Light in back of the interviewer should always be avoided. Chairs should be comfortable but high enough for an elderly person to arise easily. The examining table should be at a height to which frail elders can easily mount and from which they can dismount without hazard. Examining gowns should also be usable with arthritic hands and of an appropriate safe length. Finally, elderly individuals should be allowed adequate time to undress.

HISTORY

Several special features of history-taking from the elderly deserve mention. Rarely is there a single chief complaint from a sick old person. Even when only one disease flares up, it interacts with the ubiquitous multiple pathologies and psychosocial and economic problems of old age, guaranteeing multiple presenting complaints. Each complaint usually is rooted in a different problem, contrary to the law of parsimony. The family history is rarely relevant, but a thorough social history is required to identify recent stressful events that could possibly contribute to the presenting problems. Informal and formal supports available or operational at home give an accurate picture of resources as well as functional losses. The current functional status must be accurately assessed, and the duration and cause of deficits sought in order to identify remediable problems. An accurate diet history is relevant in those in whom disease management includes food restrictions that could interfere with nutrition, for example, diabetes, hypertension, acid peptic disease, or congestive heart failure. Although the status of polio, pertussis, and small pox immunizations are rarely relevant, tetanus, pneumococcus, and influenza vaccination histories are important. Perhaps most important in the ambulatory setting is having the patient bring all medications—prescription and proprietary—on each doctor visit.

PHYSICAL EXAMINATION

Patients at any age deserve a careful physical examination, but in the old person, certain areas require special attention. Because of the high prevalence of symptomatic hypotension when the patient is standing, blood pressure should be recorded during an initial period of standing and for several minutes. Tender or thickened temporal arteries should be sought. Sensitive and reliable testing of hearing and vision function is essential. Dentition and taste status will often determine nutrition; the oral cavity should be carefully examined for tumors after dentures are removed. Aortic systolic murmurs abound in the aged, appearing in nearly half of individuals 75 years of age and older. Although the majority of these murmurs are produced by aortic valve sclerosis—a relatively benign condition compared with aortic stenosis—clinical clues distinguishing one from the other should be sought. The rectal and pelvic or male genital examinations are essential. Deferring any aspect deprives physician and patient of the opportunity to detect and treat hemorrhoids, constipation, prostatic enlargement, rectal and genital cancers, epididymal scarring of tuberculosis, and other problems especially likely to be concealed in the history by an overly modest patient. A reliable standard mental status test should be performed and recorded annually in all elderly individuals. The Goldfarb mental status quotient

[27], although relatively insensitive, is easily done and accurate. A more recent screening test introduced in 1977 by Jacobs and associates takes only a few minutes longer to administer and is more sensitive [28]. Considering the increasing prevalence of dementing illness with age, recording a mental status test may be more useful than auscultation of the heart in ambulatory elderly individuals.

Diseases of the Elderly

The data base for learning about disease in old age exists in the medical literature of many countries. Several textbooks have been published [29,30], but few American medical schools have specifically included a study of geriatrics in their curricula [5]. Diseases in old age can be divided into two broad groups: disorders that are common only in the elderly, and diseases that occur in middle as well as old age but present unusual features in the elderly. Diseases and conditions of the first group include:

Diabetic hyperosmolar nonketotic coma
Stroke
The spectrum of diseases from polymyalgia rheumatica to giant cell arteritis
Metabolic bone disease
Osteoarthritis
Hip fracture and its rehabilitation
Dementia syndrome
Paget's disease
Gammopathies, including multiple myeloma
Chronic lymphatic leukemia
Tuberculosis, especially miliary
Herpes zoster
Basal cell carcinoma
Parkinsonism
Angioimmunoblastic lymphadenopathy with dysproteinemia
Normal pressure hydrocephalus
Decubitus ulcer
Accidental hypothermia
Neurogenic urinary incontinence
Rheumatoid arthritis
Arteriosclerotic heart disease and its complications
Gallbladder disease
Amyloidosis
Most solid tumors, especially prostate, colon, breast, and lung
Carpal tunnel syndrome
Hearing and vision impairment
Colonic angiodysplasia
Autoimmune disease

Although not strictly diseases, falls and suicide are also particular problems in the elderly.

DISEASES WITH UNUSUAL PRESENTATION IN OLD AGE
The second and much larger group of diseases requiring special attention are those that, although common in youth and middle age, behave differently in the elderly. These diseases constitute a substantial portion of a textbook of internal medicine. A fundamental principle in caring for aged individuals is that virtually any disease with a classic complex of symptoms or signs frequently presents in old age with few or none of the characteristic findings [31]. The classic presentation is often replaced by one or more nonspecific problems, the most common being refusal to eat or drink, falling, incontinence, dizziness, acute confusion, a new or worsening dementia syndrome, weight loss, and failure to thrive [25]. Certain diseases or conditions are especially likely to be enigmatic or perplexing in the elderly; some of these that present nonspecifically are depression; drug intoxication; myxedema; alcoholism; myocardial infarction; pulmonary embolism; pneumonia; malignant disease, especially of the colon, lung, and breast; "surgical abdomen"; and thyrotoxicosis, apathetic or masked. Surprising survival and recovery is another characteristic of disease in old age.

HAZARDS FOR HOSPITALIZED ELDERLY
Besides unfamiliar presentation, unexpected complications and peculiar clinical courses occur commonly in elderly patients. Predictable hazards for hospitalized patients are nighttime confusion or "sundowning," falls, fractures with no identifiable trauma, sudden appearance of decubiti, fecal impaction and urinary retention, and prolonged convalescence. Loss of his or her home during a person's hospitalization is another hazard.

Geriatric Pharmacology

Another special aspect of clinical geriatrics is pharmacokinetics and pharmacotherapeutics (see Chap. 4). The average older American fills 13 prescriptions annually and spends 20 percent of personal funds on drugs. The aged often bear the brunt of reflexive prescribing for uninvestigated symptoms. Therapeutic drug advances in many areas have led to greater opportunities for effective rational treatment, regardless of the patient's age; however, because of multiple phenomena, elderly patients are more susceptible to side effects and toxic effects of most agents [32]. Body composition and drug distribution, metabolism, excretion, and response have special features in the elderly. Most contemporary clinical drug trials and pharmacologic studies were performed in young humans. Gerontology teaches us that because octogenarians differ from their grandchildren in many ways, pharmacokinetic data about either group are not generally applicable to the other. Drug treatment standards developed in the young and applied to the old are predictably hazardous. When a drug is indicated for the treatment of a specific disease, it should not be withheld because of a patient's age, but extra thoughtfulness and extreme care in selecting drugs and dosages are required when prescribing for the elderly.

A broad and growing data base is necessary for successful clinical management of elderly patients. Knowledge of demography, health care delivery, gerontology, and clinical medicine contributes to the requisite education of health professionals treating elderly patients. Drug-prescribing for the elderly is a critical area for study. Only when the data base of geriatric medicine is taught vigorously in American medical schools can society expect improved health care for our growing population of elders. Without these changes in medical education, physicians and elderly patients are destined to continued frustrating failure within our present system, which has ignored the special character of our aging selves.

References

1. Akpom, C. A., and Mayer, S. A. A survey of geriatric education in U. S. medical schools. *J. Med. Educ.* 53:66, 1978.
2. Somers, A. R. Geriatric care in the United Kingdom: an American perspective. *Ann. Intern. Med.* 85:641, 1976.
3. Butler, R. N. Testimony before the U. S. Senate Special Committee on Aging: *Medicine and Aging: An Assessment of Opportunities and Neglect.* U.S. Government Printing Office, October 13, 1976.
4. Libow, L. S. A geriatric medical residency program: a four-year experience. *Ann. Intern. Med.* 85:641, 1976.
5. Institute of Medicine. *Aging and Medical Education.* Washington, D.C.: National Academy of Sciences, 1978.
6. Institute of Medicine. *The Elderly and Functional Dependency.* Washington, D.C.: National Academy of Sciences, 1977.
7. Comfort, A. *Ageing: The Biology of Senescence* (rev. ed.). London: Routledge and Kegan Paul, 1964.
8. Isaacs, B. *Survival of the Unfittest.* London: Routledge and Kegan Paul, 1972.
9. Kovar, M. G. *Elderly People: The Population 65 Years and Over.* DHEW Publication No. (HRA) 77-1232, 1977.
10. Health Care Financing Administration. Discussion Paper: *Long-Term Care: Background and Future Directions.* U.S. Government Publication No. (HCFA) 81-20047.
11. Rowe, J. W., et al. The effect of age on creatinine clearance in man: a cross-sectional and longitudinal study. *J. Gerontol.* 31:155, 1976.
12. Finch, C. E., and Hayflick, L. *Handbook of the Biology of Aging.* New York: Van Nostrand Reinhold, 1977.
13. Helderman, J. H., et al. The response of arginine-vasopressin to intravenous ethanol and hypertonic saline in man: the impact of aging. *J. Gerontol.* 33:39, 1978.

14. Gibson, R. M., and Fisher, C. R.   Age differences in health care spending, fiscal year 1977. *HCFA Health Note,* December, 1978.
15. Butler, R. N.   The Medicine of the Future—Geriatrics. Joseph T. Freeman Lecture. Presented at the 33rd Annual Meeting of the Gerontological Society, San Diego, CA, 1980.
16. Brody, S., Polshock, S., and Masciocchi, C.   The family caring unit: a major consideration in the long-term support system. *Gerontologist* 18:6, 1978.
17. Palmore, E.   Total chance of institutionalization among the aged. *Gerontologist* 16:504, 1976.
18. Anderson, W. F.   The prevention of illness in the elderly: the Rutherglen experiment in medicine in old age. Proceedings of a conference held at the Royal College of Physicians of London. London: Pitman, 1966.
19. Williamson, J., et al.   Old people at home: their unreported needs. *Lancet* 1:1117, 1964.
20. National Institute on Aging Task Force.   Senility reconsidered: treatment possibilities for mental impairment in the elderly. *J.A.M.A.* 244:259, 1980.
21. Costa, P. T., Jr., and McCrae, R. R.   Somatic complaints in males as a function of age and neuroticism: a longitudinal analysis. *J. Behav. Med.* 3:245, 1980.
22. Stenback, A., Kumpulainen, M., and Vauhkonen, M. L.   Illness and health behavior in septuagenarians. *Gerontologist* 33:57, 1978.
23. Isaacs, B.   The concept of pre-death. *Lancet* 1:115, 1971.
24. Wilson, L. A., Lawson, I. R., and Brass, W.   Multiple disorders in the elderly. *Lancet* 2:841, 1962.
25. Besdine, R. W.   Geriatric medicine: an overview. *Annu. Rev. Gerontol. Geriatr.* 1:135, 1980.
26. Korenchevsky, V.   *Physiological and Pathological Aging.* New York: Basel/ Karger, 1961.
27. Kahn, R. L., et al.   Brief objective measures for the determination of mental status in the aged. *Am. J. Psychiatry* 117:326, 1960.
28. Jacobs, J. W., Bernhard, M. R., and Degado, A.   Screening for organic mental syndromes in the medically ill. *Ann. Intern. Med.* 86:40, 1977.
29. Brocklehurst, J. C. (Ed.)   *Textbook of Geriatric Medicine and Gerontology* (2nd ed.). Edinburgh: Churchill Livingstone, 1978.
30. Rossman, E. (Ed.).   *Clinical Geriatrics* (2nd ed.). Philadelphia: Lippincott, 1979.
31. Hodkinson, H. M.   Non-specific presentation of illness. *Br. Med. J.* 4:94, 1973.
32. Vestal, R. E.   Drug use in the elderly: a review of problems and special considerations. *Drugs* 16:358, 1978.

2. The Biology of Aging

Barbara A. Gilchrest
John W. Rowe

The phenomenon of aging is at once obvious and extraordinarily complex. While logic dictates that one or more definable molecular processes within a living organism must underlie the aging process, numerous studies in experimental animals, isolated organ systems, and individual cultured cells and their products have failed to pinpoint the mechanism(s) by which aging occurs. This chapter presents some observations that have excited interest in gerontology and outlines the major hypotheses of aging developed during the past quarter century.

What is Aging?

For most people, the term *aging* evokes an array of clinical findings based on their own experiences and their observations of others. In the general case, aging may be considered an irreversible process that begins or accelerates at maturity and results in an increasing number and/or range of deviations from the ideal state or in a decreasing rate of return to the ideal state, or both. Kohn [1] defines aging in several contexts: (1) chemical aging, as manifested by changes in the structure of crystals or in macromolecular aggregations; (2) extracellular aging, as manifested by progressive cross-linkage of collagen and elastin fibers or by amyloid deposition; (3) intracellular aging, as manifested by changes in normal cellular components or by accumulation of substances such as lipofuscin in cells; and (4) aging of entire organisms.

Aging is inevitable and every living organism has a finite life span. Moreover, each species has a characteristic maximum attainable life span. Improved nutrition and health care have increased the *average* human life span from less than 20 years in ancient Greece to over 70 years in the United States today, but they have not altered the approximately 110-year *maximum* life span of our species.

One can consider the phenomenon of maximum life span in another way. If heart disease, currently the leading cause of death in the United States, were eliminated, the life expectancy at birth would increase only seven years; and if cancer, the second leading cause of death, were eliminated, life expectancy would increase by only three years. Indeed, if the 10 leading causes of death were eliminated, life expectancy would increase by less than 11 years. Ultimately, people do not die of pathologic processes but of physiologic processes.

It is interesting that maximum life span, which is so constant within a species, may vary tremendously even among closely related mammals, 86-fold between mice and men, for example. Relations have been determined between species life span and body weight or brain weight, basal metabolic rate, reproductive rate, and ability to repair DNA damage [2]. Although such relationships are provocative, they unfortunately provide little insight into the aging process itself.

Characteristics of Aging Populations

Figure 2-1 shows a hypothetical percentage of individuals surviving with increasing age in a population in which death is purely accidental; that is, the risk of death is independent of age and death occurs randomly. In contrast, an idealized survival curve for a population in which death is positively related to age and in which there is no accidental death is shown in Figure 2-2. In Figure 2-2 the initially trivial or absent death rate begins to increase at a certain age, after which the percentage of individuals surviving declines with increasing age. A plot of the death rate in such a population displays a normal distribution. In existing human populations, the distribution is not normal but reflects a mixture of non–age-related (premature or accidental) death (accidental not only in terms of highway deaths but in biologic terms, due to infections and so on) as well as age-related or senescent deaths.

Figure 2-3 illustrates the actual experience of various societies at different times. As one proceeds in time and, perhaps, medical sophistication, the pattern of death rate in relation to age progresses from a largely accidental pattern to the experience of Swedish females born in 1961 to 1965, the projection for whom looks almost ideal. This progress is also evident in a consideration of what happened in the United States during this century. Fifty percent of the individuals born in 1901 were dead by the time they

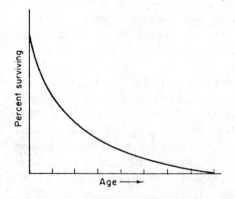

Figure 2-1. Idealized survival curve for a population in which the risk of death does not change with age, death occurring randomly. (From R. Kohn. *Principles of Mammalian Aging.* Englewood Cliffs, N.J.: Prentice-Hall, 1978. P. 13.)

were 58. For those born in 1948, 50 percent will be dead by 72; and of those born in 1975, 50 percent will be dead at 76 years. People often ask why there are suddenly so many old people. The answer is that people are really not living longer, but more people are living out the normal human life span.

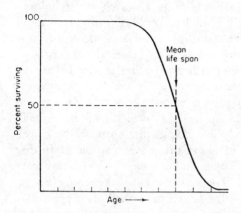

Figure 2-2. Idealized survival curve for a population in which the death rate is age-dependent. (From R. Kohn. *Principles of Mammalian Aging.* Englewood Cliffs, N.J.: Prentice-Hall, 1978. P. 11.)

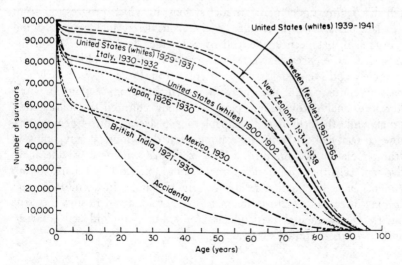

Figure 2-3. Survival curves for various human populations compared to that seen when death is accidental and not age-related. (From A. Comfort. *Ageing: The Biology of Senescence.* New York: Holt, Rinehart and Winston, 1964.)

Cellular Aging

A major experimental approach to the mystery of aging has been the study of cultured cells. Alexis Carrel, a French surgeon and cell biologist working more than 50 years ago, asked the question: Is an animal's finite life span due to limitations inherent in each individual cell or to mechanisms operative only at the level of the whole organism? Using tissue culture techniques available at that time, he found chick fibroblasts could be maintained in an actively dividing state for periods far exceeding a chicken's life span; some cells were kept in continuous culture for 34 years before the experiments were terminated. Similar results using cells from other species led to the conclusion that individual cells were immortal—only whole organisms experienced aging and death after a predetermined period. This view was later challenged by Hayflick and Moorehead [3] who found that human fetal fibroblasts had a finite, reproducible culture life span, 50 ± 10 cell generations, after which the cultured fibroblasts were incapable of further cell division and ultimately died. These findings were subsequently confirmed by many other investigators. The earlier results have since been explained in one of two ways. At the time Carrel performed his experiments, fibroblast cultures were fed with embryo extracts, and a small number of viable young cells could have been added at each feeding, enough to replenish the cell population and make it seem immortal. Other "immortal" cell lines from experiments in the 1940s and 1950s were found to be karyotypically abnormal (the in vitro equivalent of malignant cells), having undergone spontaneous transformation in culture.

Hayflick's "aging under glass" model system, in which progression from early to late passage at the cellular level is considered analogous to aging of an organism, has been challenged by Schneider and Mitsui [4] on the grounds that differences between cells from young and old donors are quantitatively and even qualitatively different from those between early and late passage cultured cells, i.e., aging in vivo differs from "aging" in vitro. Furthermore, analysis of mitotic patterns among cultured fibroblasts indicates that while the cells may be capable on an average of 50 generations, or more correctly of 50 cumulative population doublings, at any point in time the population is a mixture of "old" cells that will never divide again and "young" cells that will undergo many more mitoses [5]. Finally, recent experiments have shown that relatively minor changes in a cultured cell's milieu may increase its culture life span several-fold, again raising the issue that subtle environmental inadequacies for cultured diploid cells may be responsible for their limited survival.

RELATION OF LIFE SPAN OF CELLS IN CULTURE TO LIFE SPAN OF THE ORGANISM

Several lines of evidence suggest that the life span of normal cultured cells is related to the life span of the organism from which they are derived.

Human dermal fibroblasts and keratinocytes of adult origin have much shorter in vitro life spans than those obtained from fetuses, and when large numbers of subjects are examined, it becomes apparent that donor age and life span of cultured fibroblasts are inversely related [6]. Fibroblasts from individuals who have Werner's syndrome, progeria, and even diabetes—diseases that mimic accelerated aging clinically in some regards—have shorter culture life spans than do those from age-matched controls [7]. There is at least a rough correlation between the maximum life span of animal species and the in vitro life span of their cultured cells. Finally, to answer the nagging question that aging of cells in vitro may be an artifact of tissue culture, rather than a necessary characteristic, several investigations have serially transplanted tissue to isogenic younger animals to determine its maximal life span in vivo. Experiments with skin grafts, bone marrow cells, and mammary tissue have shown that such cells can survive for periods considerably longer than the maximum life span of the species but all die eventually. These results are thus consistent with those from tissue culture studies indicating limitation of cell life span.

Physiologic Changes with Age

Review of the physiologic changes that occur in humans as they age allows development of several principles of clinical gerontology that permit a logical approach to the changes. The first consideration that emerges is that of the phases of the normal life span. The early phase of growth and development, which is characterized by rapid increases in many functions, generally continues into early adulthood, peaking in the late twenties or early thirties. As seen in Figure 2-4, in those variables that do change with age after adulthood, the change generally begins immediately at the end of the growth and development phase and is generally linear into old age. There is no pleasant "plateau" of the middle years in which we maintain our prime functional level for 20 to 30 years.

As is seen in Figure 2-4, the loss of function of most variables that do change with age is *linear* into the eighth and ninth decade and does not increase as we become older. Thus, the rate of aging does not change in most cases—an 80-year-old is aging just as fast as a 30-year-old. The 80-year-old is more aged than his younger counterpart, having accumulated more of the changes secondary to age, but he is not losing function at a more rapid rate.

An important characteristic of age-related changes is their *variability*. There are several sources of variability, including changes within individuals from organ to organ, and changes from individual to individual in a given population. Such functions as cardiac output, glomerular filtration rate, and carbohydrate tolerance change rather dramatically, whereas others, such as nerve conduction velocity and hematocrit, undergo no significant change into the eighth or ninth decade.

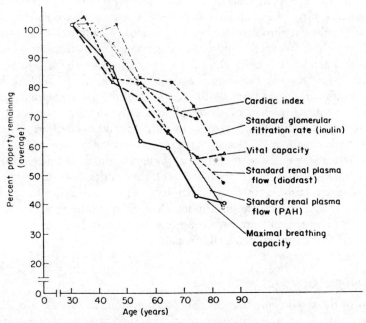

Figure 2-4. Influence of age on physiologic function in humans after the end of the growth and development stage in the late twenties and early thirties.
(From A. S. Mildvan and B. L. Strehler, A Critique of Theories of Mortality. In B. L. Strehler, *The Biology of Aging.* Copyright © 1960, by the American Institute of Biological Sciences. Reprinted with permission of the copyright holder.)

Changes in one organ are not necessarily predictive of changes with age in other organs. If an apparently healthy 60-year-old is found on serial prospective measurements to have a cardiac output that is falling at a certain rate, perhaps at the rate average for his age group, this information is of no value in predicting the rate at which his kidneys, thyroid, sympathetic nervous system, or any other organ is changing with time. This apparent failure of various organs to be synchronized in their age-related changes rules against the presence of a basic biologic clock. At present one cannot construct a variable termed *functional age* that predicts performance on a physiologic or psychologic test better than the individual chronological age.

The variability in human aging from individual to individual is also substantial. In studies of variables that undergo major changes with age the variance is always large and one can easily identify apparently healthy 40-year-olds who perform at the same level as the average 80-year-old. Likewise, many 80-year-olds can be found who perform like the average 40-year-old.

Age Versus Disease

Increasing age after adulthood is associated with an exponential increase in mortality rate, and this mortality is preceded by a similar exponential increase in the presence of pathologic changes. This has stimulated controversy about whether aging should be considered a disease state, and, if not, what is the relation of normal aging to disease-related changes. There is now general agreement that increasing age is accompanied by inevitable physiologic changes that represent normal aging and are separable from the effects of disease states that become increasingly prevalent with age. These age-related changes are the substrate onto which the effects of specific diseases are grafted. These changes have clinical importance to the physician since they influence the presentation of illness, its response to treatment, and the complications that ensue.

One fairly superficial and simple way of separating disease effects from the influence of normal aging is the inevitability of the changes. Although a change may vary from individual to individual in its age of onset or the rate of loss of function, some loss of function should be demonstrable in all old subjects if the change is due to aging. Aging is a universal phenomenon whereas many disease states, which occur with increasing prevalence as age advances, influence only a small portion of the elderly population. Evaluation of the presence of a change secondary to a disease state or some other factor not age-related in an elderly cohort would often show two populations: one with the effect and one population with no evidence of the effect. The utility of this approach in determining whether or not a change is likely to be related to age can be seen in, as an example, mental failure or senile dementia. This loss of mental function with advancing age is thought by some individuals to be characteristic of aging itself. When populations are studied in detail, however, it is shown that dementia occurs in no greater than 10 percent of elders. Thus, the presence of an intact intellect and the absence of mental failure is consistent with normal aging and is in fact the rule rather than the exception. This would indicate that the mental failure cannot be considered a normal consequence of aging but more properly represents a disease that has increasing prevalence in advanced years. This can be contrasted with the menopause, which, although variable in its age of onset, is universally present in aged women and thus is more likely to be a result of normal aging.

Theories on Aging
DNA REPLICATION THEORY

Deoxyribonucleic acid (DNA), the genetic material of all cells, figures prominently in many theories on aging. It is known that random errors occur, albeit with a very low frequency, during DNA replication. This theory states that aging results from a gradual accumulation of such errors, with eventual functional and/or reproductive death of individual cells. In support of this hypothesis, Hart and Setlow [8] have found the life span of animal species, including humans, to correlate with the ability of cultured fibroblasts to repair damage to DNA by induced ultraviolet radiation. A variant of the DNA-error–dependent hypothesis of aging suggests that the number of gene copies for certain critical genes determines the life span of a species. It is known that only 2 percent of a cell's genetic materials are in use at any time and that multiple copies of at least certain genes exist. If the cell can recognize and replace error-containing genes with undamaged copies, no detrimental effects will occur until the cell has exhausted its genetic reserves.

ORGEL'S ERROR THEORY

Orgel's error catastrophe theory states that even infrequent errors in the transcription of DNA would produce imperfect RNA molecules, each of which in turn would code for many faulty enzymes and other proteins. These proteins could accumulate rapidly within the cell and compromise its function [9]. Progressive loss of functional cells would eventually produce aging changes and death of the organism.

In support of such a mechanism, most enzyme studies to date have shown an age-dependent increase in the proportion of partially or totally inactive molecules. In representative cases a 30 to 70 percent loss of activity per antigenic unit can be measured between enzymes of young and old adults. Against this theory is the fact that it has not been possible to detect any change in charge of the altered molecules, even when utilizing techniques sufficiently sensitive to detect replacement of a single amino acid, while functionally significant transcriptional or translational errors might be expected to replace numerous amino acids. Moreover, viral infection of early and later passage human fibroblasts has failed to show a host cell age-dependent increase in production of faulty viral particles. An alternative explanation for the accumulation with age of functionless proteins without change in charge is posttranslational modification. Most amino acid modifications, such as phosphorylation, glycosylation, deamination, and hydroxylation, would again be expected to measurably alter molecular charge or chromatographic properties, but oxidation of sulfhydryl groups, an event already shown to occur in lens protein during cataract formation, would not alter the charge.

CROSS-LINKAGE THEORY

Bjorksten [10] and others have hypothesized that aging results from progressive cross-linkage of intracellular and intercellular proteins. Collagen fibers, major structural proteins for many organs, are increasingly cross-linked with age, with a resultant decrease in elasticity and tensile strength, are offered as a prototype. Age-related changes in basement membrane collagen or in the ground substance of connective tissue, are likely to impair organ function.

FREE RADICAL THEORY

Free radical reactions have been postulated to contribute to biochemical, and ultimately to clinical, aging through progressive membrane damage, protein cross-linkage, enzyme inactivation, and production of "aging pigments." Superoxide and hydroxyl radicals are generated by mitochondrial respiration by autooxidation of numerous intracellular molecules, and by the action of certain environmental agents such as ultraviolet light on biologic systems. The enzyme, superoxide dismutase, a major cellular defense against damage by free radicals, has been found to decrease as a function of age in rats; and reduced blood levels of other free radical quenchers, including vitamin C, have been measured in elderly human beings. Studies in mice, as yet unconfirmed, suggest that appropriate dietary antioxidants increase the mean life span by 20 to 45 percent and decrease the incidence of spontaneous carcinoma in genetically predisposed species [11].

"PACEMAKER" OR ENDOCRINE THEORY

Some researchers postulate that aging is controlled by a "pacemaker" such as the thymus, hypothalamus, pituitary, or thyroid gland. Either by elaborating a hormone or by ultimately failing to do so, a single organ might influence the behavior of cells throughout the body.

IMMUNOLOGIC THEORY

The immunologic theory of senescence identifies thymus-derived (T) lymphocytes as the pacemaker tissue and states that age-dependent changes in these cells are responsible for much of the pathology that accompanies aging, for example, cancer and certain forms of autoimmunity. The specific effects of age on the immune system and their clinical implications are discussed in Chapter 19.

References

1. Kohn, R. R. *Principles of Mammalian Aging* (2nd ed.). Englewood Cliffs, N.J.: Prentice-Hall, 1978. P. 240.
2. Sacher, G. A. Relation of Lifespan to Brain Weight and Body Weight in Mammals. In G. E. W. Wolstenholme and M. O'Connor (Eds.), *The Lifespan of Animals* (Ciba Foundation Colloq. on Aging). Boston: Little, Brown, 1959. Vol. 5.
3. Hayflick, L., and Moorehead, P. S. The serial cultivation of human diploid cell strains. *Exp. Cell. Res.* 37:614, 1961.
4. Schneider, E. L., and Mitsui, Y. The relationship between in vitro cellular aging and in vivo human age. *Proc. Natl. Acad. Sci. U.S.A.* 73:3584, 1976.
5. Bell, E., et al. Loss of division potential in vitro: aging or differentiation. *Science* 202:1158, 1978.

6. Martin, G. I., Sprague, C. S., and Epstein, C. J.   Replicative lifespan of culti-vated human cells. Effects of donor's age, tissue, and genotype. *Lab. Invest.* 23:66, 1970.
7. Goldstein, S., et al.   Chronologic and physiologic age affect replicative life-span of fibroblasts from diabetic, prediabetic, and normal donors. *Science* 199:761, 1978.
8. Hart, R. W., and Setlow, R. B.   Correlation between deoxyribonucleic acid excision–repair and lifespan in a number of mammalian species. *Proc. Natl. Acad. Sci. U.S.A.* 71:2169, 1974.
9. Orgel, L. E.   The maintenance of the accuracy of protein synthesis in its rele-vance to aging. *Proc. Natl. Acad. Sci. U.S.A.* 49:517, 1963.
10. Bjorksten, J.   The crosslinkage theory of aging. *Finska Kenists Medd.* 80:23, 1971.
11. Harman, D.   Prolongation of the normal lifespan and inhibition of spon-taneous cancer by antioxidants. *J. Gerontol.* 16:247, 1961.

Suggested Reading

Harman, D.   The aging process. *Proc. Natl. Acad. Sci. U.S.A.* 78:7124, 1981.
Hayflick, L.   The cell biology of human aging. *N. Engl. J. Med.* 295:1302, 1976.
Holliday, R., Huschtscha, L. I., Kirkwood, T. B. L. Cellular aging: further evi-dence for the commitment theory. *Science* 213:1505, 1981.

3. Beyond the Bedside: The Social Context of Geriatric Practice

Jerry Avorn

Perhaps more than any other part of medicine, the practice of geriatrics is enmeshed in a rich and complex social context. The historical evolution of the present status of the elderly, the sweeping demographic changes in the age structure of industrialized societies, the psychosocial environment in which the patient lives, the ornate patchwork of health and social services provided (or not provided) by society—all of these bear directly on the management of the aged patient. A thorough understanding of these factors is as crucial for the practice of good geriatric medicine as is the grasp of basic pathophysiology.

"The Demographic Imperative"

One major cause of the relatively recent upsurge in interest in the elderly is the population tidal wave now being experienced by most Western societies. In 1900, only about 1 in 25 Americans (4 percent) was over 65 (Fig. 3-1). Today that figure has risen to 1 in 9 (11 percent). Because all those who will be elderly at the start of the twenty-first century are alive today, barring any unforeseen changes in the composition of the rest of the population, it can be safely predicted that by the year 2020 about 1 in 6 Americans, or 17 percent of the nation's population, will be over 65. A more graphic way of portraying this population boom is the observation that each day about 4,000 Americans turn 65, and about 3,000 of those in the 65-plus cohort die. This results in a net gain of about 1,000 new people entering the "Medicare generation" *daily* in the United States. More than half the people who have ever lived past 65 since the dawn of history are alive today.

Within this major demographic shift is hidden another set of changes that is even more significant. The elderly population itself is "getting older," that is, the very old (over 80) are each year comprising a larger and larger proportion of the over-65 group (Fig. 3-2). This is of great importance since the relative impact on the health care system of the over-80 elderly is much greater than that of those between 65 and 80. At present, the fastest growing segment of the entire United States population is the group 85 years old and older.

A number of factors have come together to create this aging "boom." The propagation of basic public health measures (such as sanitation and sewage) and improved nutrition in the last century dramatically reduced the death rate for infants and young adults, allowing more of them to reach old age. In the middle of this century, the development of antibiotics further cut

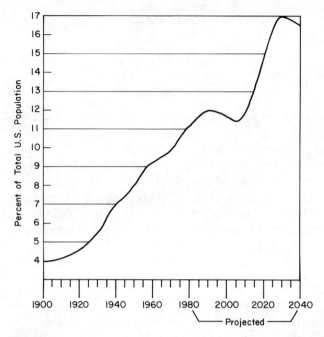

Figure 3-1. Population of the United States: percent age 65 and over, 1900 to 2040. (From U.S. Bureau of the Census. *Current Population Reports: Projections of the Population of the United States.* Washington, D.C.: U.S. Government Printing Office, 1975.)

down on the incidence of premature deaths in all age groups. More recent high technology advances such as renal dialysis and cardiac pacemakers have made the numbers of those surviving into their seventies, eighties, and nineties even greater.

Every proportion obviously has both a numerator and a denominator. In the case of the aging boom, the ratio of elderly to total population has also risen because of the slackening of the growth rate of the nonelderly population. With the end of the postwar baby boom, the birth rate has dropped markedly, thus further magnifying the relative proportion of elderly in society. Just as this baby boom accounted for much of the often exaggerated youth orientation of American culture in the sixties and seventies, so the elder boom is expected to have a major impact on American social relations at the next turn of the century.

The trend of ever-increasing proportions of elderly does not, however, extend out indefinitely through the twenty-first century. The very downturn of the birthrate at the end of the postwar baby boom will have its repercussions around 2025, when the last of those "babies" has turned 65. At that point (Fig. 3-1) the absolute and relative numbers of elderly will

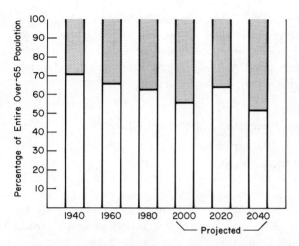

Figure 3-2. Age distribution of the United States elderly population: percentage composition of various subgroups. In each column the lower (unshaded) portion represents the proportion of those 65 and older who are in the 65 to 74 age range; the upper (shaded) portion, 75 and older. (From U.S. Bureau of the Census. *Current Population Reports: Projections of the Population of the United States.* Washington, D.C.: U.S. Government Printing Office, 1975.)

begin to decline slowly, having peaked at about one-sixth of the population.

Striking as these demographic changes are, their impact on the health care system is magnified even further because of the high rate of utilization of health care by the elderly. Currently, the average American over 65 consults with a physician on an average of 6.7 times per year, as compared with 4.8 visits for those under 65. The elderly annually spend nearly five times as many days in hospital per capita than do the nonelderly, with the figure rising progressively for each decade of age. Summing overall health care expenditures from all sources, we find that those 65 and over presently consume 30 percent of all health care resources (hospital care, nursing home care, professional services, drugs, and so on), although they represent only 11 percent of the population. Given the increasing representation of "older elderly" among the over-65 population, this nearly three-to-one multiplier effect is likely to increase further in coming decades. Thus the coming impact of the growing numbers of elderly on the health care system in the coming years will be truly enormous.

The burgeoning of geriatrics in American medicine is a response to these population trends in several ways. It is not only that the sheer weight of numbers of aged patients has had an impact on medical practice. It has also become clear to legislators that the elderly and almost-elderly participate in the electoral process with impressive regularity. Although their voting patterns are not totally predictable, advocating programs for the elderly has become a popular strategy for those seeking public office; opposing them, politically dangerous. Such initiatives have in the past met with a warm response in state and federal legislative bodies (whose members are often in the geriatric age group themselves and thus bring added sympathy to the issue), but are not immune to wide-ranging fiscal cutbacks.

Cohort Effects: Today's Versus Tomorrow's Elders

A cohort is any group of people united by a common characteristic—in this case, age. An important concept in both clinical geriatrics and policy planning is the notion of cohort differences among different groups of elderly. Economically, culturally, educationally, and medically the cohort of those in their seventies and eighties are now very different from those who will be old in the year 2000. Such differences must be taken into account in treating the elderly of today and in planning for the elderly of tomorrow.

For instance, today's elders are much more likely to have less education, come from rural backgrounds, be foreign-born, have several siblings and children, and be married, compared to the cohort that will turn 65 in 2000. Today's elders are also unique in having had their lives shaped by specific historical events such as the Great Depression, World War II, and the New Deal. Policies and approaches developed to serve this group must take such cohort factors into account, just as our vision of services for the elderly of the next century (including most readers of this book) must fit the cultural/ historical experience unique to that group.

Social Factors in the Presentation of Illness

Nonmedical aspects of the elderly patient's life can be among the most important factors determining whether or not the patient perceives symptoms as warranting medical attention at all. The process can work in either direction. Depression or loneliness can prompt numerous visits to the doctor with myriad complaints that are not susceptible to organic workup and therapy. A sensitive personal history can often reveal that the underlying pathology is psychologic rather than somatic, pointing the way to more appropriate interventions, ones that can address either the patient's environment or his or her mental status directly. The physician unable to conceptualize the chief complaint in anything but a concrete way may expend considerable effort, dollars, and risk on exhaustive biomedical investigations that ultimately prove fruitless.

Conversely, psychosocial factors can often militate *against* the patient's presenting himself to the health care system at all. The belief, widespread among patients, family, and health care professionals that illness is the "natural state" of the elderly can exert significant social pressure against seeking help for specific symptoms. Dyspnea on exertion, joint pains, and confusion are all too often mislabeled as "just getting old," when specific diagnoses and treatments could result from a straightforward workup.

Even the likelihood of institutionalization in a nursing home is heavily modulated by social factors, their impact often far outweighing that of the pathology that is cited as the cause for admission. It has been estimated that for every chronically ill elderly patient living in a nursing home, there is at least one *equally disabled* elderly person being maintained successfully in the community. Apart from age, the most important predictors of whether a given elder will be institutionalized include demographic factors such as sex, presence of spouse or other family members, and income. Compared to free-living elderly of the same age, the nursing home resident is disproportionately likely to be female, unmarried (usually through widowhood), and dependent on public welfare (even prior to institutionalization). Thus whether or not a particular 80-year-old stroke victim will require nursing home care often depends as much on the patient's social history and supports as on neuropathology or rehabilitation status.

Social Pathology as a Cause of Organic Pathology

The impact of nonsomatic factors on physical health in the elderly extends far deeper than the perception of symptoms or the likelihood of institutionalization. There is much suggestive evidence that psychosocial aspects of the aged patient's life can in fact generate physical disease.

BEREAVEMENT

Although controversial, some community-based studies have shown that the likelihood of death rises dramatically the year following the death of one's spouse. This excess mortality was significant when compared with the death rate of comparable nonbereaved subjects of the same age. If valid, it is unclear whether the findings result from disordered physiology mediated through the autonomic nervous system or endocrine system, or rather are more intentional in nature, such as poor nutrition, failure to take prescribed medications, or outright suicide. Similarly, Holmes and Rahe have developed a scale of "life change units" that, if accumulated in sufficient amounts, correlate well with the subsequent development of illness in several populations studied. Heading the list in magnitude of such dislocating life changes is death of a spouse. Also high on the list are several other transitions to which the elderly are particularly prone, such as loss of job and/or change in residence.

RETIREMENT

There is a growing literature concerning the impact of retirement on health. Being told (implicitly or explicitly) that one is no longer competent to be a productive member of society can be accompanied by the simultaneous loss of much of one's social network and income. Not surprisingly, this transition can have negative effects on self-image and mental health. On the other hand, many retirees thrive when the burden of work responsibility is removed. Considerable individual variation exists in the response to retirement, and available research bears out neither the stereotype of euphoria nor that of profound melancholy as a consistent response to the end of one's working life.

LABELING AND "LEARNED HELPLESSNESS"

Evidence is accumulating that some aspects of intellectual deterioration can be accelerated (and, in some cases, initiated) by social rather than neurologic causes. Social psychologists have long known that simply labeling an individual as inept or deficient can elicit precisely such behavior. Elderly people relegated to diminished status and insignificant social roles seem often to match this new condition with diminished intellectual ability. Some of this deterioration is undoubtedly related to depression (Chap. 6). Yet some of the mental impairment seen in the elderly (with or without underlying structural cerebral abnormality) can also be seen as culturally induced impairment of the kind frequently seen in other stigmatized groups, from concentration camp victims to schoolchildren labeled (sometimes incorrectly) as "slow." Recent controlled experiments in social psychology have replicated this performance deficit caused by labeling and role change.

Several different mechanisms have been postulated for this drop in mental performance. These include the perception of lack of control; self-induced helplessness; and loss of opportunities to practice high-level cognitive activity, practice that is probably essential for optimal mental functioning. Because of the negative labeling and reduced stimulation that often accompany institutionalization, the elderly in nursing homes are at particularly high risk for such sociogenic intellectual deterioration, above and beyond whatever organic neurologic deficits they already possess.

OPTIONS FOR PREVENTION AND TREATMENT OF SOCIOGENIC DETERIORATION

Once the problems already mentioned are conceptualized as excess morbidity and mortality due partially to social rather than physiologic precipitants, a number of interventions suggest themselves. Theoretically, at least, social interventions often seem more "do-able" than organic approaches to incompletely understood diseases. Yet, in practice, the former may be as difficult as the latter. For example, it would seem far easier for the health care enterprise to persuade people to stop smoking than for it to understand the molecular basis of bronchogenic carcinoma and develop a cure. In reality, however, we have been only minimally successful in both areas. The history of medicine and public health is littered with the intellectual corpses of those who underestimated the complexity of psychosocial causation and cure of illness.

Nonetheless, geriatrics does offer numerous challenging opportunities for progress on the front lines of nonorganic prevention and treatment. Perception and misperception of disease by the elderly can be made much more appropriate both in the single doctor-patient encounter and in large-scale public education programs. The toll taken by many common geriatric conditions, from cancer to diabetes, is much higher than it need be because of delay (in the former case) or poor self-care (in the latter)—both areas possibly responsive to more effective education of patients and public. Far from being impotent gestures, given the relatively primitive understanding we have of the genesis and cure of these diseases, it is just such nonorganic interventions that may have the greatest impact on morbidity in the coming decade.

Physicians are another potentially fruitful target for large-scale educational interventions. Because of the paucity of geriatric training in medical education, most doctors now in practice have never been exposed to systematic education on the care of the elderly. The recent changes in medical school curricula as well as new continuing education courses in geriatrics could have an important effect on the quality of care (and therefore of health) of the nation's aged. For example, numerous elderly are institutionalized and severely impaired because of mental deterioration diagnosed as "senility." Most of these in fact have Alzheimer's disease, an organic condition of unknown etiology and thus far without an effective treatment (see Chap. 7). Yet many others have undiagnosed and (at one time at least) potentially treatable thyroid dysfunction, pernicious anemia, or other somatic disorders misdiagnosed as Alzheimer's disease.

Because effective treatment of these conditions has been available for decades, one could argue that the primary lesion in these cases is a social one, in dissemination and application of existing knowledge through the health care system. It is intriguing to speculate how many other "senile" patients have neither Alzheimer's disease nor another organic cause for their mental impairment, but rather are victims of social isolation, cognitive deprivation, and "learned helplessness" as the main cause of their mental deterioration. All of these patients, however, are significantly disabled, whether the initial cause of their problem is biomedical or psychosocial.

The emerging research on psychosocial factors in geriatric morbidity and mortality offers further opportunities for averting some of the negative consequences that have been described. Although any large-scale implementation of such approaches would first require adequate experimental verification, a number of avenues are appropriate for current consideration in the clinical care of the elderly.

A systematic consideration of risk factors for socially induced pathology (mental and physical) should be part of the initial and continuing assessment of every older patient. For example, the epidemiological investigations that revealed that hypertensive, hyperlipidemic smokers are at markedly increased risk of heart disease paved the way for intervention programs that target these specific factors in the management of particular patients as well as in large-scale public programs. Similarly, an awareness of the excess morbidity which can follow bereavement, retirement, or institutionalization can alert the clinician to potential problems before they arise. Preventive programs, such as preretirement counseling, widow's groups, and attempts at restructuring some aspects of nursing home environments may prove useful in lessening subsequent deterioration. On a larger scale, accumulating evidence on the health effects of age segregation or overreliance on institutionally based long-term care may suggest changes in public policy on these issues.

The Health Care Delivery System

The elderly patient in need of care confronts a complex, often confusing maze of services, entitlements, and restrictions, and it is often the physician who must act as the patient's navigator through this maze. To perform this job effectively, one must have a sense of what the health and social service systems offer the elderly and what they do not.

The two most important pieces of health legislation affecting care of the elderly in the United States have been the Medicare and Medicaid programs. Both enacted as part of the Great Society legislation in 1965, they are the products of a deep national ambivalence about tax-supported health insurance. Both programs are the result of years of political pressure, counterpressure, and compromise between those who saw the assurance of health care as an appropriate role for government and those who felt such involvement to be misplaced. It is this conflict-ridden gestation that helps explain many of the inconsistencies and gaps in the two programs.

MEDICARE

Medicare (also known as Title XVIII of the Social Security Act) is a federally funded health insurance program covering virtually all Americans 65 and over, regardless of financial status. As a federal program, it is uniform in terms of entitlement and benefits throughout the country. The benefits are divided into two subparts, A and B. Part A, which is available at no charge, covers hospital costs primarily. In any year, the patient must pay the cost of the first day in the hospital; days 2 through 60 are fully covered. For subsequent days, the patient must pay a "coinsurance" charge. Medicare does not cover the cost of hospitalization beyond the 150th day.

Because the framers of Medicare specifically wanted to avoid the costs involved in the long-term care of the elderly, coverage of nursing home costs is strictly limited. Such care must generally follow a stay in an acute hospital and is limited to a 100-day maximum, in keeping with the concept of nursing home care as extended recuperation after an acute illness. There is a small coinsurance charge for most of this period, which must be borne by the patient. After the hundredth day, nursing home care is no longer covered by Medicare, making this program relatively insignificant in paying for long-term care for the elderly.

Similarly, because of the fear of a "bottomless pit" of demand for services, and owing to the original conception of Medicare as basically a hospital insurance plan for acute illnesses, the coverage it offers for home-based care is likewise limited. Until 1981 such care had to follow a hospital stay, although this restrictive requirement has now been dropped. Until recently home care coverage under Medicare was limited to a fixed number of visits, but this restriction was dropped in 1981. However, the greatest limitation on home care under Medicare has not been the number of visits allowed but rather the requirement that the patient needs "skilled care" in order to receive any home care benefits. Thus, many disabled elderly who need only home health aides or other nonnursing help at home cannot qualify for home care under Medicare because their condition is "too stable." Concerns about cost containment have resulted in relatively strict enforcement of the skilled care criterion. As a result, as rehabilitation proceeds (e.g., after a stroke), the closer a patient comes to a plateau of limited self-care, the closer he or she comes to termination of home care benefits. Related to the skilled care need requirement is a second restriction: that the patient be homebound. One final limitation of home care under Medicare should be noted. In keeping with the acute-care medical orientation of the program, no reimbursement is provided for homemaker help, chore services, meal preparation, or other "nonmedical" needs.

Part B of Medicare, known as Supplementary Medical Insurance, is optional at extra cost to the subscriber—an option chosen by well over 90 percent of all elderly. (The premium cost is paid by many states for poor elders.) It covers physician services not included in Part A, physical therapy, and home care, with the same limitations cited above.

Owing again to fears from the outset of uncontrolled overutilization and runaway budgets, Medicare was designed *not* to cover many other health-related services of importance to old people, such as eyeglasses, hearing aids, drugs, dental expenses, and extended periods of home health care or nursing home care. Because of these exceptions and because of the various deductible and coinsurance requirements, Medicare now covers only about a third of the health care costs incurred by the nation's elderly. In fact, the amount spent by elders out of pocket on health care is now higher than it was before the advent of Medicare. Many middle-class and affluent elderly attempt to make up for the inadequacies of Medicare by purchasing supplementary private insurance to cover what Medicare does not (known colloquially as "Medigap" insurance). Poorer elders do without the noncovered care or, if poor enough, may qualify for Medicaid to meet their needs.

MEDICAID
While Medicare is a federally funded, nationally uniform program of health insurance for the elderly, its sister program, Medicaid (Title XIX of the

Social Security Act), differs from it in several important ways. Also passed in 1965, Medicaid was an attempt to provide health coverage to the nation's poor, regardless of age. However, national consensus on this goal was much spottier than it was for the aims of Medicare. As a result, Congress decided to let each state determine the eligibility and benefits that would apply to its own Medicaid program. Some states, such as Arizona and Alaska, chose to have no Medicaid program at all. Others, particularly in the South, devised "tough" programs with high eligibility criteria and low benefits. Still others, such as New York, California, and Massachusetts, put together relatively generous Medicaid programs that were easier to qualify for and more open-handed with reimbursement. All Medicaid programs require that the recipient prove indigency in order to qualify for benefits.

Like Medicare, Medicaid covers hospital charges and physician services. But unlike Medicare, Medicaid also (generally) covers drugs, some ancillary services, and—most important in the present context—nursing home care.

Although it was designed primarily for the poor, the Medicaid program has become of central importance to the elderly, primarily because of its provision for the reimbursement for nursing home care. If a Medicaid-eligible patient requires long-term institutional care, Medicaid will pay for that care for as long as it is needed. Because of the very high cost of nursing home care ($12,000 and up per year), many nonpoor elderly who need long-term care quickly find themselves impoverished after admission to a nursing home; they then join the ranks of the medically indigent, becoming eligible for assistance. This is known as the "Medicaid spend-down." In paying hospital or nursing home charges, a patient is expected to exhaust nearly all of his or her assets (often including savings, house, and car) to a state-determined level (usually a few thousand dollars), after which he or she is eligible for Medicaid. One of the many problems raised by this spend-down procedure is that an elderly patient in a nursing home may be forced to give up the very things (house, car, savings) that would make eventual return to the community possible. A further complication of the spend-down requirement arises when one spouse requires Medicaid-supported nursing home care but the other spouse wants to continue living in the community.

So great is the extent of long-term care reimbursement that fully 40 percent of the entire Medicaid program budget for all age groups is spent on nursing home care for the elderly. Similarly, about half of all nursing home charges in the United States are paid for by Medicaid.

With such a great annual investment in nursing home care, it might seem that comparable expenditures would be made annually in the Medicaid program for home-based health care for the disabled elderly. This is not the case. Against about $10 billion spent by all sources on nursing home care in 1978, the Medicaid program spent about half, or $5 billion. Yet less than two percent of the Medicaid long-term care budget was allocated for home-based geriatric health services. As with Medicare, the difference seems to stem from an unwillingness by legislators to begin covering services that they feel could be limitless in use. Recent federal decisions to reduce spending on human services, particularly imposing "caps" on Medicaid expenditures, jeopardize the extent and quality of services in all forms of long-term care.

POLICY CONSIDERATIONS IN LONG-TERM CARE
One result of the reluctance by the planners and administrators of Medicaid to reimburse for home-based services for the elderly has been a heavy reliance on institutional alternatives. At any given time, about 5 percent of the nation's elderly are institutionalized, although considerable evidence suggests that many of these people could be successfully maintained in the community if a more flexible continuum of care were available and covered by tax-supported insurance.

For example, a 75-year-old widow who suffers a stroke that leaves her with a mild hemiparesis may be unable to return to her fourth-floor walk-up apartment and may have some difficulty with cooking. Were congregate housing for the elderly available to her, incorporating a barrier-free environment, some chore services, and perhaps a hot meal program, she would not require institutionalization. But in the absence of such alternatives, she may well become a placement problem and require a nursing home "bed." For such patients, their eventual institutionalization is a result more of a lesion in the care delivery system than of pathophysiology.

There appears to be an increasing understanding of these notions in policymaking circles, and some progress is being made toward establishing (and funding) more community-based services such as homemaker help, chore services, and specialized housing. However, the lack of a workable "gatekeeper" function to allocate services continues to limit full expansion of these options. There is considerable fear that coverage of such services would, because of overutilization and the existence of a huge reservoir of real unmet need, consume far more public money than it would save. In an era of cost containment in the public sector, that is a price we may as a nation be unwilling to pay.

OTHER FEDERAL PROGRAMS THAT IMPACT ON THE ELDERLY
In addition to Medicare and Medicaid, several other programs attempt to address the needs of the elderly, albeit with much smaller budgets. A continuing challenge for those providing health care for the aged is the discovery, utilization, and coordination of these multiple services that generally operate in isolation from one another.

Title XX is the amendment to the Social Security Act that provides for selected social (as opposed to medical) services outside of institutions, such as homemaker assistance. As is the case for Medicaid, eligibility and scope of services are determined separately by each state and vary widely. Because many states restrict eligibility to the poor, and because the bulk of Title XX funds go to other age groups, the benefit this program holds for the aged is at present limited.

The *Older Americans Act* funds senior citizen centers and congregate hot-lunch programs for the elderly. It also supports local area Agencies on Aging and training, research, and demonstration programs related to aging.

Social Security is the term used to describe the federal retirement benefits program. This program was never conceptualized as a means of total financial support for the elderly, and in fact does not come close to this goal. In 1977, the average payment was $2,900 per year for an individual and $4,800 per year for a couple (if both received benefits). Since these are averages, the actual Social Security check for a given recipient may be much lower or higher, depending on the amount of lifetime earnings paid in to the Social Security account. Women with minimal out-of-home work time or people with histories of low-paying or noncovered jobs receive no Social Security or much smaller monthly amounts. Despite recently mandated cost-of-living adjustments in benefits, about a third of the elderly in the United States receive Social Security checks that, if not supplemented by other sources of income, place them below the federally defined poverty level ($2,730 for an individual in 1978). The Senate Special Committee on Aging has named inadequate income as the most important problem facing the nation's elderly.

Despite the limitations in benefits paid through the Social Security system (especially in contrast to other industrialized nations) the demographic changes discussed earlier, combined with inflation, have cast great doubt on the ability of the Social Security system to remain solvent even into the next century. (Further discussion of income maintenance and the elderly, although it impacts heavily on health and illness, is beyond the scope of this chapter.)

Housing represents a cornerstone of services for the elderly in many developed nations, but in the United States thus far, federal, state, and local governments have been slow in building this component of the care continuum. As noted earlier, adequate purpose-built housing could prevent institutionalization in many instances. Construction of specialized housing for the elderly is increasing at a modest pace, but the demand at present so far outstrips the supply that applicants often face waiting lists comparable in length to their remaining life expectancy.

THE INFORMAL SUPPORT NETWORK

Emphasis on governmental and professional programs for the elderly should not obscure the fact that an enormous amount of care for the elderly is provided by families, friends, and neighbors, often totally apart from the formal network of services. As noted, these informal supports often maintain in the home very frail elders who are fully as disabled as many institutionalized aged. Families (usually daughters or daughters-in-law) may run what have been termed "one-bed nursing homes" that often receive little or no support from official programs designed for the elderly.

In considering the total management of the geriatric patient, it is critical to assess systematically the nature and extent of the informal support network that exists or could be mobilized around the patient. Attention to this oft-neglected mode of care can enable the health care team to maintain patients in noninstitutional environments in many instances. A careful social history and interviews with the family or neighbors is the best way to define the potential for this aspect of patient care.

Like other forms of support, the informal support network is constantly buffeted by the winds of social change and health policy. Throughout the late 1960s and 1970s, many aspects of health legislation were put into place that impinged on the functioning of informal supports. Health care, round-the-clock supervision, and room and board for a parent or grandparent could be totally paid for (after the spend-down period) by Medicaid, but the family willing to undertake responsibility themselves could expect very little financial or service assistance. (This contrasts starkly with the policy in Scandinavian countries to reimburse for in-home care of frail elderly even if such care is provided by family members.) The health care delivery system thus has created strong incentives against in-home care of frail aged family members.

On the other hand, as cost containment becomes the rallying cry of health planners, in-home care using informal supports has begun to look much more attractive. Here, however, a conflict arises with another important development of the last two decades: the changing role of women. With the proportion of women in the labor force now exceeding 50 percent, family care (generally "daughter care") faces a new obstacle. Smaller families, more geographic mobility, and more divorce in each succeeding cohort of elders makes the likelihood of extensive family-based care recede even further with each passing year. Devising health and social policy to accommodate these diverse trends will be a major challenge of the next 20 years.

Suggested Reading

de Beauvoir, S. *The Coming of Age*. New York: Putnam, 1972.

Binstock, R., and Shanas, E. *Handbook of Aging and the Social Sciences*. New York: Van Nostrand Reinhold, 1976.

Butler, R. *Why Survive? Being Old in America*. New York: Harper & Row, 1975.

Estes, C. *The Aging Enterprise*. San Francisco: Jossey-Bass, 1980.

Haynes, S., and Feinleib, M. *Second Conference on the Epidemiology of Aging*. NIH Publication No. 80-969. Washington, D.C.: U.S. Government Printing Office, 1980.

Holmes, T. H., and Rahe, R. H.   The social readjustment rating scale. *J. Psychosomatic Res.* 11:213, 1967.

Kane, R. L., and Kane, R. A.   Care of the aged: old problems in need of new solutions. *Science* 200:913, 1978.

Master, R. J., et al.   A continuum of care for the inner city. *N. Engl. J. Med.* 302: 1434, 1980.

Sourcebook on Aging. Chicago: Marquis Academic Media, 1979.

Vladeck, B.   *Un-Loving Care: The Nursing Home Tragedy.* New York: Basic Books, 1980.

4. Drug Therapy

John W. Rowe
Richard W. Besdine

As people age they accumulate disease, doctor visits, and disability. These events, coupled with appropriate anxiety about their health, make the aged use an excess proportion of the prescription and over-the-counter drugs consumed in the United States. Although our 25 million citizens over 65 years of age represent less than 12 percent of our population, they purchase 25 percent of the drugs sold in America, spending nearly 20 percent of their personal funds. In Great Britain outpatients over 75 years old take three times as many medicines as the national average, with women consuming twice as many drugs as men. This excess consumption of medicines is accompanied, not surprisingly, by excess rates of adverse reactions. Of equal importance is that when older people consume the same drugs with the same frequency as the young, toxicity is more frequent and severe in the elderly. Several factors contribute to this special vulnerability of the elderly: body composition; drug distribution, metabolism, and excretion; and tissue sensitivity. Standards for the use of most current therapeutic agents were obtained in young adults, and applying these guidelines to the elderly is often hazardous.

Because the prevalence of disease rises sharply with age, a sick old person is likely to have several associated disorders, and multiple organ-system dysfunction also increases the risk of adverse drug reaction. When the high prevalence of cognitive and visual impairment in the elderly is juxtaposed to the similar size, shape, texture, and color of many medicines, errors involving drugs are especially likely. A better understanding of the special features of drug use in the elderly is necessary to reduce excess toxicity.

Drug Use in the Elderly
ADVERSE REACTIONS

Numerous studies have documented that old people have more trouble with drugs than do their descendants. As many as one-seventh of all hospitalizations result from adverse drug reactions, and elderly people comprise nearly half the hospital admissions caused by drug intoxication [1]. Rates of adverse drug reaction rise steadily after age 50, and patients over 60 years old are twice as likely to suffer an adverse drug reaction as younger patients [2]. Those over 80 years have a one in four risk of drug intoxication, twice the rate seen in patients under 50 years. Hospital stay is prolonged for all patients with adverse reactions, but older patients remain hospitalized longest [3]. Two age-related phenomena, impaired kidney function and multiple drug use, are major risk factors in adverse reactions [4].

COMPLIANCE

When a patient fails to improve with a prescribed therapeutic regimen, suspicion of medication failure or worsening disease, or both, often impel the physician to change drugs. The possibility of noncompliance with the prescribed medication regimen may be overlooked unless the patient manifests obvious psychopathology. Noncompliance can occur in four ways:

1. Omission: the drug is not taken.
2. Commission: unprescribed drugs are taken.
3. Scheduling misconception: a prescribed drug is taken without knowledge of the correct schedule.
4. Scheduling noncompliance: a prescribed drug is taken incorrectly with knowledge of the correct schedule.

When compliance has been studied, half the patients are found not to take medication as prescribed. One-quarter to one-half of patients fail entirely to take a prescribed drug, and still more take them incorrectly. One drug error increases the risk for many errors. At risk for noncompliance are those patients with chronic illness, a low socioeconomic and educational level, language difficulty, multiple drug treatment (greater than three drugs), drugs requiring frequent doses, drugs with frequent side effects, and complicated drug regimens. In most studies noncompliance was highest among elderly patients and was related to the preceding risk factors as well as to the following age-related characteristics: (1) poor vision, (2) poor hearing, (3) unusable childproof containers, (4) dementia, and (5) difficulty swallowing large pills.

Some suggestions for generating better compliance, especially by the elderly, are listed here:

1. Carefully explain the disease and the medication being prescribed for it, including the precise regimen.
2. Use large type and simple directions on the label.
3. Use texture codes on medicine containers.
4. Provide preloaded multicompartment containers providing a week's schedule of medication.
5. Provide a medication calendar that allows tearing or marking off as drugs are taken.
6. Use easily opened containers.
7. Avoid very large or very small pills.
8. Use liquid formulations liberally.
9. Give simplified dosage regimens related to daily routine events.
10. Ask the patient to bring periodically all medications for the doctor's inspection.

Improved compliance, especially for the elderly, can only be expected if the special problems related to drug treatment are known and considered in the design of drug regimens.

Age-Related Changes
PHYSIOLOGIC CHANGES
Normal aging, in the absence of disease, is associated with physiologic changes that have important clinical influence. These changes form the substrate of the impact of aging on the presentation, response to treatment, and complications of a variety of acute and chronic illnesses. The coexistence of age-related normative changes and the physiologic toll of diseases prevalent in old age generate the special vulnerability of the elderly to adverse drug reactions.

CHANGES IN BODY COMPOSITION
The well-documented changes in body composition with age are primarily reflected in a decrease in the amount of muscle and an increase in the amount of fat per pound. Thus, a 150-pound 80-year-old has less muscle and more fat than a 150-pound 30-year-old of the same height. Accordingly, the same dose of a non-lipid–soluble medication would give the old person more drug in proportion to lean body mass and more drug effect. This alteration in the volume of distribution of many drugs needs to be considered in prescribing medications for the elderly.

LOSS OF FUNCTION OF SPECIFIC ORGANS
The major age-related physiologic changes that influence drug prescribing are the progressive losses after maturity in individual organs, especially the heart and kidneys. These losses in function are accompanied by a reduced capacity of the elderly to dispose of drugs, either through metabolism to inactive compounds or elimination in the urine. The most important physiologic change, in terms of drug therapy, is the alteration in kidney function, since many medications are eliminated in the urine. Normal elderly individuals have glomerular filtration rates significantly less than those of young individuals [5]. In general there is a nearly 50 percent reduction in renal function between age 30 and age 80 years. The clinical impact of this decrease is augmented by the lack of change in the serum creatinine concentration despite the decrease in renal function. Serum creatinine is generally used as a guide to renal function since it is easier to obtain than a 24-hour creatinine clearance and more reliable than the blood urea nitrogen (BUN). However, since creatinine is produced in muscle, and muscle mass decreases with age in parallel with renal function, the decreased renal function in the elderly is not reflected in an increase in serum creatinine. An elderly individual with half the renal function of his or her 30-year-old counterpart will actually have the same serum creatinine as the younger person. Thus,

because serum creatinine can be said to overestimate renal function in the elderly, advanced age calls for reduced dosages of drugs excreted primarily via renal mechanisms, such as digitalis or aminoglycoside antibiotics (gentamicin or kanamycin), even in the presence of a "normal" serum creatinine.

ALTERED TISSUE SENSITIVITY TO DRUGS
The tissues of elderly individuals are frequently more sensitive to a drug than are the tissues of a young individual, and even if a lower dose is given, a greater or, in some cases, paradoxical effect of the drug may be seen. Morphine follows this pattern, producing greater analgesic effect per milligram in old patients than in healthy young individuals.

Principles of Drug Therapy in the Elderly
The following principles should always be followed when drugs are given to elderly patients.

1. Before prescribing new drugs, thoroughly review all medication the patient is presently taking.
2. Before prescribing a drug for a specific symptom, consider the possibility that the symptom is an adverse reaction to a medication. In general, stopping a drug is more beneficial than starting one.
3. Before prescribing a drug, consider the patient's age and the presence of any specific disease states, particularly cardiac disease and impaired renal function.
4. Keep drug regimens as simple as possible.
5. Use the lowest effective dose and increase the dose slowly.
6. Do not withhold drugs because of age.
7. Assess therapeutic response frequently and discontinue unneeded drugs.
8. Perform thorough, frequent reviews of the medication regimen.
9. Consider the cost of medications and use generic preparations when appropriate.

Pharmacotherapy of Specific Disease States or Medical Problems
In this section we will try to provide only a general overview of the approach to pharmacotherapy of general categories of disease. A detailed review of the pharmacologic management of specific disease states is provided in the chapters of this book devoted to particular organs or organ systems and the diseases thereof.

CARDIOVASCULAR DISEASES
Cardiovascular diseases are very prevalent among the elderly. In long-term care facilities, as many as 80 percent of individuals have organic heart dis-

ease, and half the residents show evidence of congestive heart failure. In evaluating the possible presence of heart disease in elderly patients, one must consider that disease presentation is often markedly influenced by age. As many as 70 percent of old patients with acute myocardial infarction may present without chest pain, showing instead shortness of breath, confusion, syncope, dizziness, or weakness [6].

Digitalis Preparations

When prescribing digitalis preparations for elderly patients with congestive heart failure, several important points must be kept in mind:

1. Digoxin is excreted primarily via renal mechanisms, and excretion will be impaired in elderly individuals. Because the clearance rate of digoxin from plasma is decreased by as much as 40 percent in the elderly, lower maintenance doses are often needed [7]. In addition to lower maintenance doses, a decrease in loading dose should be considered in small elderly patients with low lean body mass. Digitoxin excretion is more dependent on hepatic than renal mechanisms, and in the presence of renal insufficiency it may be more conveniently used than digoxin preparations.

2. Studies in patients with atrial fibrillation have failed to show an effect of age on the sensitivity of the heart rate to digitalis. Therefore, heart rate can be controlled in elderly patients with atrial fibrillation with the same blood levels of digitalis as are necessary in young individuals.

3. In addition to atypical presentation of ischemic heart disease, congestive heart failure may also present peculiarly. Insomnia may be an early unrecognized symptom of congestive heart failure in the elderly, and digitalis toxicity may paradoxically present as heart failure.

4. Digitalis toxicity is increased in the presence of potassium depletion. This is especially common in elderly patients on diuretics who have a markedly diminished dietary intake of potassium or who have chronic vomiting or diarrhea.

5. The elderly appear particularly susceptible to several consequences of digitalis overdose, including confusion and disorientation. Gynecomastia in elderly men can occur with appropriate dosage and therapeutic blood levels and is therefore not a manifestation of toxicity.

6. Many elderly individuals on chronic maintenance digoxin for control of congestive heart failure can be safely withdrawn from the medication. Digitalis is often begun when cardiac decompensation develops in association with arrhythmias, marked volume expansion, or acute myocardial infarction; after the acute illness passes the digitalis may no longer be required. This view is supported by an interesting study by Dall [8], showing that

75 percent of elderly patients on digoxin for congestive heart failure could be safely withdrawn from the treatment.

Diuretics

Elderly individuals are more likely to develop complications secondary to diuretics, whether prescribed for heart failure or hypertension. Diuretics that deplete potassium (thiazides, furosemide, and ethacrynic acid) are particularly likely to produce hypokalemia in the elderly since they may not have an adequate dietary potassium intake. Diuretics that spare potassium (triamterene and spironolactone) may be useful in conjunction with thiazide diuretics to prevent the development of hypokalemia. Such combinations, however, may also result in the development of life-threatening elevations of serum potassium, particularly in elderly individuals with renal disease, and, therefore, they should be used with great caution, if at all, in such individuals. Supplemental potassium is best avoided when potassium-sparing drugs are administered. Hypercalcemia, an additional electrolyte abnormality occasionally unmasked by thiazide diuretics, often presents in elderly individuals as confusion.

A major complication of diuretic therapy in elderly individuals is volume depletion. The normal tendency for old patients to become salt- and water-depleted during an acute illness complicated by fever, vomiting, diarrhea, or dramatic reduction in fluid intake is augmented by the concurrent administration of diuretics. The severe volume depletion that may result will induce mental changes, prerenal azotemia, and may aggravate the orthostatic hypotension found in elderly individuals who spend most of their day in bed or in the chair.

A frequent complication of diuretic use in the elderly is exacerbation of previously inapparent or mild diabetes mellitus. Because this effect is related, at least in part, to potassium deficiency, potassium replacement may be helpful in this diabetogenic effect of diuretics.

Many complications of diuretic therapy can be eliminated if diuretics are prescribed more sparingly. Diuretics are frequently unnecessarily administered to elderly patients with modest degrees of dependent peripheral edema, often associated with venous insufficiency without congestive heart failure, and result in intravascular volume contraction and orthostatic hypotension. Mild heart failure is often treated satisfactorily with digitalis alone—without the administration of diuretics—thus avoiding the adverse effects of the diuretics themselves and lessening the risk of hypokalemia and digitalis toxicity.

Drugs for Hypertension

Postural hypotension is common in the elderly, especially in those who are not ambulatory, and is aggravated by the use of antihypertensive agents [9]. Appropriate use of hypotensive agents is clouded by the uncertainty regarding the management of the so-called normal systolic hypertension of old age. Systolic blood pressure rises with age, and the age-corrected cutoff point for the appropriate institution of antihypertensive therapy is not known. It is known, however, that pathologic systolic or diastolic hypertension is a striking risk factor for cardiovascular and central nervous system vascular disease in the elderly, though risk reduction by treatment has not been proved. The important point is that when treating hypertension in the elderly special caution must be exercised to avoid side effects that may be as dangerous as the hypertension itself.

Diuretics are the most frequently used first-line drugs for hypertension in young and old patients, and special considerations in their use for the elderly have already been discussed. Another common antihypertensive agent used is methyldopa, which can produce central nervous system depression, particularly in elderly individuals, as a major side effect. Propranolol is commonly used for the management of hypertension as well as for treatment of cardiac arrhythmias, this drug has a higher level of toxicity in elderly patients than in younger patients [10]. The most common adverse reactions from propranolol are bradycardia, congestive heart failure, and hypotension.

Drugs for Arrhythmias

In general, the type and dose of medications for arrhythmias is the same for elderly individuals as for younger individuals. Of particular interest is the apparent increased toxicity of lidocaine, particularly manifested as central nervous system (CNS) symptoms such as confusion, lethargy, and dysarthria, in the elderly [11]. Because of the short half-life of lidocaine and the fact that it is usually administered intravenously, however, this problem is generally easily managed, once recognized, by reduction in the infusion rate. Quinidine, which is commonly used in the management of arrhythmias, has a decreased disposal rate in the elderly and may cause disturbing tinnitus, vertigo, visual disturbances, headache, confusion, or diarrhea. It even has been shown to lead, on occasion, to the development of a psychosis that can be mistaken for dementia [12].

PAIN

Analgesics are frequently used by the elderly for arthritis, headaches, and nonspecific complaints. Age influences the response of individuals to analgesics, and dosage alterations are often necessary in the elderly. An important principle in the treatment of pain is avoidance, when possible, of administration of analgesics on an as-needed basis. When pain is predictable it is more advisable to prescribe analgesics on an around-the-clock schedule to prevent pain than have the patient self-medicating in response to pain. Advancing age is associated with increased sensitivity to parenterally administered narcotics, and lower doses are required for adequate analgesic effects in old patients. This is particularly important postoperatively, when excess sedation associated with narcotics may lead to excessive lethargy, confusion, delirium, or aspiration [13].

Among nonnarcotic analgesics, aspirin has a deserved reputation for therapeutic efficacy. The frequency of gastrointestinal blood loss and resulting anemia in the elderly, however, is sufficient to justify careful monitoring. Tinnitus and confusion are manifestations of acute toxicity. Acetaminophen is not as effective an analgesic as aspirin but does not cause gastrointestinal bleeding. There appears to be no influence of age on toxicity associated with acetaminophen. Propoxyphene has potent brain side effects and can lead to giddiness, confusion, lethargy, and occasionally chronic dementia in the elderly. Codeine, while as effective in the elderly as in young individuals, has a strong tendency to aggravate preexisting constipation. This represents a serious drawback in debilitated elderly patients, and prophylactic laxative use may be indicated.

ARTHRITIS AND INFLAMMATION

Arthritis and musculoskeletal complaints are very common in the elderly, and antiinflammatory medications are universally used in chronic care facilities. Aspirin is an effective antiinflammatory agent as well as an analgesic, and can be used safely in the elderly, providing patients are monitored for asymptomatic gastrointestinal bleeding. The usual symptoms associated with salicylism—tinnitus, decreased hearing, and toxic CNS effects such as delirium and psychosis—can occur at relatively low doses. In some patients toxicity develops without first producing tinnitus. The newer, nonsteroidal agents have gastrointestinal side effects similar to those of aspirin (dyspepsia, occult bleeding, and so on), although they occur much less frequently. Alterations in mental status or fluid retention develop in occasional patients, but this is somewhat unusual.

Phenylbutazone, a potent antiinflammatory, antirheumatic drug, sometimes causes aplastic anemia when administered for long periods of time and can lead to acute peptic ulceration and salt and water retention. Since salt and water retention may aggravate underlying heart disease, this agent should probably not be used in elderly individuals with congestive heart failure. Indomethacin is a useful drug for arthritis but frequently causes confusion or psychosis in elderly patients. The incidence of gastrointestinal distress and bleeding in the elderly is also considerable.

Aspirin, phenylbutazone, indomethacin, and the newer agents have antiplatelet effects; consequently these drugs should not be given to patients with bleeding problems or to individuals who are on anticoagulants. In this instance a nonacetylated salicylate (such as salsalate or choline salicylate), which does not interfere with platelet function, is indicated.

Corticosteroids are potent antiinflammatory agents that should be prescribed only for specific reasons and whose use must be monitored closely in all patients. Because many diseases that are more prevalent in the elderly, such as hypertension, diabetes, and osteoporosis, are aggravated by corticosteroids, elderly patients are at a risk for excess morbidity from these medications. While the acute psychosis or confusional state seen occasionally with high-dose steroids occurs in patients of all ages, old patients may also develop a chronic dementing syndrome secondary to these drugs. All antiinflammatory drugs should be taken after meals or with an antacid to minimize gastro-intestinal toxicity.

INFECTIONS

The issue of compliance—the tendency of the elderly to noncompliance—is particularly important when prescribing antiinfective agents. Since many classes of antibiotics, particularly aminoglycosides (kanamycin, gentamicin, amikacin, tobramycin), are excreted via renal mechanisms, a reduction in dose of these agents must be considered even in elderly people without renal disease. The aminoglycosides are particularly hazardous since accumulation in serum may rapidly cause renal failure and auditory nerve toxicity. These antibiotics should always be given cautiously and in reduced dosage proportional to creatinine clearance in elderly patients. In general, once a diagnosis is established, neither the choice of antibiotic, nor the dose is influenced by age, with the exception of the adjustment for renal function. The incidence of pseudomembranous colitis in patients receiving clindamycin increases with age, and elderly patients on this medication should be monitored closely for the development of diarrhea.

THROMBOTIC DISORDERS

Aspirin is finding increasing clinical use as an anticoagulant, and its effectiveness in decreasing platelet aggregation is not known to be affected by age. Use of the more potent anticoagulants, warfarin and heparin, carries an increased risk of bleeding in old age. Similar blood concentrations of warfarin in young and old patients result in a greater prolongation of the prothrombin time in the elderly [14,15]. Elderly individuals thus require a lower warfarin dose to maintain the prothrombin time in the therapeutic range and are at greater risk for the development of warfarin intoxication. The risk of bleeding while on heparin increases with age, particularly in women, and careful monitoring of stool, urine, and hematocrit should be performed in order to detect bleeding as early as possible [16]. Anticoagulants, nevertheless, can be used safely in the elderly, and these patients should not be denied their benefits when indicated.

DIABETES

The use of oral anti-diabetic drugs in old people is hazardous because delayed excretion results in markedly prolonged hypoglycemia with a spectrum of mental changes. Even when the patient is treated acutely with oral or intravenous sugar, hypoglycemia often recurs because of drug persistence. Chlorpropamide, which persists up to five days or more in elderly patients, may also increase an antidiuretic hormone effect and induce hyponatremia, particularly in old age. Phenformin has been withdrawn from clinical use because of its propensity to produce life-threatening lactic acidosis, especially in elderly patients.

PARKINSON'S DISEASE

L-dopa is a remarkable breakthrough in the therapy of parkinsonian rigidity and akinesia, but its side effects are also substantial. More than 20 percent of the elderly taking it become confused, demented, depressed, or psychotic. In the presence of underlying dementia, problems are even more common. Facial grimacing and other involuntary movements, although rarer side effects, may appear to be voluntary and behavioral rather than drug-related and provoke more L-dopa or the addition of a psychotropic agent. Administration of L-dopa in combination with carbidopa, a substance blocking the enzyme that degrades L-dopa in the body, allows a reduction of the dose and produces less frequent side effects. L-dopa has no effect on the parkinsonism produced by the neuroleptic (phenothiazines and such) drugs, and in fact the two negate each other's therapeutic effects.

Anticholinergic drugs, although less effective than L-dopa, can be useful in certain patients. Especially common or troublesome side effects include constipation, urinary retention, confusion, psychosis, and glaucoma. These drugs are useful in managing the parkinsonism induced by neuroleptic agents.

SLEEP DISTURBANCES

Even though hypnotics are used almost universally in institutionalized old people, when a sleep disturbance is documented, a cause should always be sought. Often all that is required is reassurance to the patient that the observed change in sleep pattern is within normal limits. Pain, depression, anxiety, early dementia, intoxication by another drug(s), urinary frequency, or even a strange bed can all provoke sleep disorder. Each cause should be specifically evaluated and treated. Temporary use of a sleeping pill may be indicated, and many are available. The few controlled studies that have been done do not identify any one agent as being more effective than others. The common belief that barbiturate excitation and hangover are more common and intense in the elderly has not been verified. All hypnotics produce hangover and decrease early-morning performance. Flurazepam is particularly likely to result in prolonged drowsiness in the elderly when given in doses greater than 15 mg daily [17]. Sleep medications are generally not effective for long periods of time and may need to be changed periodically.

PSYCHOSIS

Antipsychotic or neuroleptic drugs include phenothiazines, the butyrophenones, and the thioxanthenes. They are indicated in treatment of severe agitation, psychosis, and bizarre, disordered behavior. All are similar in therapeutic effect but differ greatly in side effects. They deposit in tissues and have a clearance time of a month or more. All can produce jaundice, cardiac arrhythmias, agranulocytosis, and photosensitivity in all age groups. They potentiate hypnotics and tranquilizers, as well as antihypertensives, and the hypotensive effects of other drugs. Important side effects in old people are sedation; confusion; hypotension; extrapyramidal syndromes, including parkinsonism, dystonic reactions, akathisia (motor restlessness), and tardive dyskinesia (facial grimacing); and anticholinergic effects of urinary retention, glaucoma, and atonic colon.

Side effects of neuroleptic agents are usually in one of two categories. Those drugs that produce intense sedation and hypotension are relatively free of extrapyramidal syndromes, and vice versa. Chlorpromazine is known for its sedating effects, which can be severe in the elderly even when given in small doses; haloperidol is known for its propensity to produce extrapyramidal syndromes, including frequently irreversible tardive dyskinesia. Thioridazine, of all drugs in the group, produces fewest and least severe extrapyramidal syndromes, and provides mild to moderate sedation, frequently a desirable side effect in agitated elderly patients behaving in a bizarre manner.

A particularly common situation calling for the appropriate use of an antipsychotic drug is the nocturnal emergence of sudden bizarre, violent, or self-destructive behavior in an acutely ill, elderly hospitalized patient, the "sundowning syndrome." Risk factors for sundowning include advanced age, mild preexisting cognitive loss, acute medical illness, sleep deprivation, visual or hearing loss, sensory deprivation, pain, and environmental dislocation. After remediation of risk factors for these most difficult patients, there often still exists the need for pharmacologic intervention. In such situations a rapid-acting drug with both sedating and antipsychotic effects is most desirable. When the patient will take an oral medication, a small dose (10–25 mg) of thioridazine concentrate will often be effective, acting within 30 minutes. When a parenteral drug must be used, mesoridazine, the active metabolite of thioridazine, can be given in a low dose. It is more likely to produce extrapyramidal side effects than its parent compound.

DEPRESSION

Antidepressants are effective in treating or maintaining young or old patients with affective disorders. There are three groups of antidepressants.

Monoamine Oxidase Inhibitors

These antidepressants, although effective, interact with a variety of foods and drugs to produce life-threatening hypertension. They probably should not be used in old people except in highly supervised situations after other therapeutic agents have been tried and have proved to be unsuccessful.

Tricyclic Antidepressants

The tricyclic antidepressants share their basic chemical structure with phenothiazines, as well as many of the same side effects, including hypotension, excess sedation, and cardiac arrhythmias. They frequently cause an acute confusional state in old people. Maximum therapeutic effect may not be achieved until after two to six weeks of treatment, but toxicity can appear in days. The potential to produce excess sedation and a confusional state generally parallels the anticholinergic effects of the drug. The order of anticholinergic potency for the commonly used tricyclics is amitriptyline, imipramine, doxepin, nortriptyline, and desipramine. Usually the less anticholinergic, less sedating antidepressants are more beneficial for elderly depressives; when agitation and sleeplessness dominate the disease, however, one of the more anticholinergic drugs may be chosen. Recent evidence suggests that, at least with nortriptyline, cardiac arrhythmias only occur at toxic blood levels. There is no complete therapeutic overlap with these drugs, so failure with one agent may reasonably be followed by a trial with another.

Lithium

Lithium is a valuable drug in the maintenance of young and old patients with manic-depressive illness. It appears to be effective in the elderly at both a lower daily dose and lower serum level. It has major effects on sodium economy in the body and is difficult to use in patients receiving diuretics.

ANXIETY

Antianxiety drugs in common use fall into three classes: propanediols, barbiturates, and benzodiazepines.

Propanediols

The propanediols, represented by meprobamate, should not be used in old people. They are questionably effective, addicting, and produce drowsiness and withdrawal seizures. Overdose can be fatal.

Barbiturates

Both short- and long-acting barbiturates produce mild to moderate daytime sedation with attendant relief of anxiety. A high incidence of addiction, withdrawal seizures, and excess drowsiness, however, make them poor drugs for old people. The classically described paradoxical excitation is uncommon but very unpleasant.

Benzodiazepines

Benzodiazepines are the most useful group of antianxiety drugs in treating old people. They are represented by chlordiazepoxide, diazepam, oxazepam, and lorazepam. Chlordiazepoxide has been shown to be safer and more effective than barbiturates in the control of anxiety. Its major problem is excess sedation. Diazepam has the additional effect of skeletal muscle relaxation and is more potent than chlordiazepoxide. It induces sleep, and side effects are more marked, with a propensity to postural hypotension, especially in the elderly.

The major problem with both chlordiazepoxide and diazepam, however, is marked persistence in the body because of a complex multistep degradation process that produces many active metabolites [18]. Clearance of diazepam can take 40 to 90 hours. Oxazepam, the shortest acting and probably safest benzodiazepine for elderly patients, has little or no tendency to accumulate and is an effective sedative.

SKIN DISORDERS
Decubitus Ulcers
Decubitus ulcers are extremely common in elderly bedridden individuals. Prevention requires frequent redistribution of body weight by turning, use of air mattresses, and protection of pressure points with lamb's wool pads, foam "doughnuts," or similar devices. Once skin is broken down, avoidance of pressure is mandatory for healing. In addition, the area should be kept clean and dry. Benzoyl peroxide 20% lotion, both bactericidal and drying, can be applied to the ulcer base as a thin film four times a day. To obtain a 20% concentration, two packets of loroxide powder are mixed with one vial of its lotion base. Maalox or other antacids can be used in the same manner.

Stasis Dermatitis
Stasis dermatitis usually produces marked erythema, hyperpigmentation, and pruritus of the lower legs. Excellent symptomatic relief is obtained by use of a fluorinated steroid ointment with occlusive wraps for four to eight hours a day. Once improvement occurs, a less potent steroid should be substituted to prevent cutaneous atrophy and possible ulceration. Topical antibiotics and antihistamines should be avoided because of their potential for allergic sensitization.

Pruritus
Generalized pruritus in the absence of a primary dermatitis is common in the elderly. Mild cases often respond to frequent application of a topical emollient. Moderate sun exposure may be helpful. Oral antihistamines or minor tranquilizers may decrease awareness of discomfort, but they will occasionally produce excessive somnolence or paradoxical restlessness. Patients with severe, persistent pruritus should be evaluated for occult malignancy, biliary obstruction, hyperthyroidism, or the possibility of drug allergy.

ASTHMA

The major indication for the use of bronchodilators is bronchospasm, manifested clinically by wheezing. Dose modification of these drugs in elderly patients is needed in the presence of coexisting heart and liver disease.

Epinephrine and the synthetic agent terbutaline are the mainstays of therapy for acute bronchospasm. On pharmacologic grounds terbutaline is preferred because of its specificity for noncardiac β_2 receptors and the decreased risk of cardiac side effects; however, it can lead to marked increases in heart rate secondary to peripheral vasodilatation. In acutely asthmatic patients over the age of 50, it is best to use terbutaline and to start with a low dose (1.25–2.5 mg by mouth or 0.125–0.25 mg subcutaneously).

Aminophylline, used frequently in chronic asthma, is well absorbed after oral administration, is metabolized by the liver, and can be given intravenously in the emergency setting. Patients with preexisting heart or liver disease, older patients (i.e., over 50 years), and patients on digoxin or erythromycin all require reductions in dosage. Aminophylline has a relatively narrow therapeutic to toxic ratio, with the earliest toxic side effect being nausea. Nausea can be precipitated by concomitant digoxin therapy and calls for reduction in dosage of the aminophylline. The major pharmacologic effects of aminophylline in addition to bronchodilation are stimulation of the heart, gastrointestinal system, and central nervous system. The major toxic side effects are related to these pharmacologic effects and include: nausea and vomiting, arrhythmias, and seizures. All can be avoided with careful dosage schedules [19,20].

PEPTIC ULCER DISEASE

The treatment of peptic ulcer disease is essentially the same in elderly patients as in young adults with one important exception. Cimetidine, a histamine antagonist used for inhibition of gastric acid secretion in duodenal ulcer disease, is more likely to cause adverse reactions in old patients. This is particularly true of the central nervous system effects of cimetidine, the most common of which are confusion and hallucinations. Cimetidine remains an effective agent for the treatment of duodenal ulcer and should be used in elderly patients when indicated, but at a low dose and with careful monitoring for the development of central nervous system toxicity [21,22].

References

1. Caranasos, G. J., et al. Drug induced illness leading to hospitalization. *J.A.M.A.* 228:713, 1974.
2. Stewart, R., and Cluff, L. A review of medication errors and compliance in ambulant patients. *Clin. Pharmacol. Ther.* 13:463, 1972.
3. Seidl, L. G., et al. Studies on the epidemiology of adverse drug reactions. III. Reactions in patients on a general medical service. *Bull. Johns Hopkins Hosp.* 119:299, 1966.

4. Smith, J. W., et al. Studies on the epidemiology of adverse drug reactions. V. Clinical factors influencing susceptibility. *Ann. Intern. Med.* 65:629, 1966.
5. Rowe, J. W., et al. The effect of age on creatinine clearance in man: a cross-sectional and longitudinal study. *J. Gerontol.* 31:155, 1976.
6. Pathy, M. S. Clinical presentation of myocardial infarction in the elderly. *Br. Heart J.* 29:190, 1967.
7. Ewy, G. A., Kapadia, G. G., Yao, L., Lullin, M., and Marcus, F. I. Digoxin metabolism in the elderly. *Circulation* 39:449, 1969.
8. Dall, J. L. C. Maintenance digoxin in elderly patients. *Br. Med. J.* 2:705, 1970.
9. Caird, F. I., Andrews, G. R., and Kennedy, R. D. Effect of posture on blood pressure in the elderly. *Br. Heart J.* 35:527, 1973.
10. Castleden, C. M., Kaye, C. M., and Parsons, R. L. The effect of age on plasma levels of propranolol and practolol in man. *Br. J. Clin. Pharmacol.* 2:303, 1975.
11. Pfeifer, H. J., Greenblatt, D. J., and Koch-Weser, J. Clinical use and toxicity of intravenous lidocaine. *Am. Heart J.* 92:168, 1976.
12. Ochs, H. R., et al. Reduced clearance of quinidine in elderly humans (Abstract). *Clin. Res.* 25:513A, 1977.
13. Belleville, J. W., et al. Influence of age on pain relief from analgesics. A study of postoperative patients. *J.A.M.A.* 217:1835, 1971.
14. Shepard, A. M. M., et al. Age as a determinant of sensitivity of warfarin. *Br. J. Clin. Pharmacol.* 4:315, 1977.
15. O'Malley, K., et al. Determinants of anticoagulant control in patients receiving warfarin. *Br. J. Clin. Pharmacol.* 4:309, 1977.
16. Jick, H., et al. Efficacy and toxicity of heparin in relation to age and sex. *N. Engl. J. Med.* 279:284, 1968.
17. Greenblatt, D. J., Allen, M. D., and Shader, R. I. Toxicity of high dose flurazepam in the elderly. *Clin. Pharmacol. Ther.* 21:355, 1977.
18. Greenblatt, D. J., Harmatz, J. S., and Shader, R. I. Factors influencing diazepam pharmacokinetics: Age, sex, and liver disease. *Int. J. Clin. Pharmacol.* 16:177, 1978.
19. Josko, W. J., et al. Intravenous theophylline: nomogram guidelines. *Ann. Intern. Med.* 86:400, 1977.
20. Piafsky, K. M., et al. Theophylline kinetics in acute pulmonary edema. *Clin. Pharmacol. Ther.* 21:310, 1977.
21. McMillen, M. A., Ambis, D., and Siegel, J. H. Cimetidine and mental confusion. *N. Engl. J. Med.* 298:284, 1978.
22. Delaney, J. C., and Raney, M. Cimetidine and mental confusion. *Lancet* 2:512, 1970.

5. Neurology

Louis R. Caplan

Normal Aging and the Central Nervous System

Pathologic and electrophysiologic studies of neurologically normal aged adults have documented changes at all levels of the nervous system. At times it is difficult to differentiate the changes of aging from common conditions that are statistically more likely to occur the longer one lives. For example, pathologic examination of skeletal muscle in older patients reveals some degree of group atrophy of muscle fibers, loss of single muscle fibers, clusters of muscle nuclei without cytoplasm, and a widened range of fiber size [1]. These findings could be due, at least in part, to minor trauma (bruising, stretching, or rupture of fibers), excessive use of unconditioned muscles, simple disuse, as well as minor pressure or entrapment of the peripheral innervation of the muscle, all factors increasingly likely in the elderly. A gradual decrease in size of individual muscle fibers and muscle bulk is more certainly a phenomenon related to aging. The changes in muscle seen with aging do not produce clinically symptomatic muscle weakness.

The peripheral nerves of elderly subjects contain degenerated axons; a diminution in the density and number of nerve fibers, with disproportionate loss of larger fibers; and an increase in the connective tissue content of nerves. The electrical counterpart of these changes is slowing of nerve conduction velocity, a measurement that largely reflects the rate of conduction in the largest nerve fibers. Motor conduction slows 0.15 m/sec/year and sensory conduction decreases by 0.16 m/sec/year [2]. These pathologic and electrophysiologic alterations are not associated with a symptomatic neuropathy, but in older subjects decreased vibration and touch sensation in the feet and decreased deep tendon reflexes at the wrist and ankle are common findings.

In the spinal cord, the number of motor neurons in the anterior horn cell region decreases progressively with age. These cells are the source of innervation of skeletal muscle. The pathologic changes in muscle, peripheral nerve, and spinal cord are responsible for the gradual loss of agility, strength, and athletic capabilities that begins in the fourth decade of life.

Beginning in the third decade, brain weight declines; in men, by age 70 there has been a 10 percent decline, and a 17 percent decrease by age 80. The comparable figures for women are 5 percent decline at 70 and 16 percent by age 80 [3]. The convolutions become smaller, sulci wider, ventricles larger, and leptomeninges thicker with advancing age. Histologically, loss of nerve cells, shrinkage of neurons, storage of lipofuscin in neurons, senile plaques, and the presence of spheroid-shaped enlargement of central axons are present. Loss of nerve cells is not uniform but is most apparent in the Purkinje cells of the cerebellum, and in the second and fourth layers of the cerebral cortex, affecting some cortical regions more than others [4]. Total protein and lipid content of the brain decreases slightly with advancing age. Atherosclerosis and hyalinization of the media of cerebral vessels are also more common in the elderly. Tests that provide an anatomic display of cranial contents (computed tomography or pneumoencephalogram) reveal enlargement of the cerebral ventricles and prominence of sulci after the sixth decade. Some carefully studied adults with normal intellectual function show an anatomic pattern on computed tomography (CT) scan indistinguishable from atrophy. A partial explanation for this abnormal anatomy may be that it is produced by alterations in connective tissue matrix or cerebrospinal fluid mechanics, changes that may have little reflection in brain function.

The cerebral metabolic rate of oxygen consumption decreases gradually with age beginning in the third decade. By age 70, the cerebral metabolic rate for oxygen ($CMRO_2$) is 9 percent below the third decade level [5]. There is also a concomitant fall in cerebral blood flow irrespective of the methodology used (inhalation [6], or Kety-Schmidt [7], or intracarotid injection of ^{133}Xe). Considerable controversy of the chicken–egg type surrounds the interpretation of the relationship of decreased blood flow to decreased metabolism of oxygen. Is the decreased flow responsible for less supply of oxygen and nutrients and thus the cause of the decreased metabolic rate, or is decreased flow merely a reflection of less functioning tissue and less requirement for blood. The close correlation of decreased $CMRO_2$ with abnormal mental function in patients with senile dementia, and the absence of severe pathologic changes in cerebral vessels in these patients, support the view that the reduced blood flow is a consequence of the diminished requirements and not the cause.

Atherosclerosis affects cerebral vessels in a nonuniform fashion, producing severe narrowing of some vessels in certain regions and leaving other vessels relatively unscathed. Clinically this is associated with focal disturbances of brain function, such as transient or lasting hemiparesis, aphasia, hemianopsia. More general symptoms, for example, lassitude, lethargy, lightheadedness, wooziness, lack of confidence, irritability are often falsely attributed to cerebrovascular disease but are instead usually due to a variety of psychologic and metabolic factors. The slight alteration of cerebral blood flow with age probably produces no important clinical symptomatology.

Cerebrovascular Disease
Cerebrovascular disease is a complex topic. Since a full review would be far beyond the scope of a single chapter, this section will focus on general principles and emphasize only those aspects particularly relevant to the geriatric patient.

THROMBOTIC STROKE
Included under the general category of thrombotic cerebrovascular disease are a heterogeneous group of conditions with varying etiologies, prognoses,

and treatment. Etiology of occlusive disease includes (1) atherosclerosis with luminal and subintimal accumulation of lipid-rich plaques and superimposed clot; (2) hypertrophy of the media of small vessels secondary to hypertension; (3) coagulopathy with spontaneous clotting of vessels; (4) spontaneous or traumatic dissection of vessel walls; (5) aneurysm formation causing clot within the aneurysm, blocking the orifices of vessels branching from the parent vessel in the region of the aneurysm; (6) inflammatory arteritis or phlebitis; (7) "migrainous" vascular dysfunction with vascular spasm; and (8) fibromuscular dysplasia. The major mechanism for associated brain damage is either reduced flow due to narrowing and occlusion of a proximal blood vessel or emboli originating in a more proximal plaque or blood clot blocking a more distal vessel (intraarterial emboli). Prognosis and treatment depend on two things: (1) the degree of occlusion (for example, complete occlusion of the internal carotid artery is associated less often with future strokes than is stenosis of the same vessel), and (2) the location of the occlusive process (for example, hypertensive narrowing of a small penetrating artery is managed much differently from stenosis of the larger, more proximal internal carotid artery).

There is no uniform therapy for all patients with occlusive disease. In order to institute optimal treatment of the individual patient, it is necessary to identify the location and severity of the underlying vascular disease, as well as the status of the patient's deficit, whether transient without residue, progressing, or a fully developed, fixed, clinical deficit. In this section we will first review the major features and suggest a modus operandi for the evaluation and management of elderly patients with occlusive vascular disease.

Lacunar Infarction
Small, deep cerebral infarcts [8], called lacunes, are the most common cerebrovascular lesion identified at postmortem examination. Lacunar strokes accounted for 19 percent of all cerebrovascular lesions among the greater than 800 patients included in the Harvard Stroke Registry [9]. The underlying vascular lesion is lipohyalinitic transformation of the media of penetrating cerebral arteries, producing progressive occlusion or disruption of the vessel with subsequent infarction of its area of supply. The vascular pathology is the result of systemic hypertension. These vascular lesions are especially common in the geriatric population. The diagnosis of lacunar infarction is important since treatment is simple and consists solely of controlling hypertension after the acute ischemic period has passed. The intensive or invasive investigation or treatment commonly applied to disease of larger cerebral vessels can usually be omitted.

The clinical course of lacunar infarction usually evolves over a short period (hours, days, or one week) as contrasted with disease of larger vessels, in which the full deficit may take weeks or months to accumulate fully. The clinical signs usually correspond to dysfunction of deep regions of the brain, for example, the internal capsule: paralysis of the face, arm, and leg on one side of the body without sensory, visual, or intellectual dysfunction [10]; thalamus: tingling, and subjective numbness of the face, arm, and leg on one side of the body without weakness or accompanying signs; or pons: ataxia and weakness of one side of the body [11], or slurred speech associated with clumsiness of one hand [12]. Because the lesions are small and deep they do not disturb alertness and are not usually associated with headache or electroencephalographic abnormalities.

Laboratory evaluation in patients with lacunar strokes usually reveals a normal brain scan and normal or symmetrically abnormal EEG, and a CT scan may or may not show the lesion (the lesions are often too small for resolution). Arteriography is not necessary unless the clinical picture is sufficiently atypical. Treatment consists of bed rest while the deficit is changing, vigorous physical therapy, and careful control of systemic blood pressure after the ischemic period has passed (two to four weeks). The prognosis for return of useful function is good.

Disease of the Internal Carotid Artery and Its Tributaries
Carotid artery disease is common (20 percent of Harvard Stroke Registry patients [9]). It is especially important to diagnose because of the possibility of effective treatment that can prevent subsequent stroke.

The most important clue to the carotid origin of stroke or transient ischemic attacks is transient monocular visual loss, amaurosis fujax. The ophthalmic artery is the first major branch of the internal carotid artery. Narrowing of the internal carotid artery proximal to the origin of the ophthalmic artery, most commonly at the bifurcation of the carotid artery in the neck, produces decreased blood flow to the eye, or may serve as the origin of emboli that temporarily block the ophthalmic circulation. The accompanying visual loss is usually described as a dark shade that gradually descends, blocking vision in one eye. The shade may "drop" from above or cross the eye from the side like a stage curtain. The visual obscuration usually lasts seconds to minutes and clears in the same manner it began, with the shade gradually lifting or crossing, leaving no residual visual loss. Ischemic transient monocular blindness is distinct from the more common migrainous visual obscuration. Migraine produces brightness, sparkling, scintillations and movement within the visual field as opposed to the darkness of arteriosclerotic ischemia [13].

Occlusive disease of the internal carotid artery sometimes develops over a year; symptoms may occur intermittently during a period of 1 to 12 months, as contrasted with the lacunar stroke in which the onset is measured in hours and days. Transient ischemic episodes are often multiple and variable; for example, in one episode the patient may note weakness of a leg, in another numbness of a hand, and weakness and numbness of an arm and leg in still another episode. Patients may not relate symptoms in a hand to prior transient phenomenon in the same leg or the eye. The physician must ask directly about specific symptoms and not leave it to the patient to spontaneously report phenomena that they may not connect with the episode for which they sought medical attention.

As the carotid artery is occluded, collateral circulation develops, with distention of alternate arterial pathways. This vascular distention frequently is associated with headache. Unusual frequency and severity of headache in the company of a transient ischemic episode may be a clue to the large artery origin of the lesion. With progressive narrowing of the carotid artery, ischemic episodes often become more frequent. When occlusion becomes complete, a critical situation develops. If adequate collateral circulation is established, the patient may not acquire a fixed deficit. At the time of occlusion, embolization from the clotted vessel is common. After a period of two to four weeks, stabilization of collateral circulation occurs, and adherence and fibrosis of the clot make subsequent embolization less common. Symptoms recurring more than six weeks after carotid occlusion are uncommon even in the absence of treatment.

A careful physical examination of the neck, facial pulses, and eye may provide clues as to the carotid origin of the transient ischemic attack (TIA) or stroke. These findings are tabulated in Table 5-1.

Many noninvasive laboratory tests are now available that provide information regarding the patency of the internal carotid artery. These tests are of two types: (1) tests that yield physiologic information concerning the ade-

Table 5-1. Physical Findings in Internal Carotid Artery Disease

Neck
 Bruit ipsilateral to the stenosis: focal, high-pitched, and long
 Bruit contralateral to stenosis due to increased flow: lower pitched and more
  widely radiating

Face
 Increased collateral circulation around the orbit [14]
 Reversal of flow in the frontal artery [15]
 Coolness to palpation of ipsilateral supraorbital region

Eye
 Bruit over ipsilateral orbit
 Reduced retinal artery pressure on side of lesion
 Irregular or nonreactive pupil on the side of the lesion (due to iris ischemia)
 White fluffy retinal infarcts or cholesterol, lucent emboli within retinal vessels
 Asymmetric hypertensive retinopathy with lesser changes on the side of carotid
  stenosis
 Horner's syndrome, ipsilaterally
 Venous stasis retinopathy: dilated veins, microaneurysms due to low retinal
  artery pressure

quacy of flow in the ophthalmic, intracranial, and facial arteries distal to the region of block, including Doppler directional testing, oculoplethysmography (OPG), thermography, ophthalmodynamometry (ODM), and dynamic "flow" brain scans; and (2) tests that yield more direct information concerning the anatomy of the carotid bifurcation, including phonoangiography, a technique that analyzes the sound characteristics of a bruit to calculate lumenal diameter, and a real-time echo scan of the neck that is capable of displaying an anatomic picture of the common carotid artery and its tributaries. These tests are safe and are generally available in larger diagnostic centers on an outpatient basis. They are effective in screening the patient for an obstructive lesion in the internal carotid artery, but they may fail to reveal a nonstenosing plaque that may act as the source of intraarterial emboli. Cerebral angiography remains the only definitive test that accurately depicts the anatomic detail of the entire carotid artery. It alone at present has the capability of defining the intracranial carotid artery and its middle and anterior cerebral branches.

Advancing age is never an absolute contraindication to aggressive treatment of lesions of the carotid artery. Although anticoagulation and surgical intervention are each associated with a higher complication rate in the elderly, stroke in the older age group is frequently disabling and is less easily overcome or compensated for. Aspirin and other drugs that affect platelet aggregation (e.g., dipyridamole and sulfinpyrazone) are now used widely for patients with nonstenosing plaques in an attempt to reduce embolization from these lesions. In patients with a narrowed internal carotid artery bifurcation (less than 1.0 mm residual lumen) and transient episodes or a minor fixed deficit, endarterectomy is the preferred treatment. In patients with complete occlusion of the carotid artery, a period of bed rest (one to two weeks) and physical therapy is often adequate treatment.

Stenosis of the carotid artery at the siphon, or narrowing of the middle cerebral artery or anterior cerebral artery branches, is less common than disease of the carotid artery in the neck. Recurrent transient episodes occur but the physical signs of carotid disease are absent, and noninvasive screening yields normal results. Anticoagulation with warfarin derivatives is commonly used for patients with TIAs or minor deficits when surgical correction of severe vascular narrowing is not feasible, although no controlled studies are available that document the utility of anticoagulation in this setting. In some patients with recurrent episodes not responding to anticoagulation, surgical creation of a shunt between the superficial temporal and a middle cerebral artery branch can be effective. Most authorities agree that anticoagulants should not be used for patients with severe fixed neurologic deficits.

Vertebrobasilar Territory Ischemia
Occlusive disease of the posterior circulation is associated with symptoms and signs of brain stem, cerebellar, or posterior cerebral hemisphere dysfunc-

tion. Diagnostic symptoms include dizziness, double vision, bilateral limb weakness or numbness, bilateral visual loss, or alternating hemiplegia. Nystagmus, bilateral weakness and pyramidal tract dysfunction, extraocular muscle weakness, or cerebellar system abnormalities are corroborative physical findings in posterior circulation disease.

As in the carotid circulation, vertebrobasilar dysfunction can be due to a wide variety of vascular pathologies, ranging from occlusion of small penetrating vessels to severe occlusion of the larger vertebral or basilar arteries. However, unlike the situation in carotid disease, surgical correction of the vascular lesion in the extracranial vertebral arteries is usually not practical. Noninvasive testing at present adds little useful information concerning the anatomic configuration of the posterior circulation blood supply. The only effective investigation is vertebral angiography [16]. This technique can differentiate small from large vessel disease and, surprisingly, is associated with a lower complication rate than angiography of the carotid circulation [16,17]. Agents that reduce platelet agglutination can be used in patients with nonstenosing plaques and the clinical picture of vertebrobasilar insufficiency. Warfarin anticoagulation is probably best reserved for those patients with more severe occlusive disease of the posterior circulation. The creation of an artificial shunt from the extracranial occipital artery to cerebellar branches has promise for those patients who continue to have vertebrobasilar dysfunction with more conservative treatment.

The three subdivisions of occlusive cerebrovascular disease already described share the clinical tempo and course of thrombotic stroke, that is, either TIAs or progressive, fluctuating, or stepwise accumulation of clinical deficit. The responsible physician should attempt to define the location of the deficit (carotid or vertebrobasilar system) and whether the lesion is likely to involve small penetrating arteries or larger blood vessels. The diagnosis of small vessel disease (lacunar infarctions), should be made only if the patient is, or has been, hypertensive. The physician should not be misled by the gravity of the clinical deficit. Unlike the situation with some other organ systems, patients with only warning episodes or minor dysfunction deserve the most intense evaluation, since stroke frequently can be prevented. Treatment after the stroke has occurred is much less effective. In patients with a clinical picture not typical of lacunar stroke, investigation using noninvasive procedures, EEG, and CT scanning may be helpful. Long-term warfarin anticoagulation should not be undertaken without angiographic confirmation of the nature of the arterial lesion.

MIGRAINE ACCOMPANIMENTS

The diagnosis of migraine is usually considered seriously only in patients in the second to fourth decade of life who complain of severe headaches. More accurately, migraine includes a wide spectrum of clinical dysfunction characterized by recurrent, transient altered vascular physiology. Headaches occur when vessels are distended; central nervous system symptoms are a manifestation of reduced blood flow and vessels undergoing "spasm." Many patients have transient episodes of all the migraine symptoms except the headache; in other words, migrainous accompaniments. Migrainous dysfunction can occur in the elderly, in whom it is often misdiagnosed as occlusive vascular disease [13,18]. The central nervous system disturbance of migraine usually lasts 15 to 30 minutes. Positive or excitatory phenomena (e.g., bright visual sparkling or prickling paresthetic feelings) commonly begin the episode, whereas in occlusive disease negative symptoms of loss of function predominate (e.g., loss of vision, numbness, and so on).

As the migrainous episode progresses, the positive phenomena usually move or spread within the original sensory modality (e.g., vision or tactile sensation), producing sparkling, which traverses the visual field, or prickling, which gradually spreads from distal hand to shoulder. The spread is often slow and may be from one digit to another. This feature is not seen in patients with arteriosclerotic ischemia, in whom the deficit is noted all at once or evolves at a different pace, either more quickly or much more slowly in a stepwise fashion over hours or days. As the positive phenomena move, left in their wake are "negative" symptoms (e.g., as the prickling spreads proximally, the distal parts begin to feel numb, that is, devoid of feeling; or the portion of the visual field that was bright now becomes a dark void). In addition, spread often occurs from one modality to another. A migrainous accompaniment may begin with visual sparkling, which progresses in 5 to 10 minutes; as the sparkling and subsequent scotoma clear, paresthesia begin in the fingers and spread slowly. After the somesthetic sensory disturbance has normalized, speech loss may begin. The pace and nature of a migrainous accompaniment is thus seen as characteristic and often separable from arteriosclerotic ischemia if a detailed history is taken.

In addition, migrainous episodes may involve widely varying anatomic regions; for example, right visual field in one episode, left paresthesia in another, and left visual field in the third, whereas TIAs are most frequently limited to one vascular territory. Most patients with central nervous system migraine after the sixth decade have had a history of headache or visual sparkling in youth that was attributed by their families or doctors to "sinus" or "nerves." Arteriography of patients with migrainous accompaniments usually reveals no pathology and carries with it a higher risk than in the nonmigrainous subject. Anticonvulsants, especially diphenylhydantoin, and propranolol are often effective when used prophylactically to prevent migrainous accompaniments of the elderly.

CEREBRAL EMBOLI
In times past, the diagnosis of cerebral embolization was made only in patients with a sudden onset of a neurologic deficit who had systemic embolism and a cardiac source in the form of a recent myocardial infarction or rheumatic mitral stenosis with atrial fibrillation. Recent experience in patients

with rapid-onset deficits has revealed angiographic evidence of embolisms (blockage of multiple distal blood vessels not affected by atheroma) that usually clear by 48 hours [9]. Embolism is much more common than formerly appreciated, and sources of emboli are more heterogeneous. Cerebral embolization is not always associated with a sudden-onset deficit; stepwise accumulation over a 24-hour period is also common [9,19].

The cardiac sources of embolism may be occult. Several recent reports clearly and unequivocably document a marked increase in incidence of cerebral embolization in patients with atrial fibrillation [20–22], even when the fibrillation is chronic [21,22] and when no other obvious cardiac disease is present [20]. Constant cardiac monitoring of patients with stroke has documented a surprisingly high incidence of intermittent cardiac arrythmias that could be the source of cerebral emboli. Barnett and colleagues [23] have called attention to the high incidence of stroke in patients with mitral valve prolapse. Bacterial endocarditis may present as stroke and may be difficult to diagnose in the elderly because of lack of fever or systemic response to infection [16].

All patients with ischemic (nonhemorrhagic) stroke deserve careful evaluation of their cardiac status. Many patients with cerebrovascular disease finally succumb, not to their stroke, but to coronary artery disease. A cardiac evaluation then is important not only to identify an occult embolic source but to attempt to treat or anticipate disability related to coronary disease. The evaluation should include chest x-ray, echocardiography, cardiac monitoring, and blood cultures when indicated.

Intraarterial sources of embolization are common. Arteriosclerotic plaques (e.g., in the carotid or vertebral arteries) can form a nidus for subsequent platelet aggregation and adherence, and thrombin may be layered over the plaque. Platelet clusters, thrombin fragments, or cholesterol crystals all have the potential for breaking loose and discharging themselves into the cranial circulation where they lodge distally. Use of agents that decrease platelet aggregation, warfarin, and surgical removal of plaques have all been suggested as beneficial, but at present there is no convincing proof of the superiority of one form of therapy over another. Endarterectomy is commonly reserved for plaque lesions that produce stenosis of the vessel or lesions that continue to be symptomatic despite medical therapy. Other intracerebral lesions (e.g., dissecting or congenital aneurysms [24]) may also serve as a source of emboli.

INTRACEREBRAL HEMORRHAGE

Computed tomography (CT) has led to widespread reevaluation of our concepts of intracerebral hemorrhage. Even very small hemorrhages produce radiodense lesions easily identified on a CT scan. Previously, only larger hemorrhages, with their propensity to cause severe paralysis, loss of consciousness, bloody spinal fluid, and frequently death, were diagnosed. The availability of this accurate diagnostic tool has revealed the wide spectrum of clinical presentation in patients with intracerebral hemorrhage.

Intracerebral hemorrhages [25,26] most commonly arise from arterioles previously damaged by hypertension. Lipohyalinosis of the vascular media can lead to occlusion of the vessel and ischemic infarction (lacuni); in addition, weakness of the wall, with microaneurysm formation, can lead to hemorrhage from the penetrating vessels. The initial symptoms are those of parenchymatous dysfunction of the area into which the blood has leaked (e.g., in a putaminal hemorrhage, the patient might first notice weakness of the hand or leg). Leakage is generally gradual and may take minutes, hours, or, less often, days to be complete.

As the hematoma grows, satellite blood vessels break, producing an avalanche-like effect. Increase in intracranial and local tissue pressure are factors acting to stop the hemorrhage. As the hemorrhage accumulates, there is a local mass produced in the brain, which leads to vomiting, headache, and loss of consciousness if the lesion becomes sizable. Many hemorrhages remain small and do not produce headache or altered consciousness [25]. The hematoma may discharge itself into the subarachnoid space on the surface of the brain or leak into the cerebral ventricles; this decompresses the lesion and is the source of blood in the spinal fluid. Small lesions that do not reach the surface or ventricle do not leak blood into the spinal fluid.

Hypertensive cerebral hemorrhages occur at any age, including the seventh to ninth decades. Blood pressure need not be exceedingly high and may be only slightly elevated. In the Harvard Stroke Registry series of patients with intracerebral hemorrhage, 59 percent were age 60 or over; 37 percent had a diastolic pressure less than 100 mm Hg and 31 percent had a systolic blood pressure less than 180 mm Hg at the time of the hemorrhage. Other important causes of intracerebral hemorrhage include (1) trauma, (2) bleeding diathesis, (3) arteriovenous malformations (usually a disorder of younger age groups), (4) oral or intravenous use of amphetamine compounds, and (5) anticoagulation. Evidence continues to accumulate that amphetamines, even when used orally or in combination (e.g., Dexamyl), can lead to vascular damage and intracerebral hemorrhage. These drugs are used routinely by some physicians for depression or "pepping up" the elderly, a practice that is to be vigorously discouraged. The anticoagulant drugs are the second most common cause of intracerebral hemorrhage. Anticoagulant hemorrhages are frequently in atypical locations, develop indolently, and are very difficult to stop. It is a useful axiom that any cerebral event occurring in a patient taking an anticoagulant drug should be diagnosed as hemorrhage until proved otherwise. At the time of the diagnosis of anticoagulant hemorrhage, warfarin or heparin should be stopped immediately and the effects of the anticoagulant reversed as quickly and safely as possible.

Intracerebral hemorrhage most commonly affects the basal ganglia region (50 percent). Other common sites are thalamus (15 percent), pons and cerebellum (8 percent each), and cerebral hemispheres (15 percent). Hematomas separate brain tissue and are not as destructive as an infarction of the same size. If the patient survives an intracerebral hemorrhage, his clinical deficit is usually less than that in a patient with a comparable size infarction. Treatment consists of reducing systemic blood pressure (but not to hypotensive levels) and discontinuing any agent that adversely effects blood coagulability. Surgical drainage of a sizable hematoma can be lifesaving. Hemorrhages located in the right basal ganglia, cerebellum, and cerebral hemisphere are particularly benefited by drainage. If the hemorrhages are in these regions, the residual postoperative deficit may be small. A full analysis of the various clinical signs present in hemorrhages at specific locations is contained in recent reviews [25,26]. The CT scan provides an accurate means of defining the size and locale of intracerebral hemorrhages.

The gradual onset of deficits in patients with intracerebral hemorrhage can be easily mistaken for the progressive course of large vessel occlusion. Patients with a gradually progressive course should not be given anticoagulant therapy unless the diagnosis of intracerebral hemorrhage has been excluded. Usually this will require computerized axial tomography.

CHRONIC DEMENTIA OF VASCULAR ETIOLOGY
Hardening of the arteries is a general term used by physicians and laypeople alike to describe the intellectual deterioration that so often accompanies aging. Actually, most patients with senile or presenile dementia do *not* have a vascular cause of their symptoms but instead have neuronal degeneration. There are, however, four groups of patients with different types of vascular dementia, all sharing a history of acute strokes and prominent pyramidal, motor, and pseudobulbar dysfunction paralleling in severity their intellectual decline. In cerebral atrophy of senility or the pre senium, intellectual loss precedes motor phenomena by years. The four types of vascular dementia are (1) "état lacunaire," (2) multiinfarct dementia, (3) subcortical arteriosclerotic encephalopathy, and (4) border zone ischemia.

"État Lacunaire"
Multiple lacunes in basal ganglia, brain stem, and cerebral white matter eventually decimate the function of basal gray structures and interrupt afferent and efferent cortical pathways in cerebral white matter. These patients usually have a parkinsonian aspect with stooped posture, slow shuffling gait, and apathetic facies. In addition, motor weakness, hyperreflexia, and extensor plantar responses are present (in contrast to the patient with nonvascular Parkinson's disease). The bilateral dysfunction of pyramidal and extrapyramidal pathways produces a syndrome called pseudobulbar palsy, in which dysarthria, dysphagia, drooling, and exaggerated emotional output with facile laughing and crying are prominent.

Loss of intellectual function is present, but the patient's lack of responsiveness and altered emotional output may give a false facade of simplemindedness. Frequently some aspects of higher cortical function (e.g., memory or speech) may be well preserved. One can usually obtain a history of multiple, acute small strokes in this group of patients. Hypertension and diabetes reflect the presence of a diathesis for a small vessel disease and are instrumental in producing the arteriopathy underlying lacunes. CT scan or pneumoencephalogram (PEG) reveals large ventricles with reduced white matter, sometimes without cortical atrophy. The larger cerebral vessels are usually normal angiographically. Treatment consists of control of blood pressure.

Multiinfarct Dementia

The term *multiinfarct dementia* is generally used when patients have multiple strokes of large vessel origin. Sequential loss of segments of brain, particularly cerebral cortex, summate to produce a loss of intellectual capability in addition to motor, visual, and sensory disturbances. The intellectual dysfunction is "patchy": severe aphasia, memory loss, or visual-spatial deficits may occur in isolation, with other higher functions surprisingly preserved. Motor, visual, and sensory signs are always present. Patients with multiinfarct dementia should be screened for treatable extracranial occlusive disease and for cerebral embolization.

Subcortical Arteriosclerotic Encephalopathy

Subcortical arteriosclerotic encephalopathy [27] is a term that describes diffuse scarring in cerebral white matter or basal gray structures due also to chronic small vessel disease. The clinical picture is similar to the lacunar state except that in patients with subcortical encephalopathy a mounting focal deficit frequently develops over weeks or months. Ventricular enlargement and prominent motor dysfunction with pseudobulbar palsy is similar to état lacunaire. The disorder is chronic with long plateau periods. Treatment consists of careful control of systemic blood pressure.

Border Zone Ischemia

Some patients develop multiple infarction, not due to intrinsic disease of the cerebral vessels, but related to recurrent hypoperfusion often secondary to recurrent or prolonged arrythmia or decreased cardiac output. Lesions are in the boundary zones between major cerebrovascular territories. Symptoms include poor memory, altered visual function, and weakness, usually greater in the shoulder and thighs. Speech is usually preserved. Signs are roughly symmetrical but preexisting vascular disease may lead to asymmetry. The recognition of decreased cardiac output is important, with treatment aimed at improving perfusion.

Central Nervous System Trauma

Head trauma is an important problem in the elderly. An enlarged subarachnoid space, increased vascular fragility, and decreased supportive tissue lead to an increased vulnerability in the elderly for hematoma formation, particularly in the subdural space. Trauma is often remote, considered insignificant, or not recalled by the patient. A history of trauma may be hidden by friends, attendants, or assailants because of their own feelings of guilt, negligence, or complicity. In addition, head trauma may be overshadowed by other primary disorders, for example, Adams-Stokes attacks with falling, or hip fracture; neurologic dysfunction may be blamed on the primary disorder causing the fall without taking the head injury into consideration.

Concussion refers to transient loss of consciousness due to head trauma. It is often associated with retrograde amnesia (failure to recall events prior to the trauma) and posttraumatic amnesia (failure to make enduring memories of events in the minutes or hours after the trauma). Concussive dysfunction is usually transient but may be followed by months of lassitude, decreased attention span, and headache. Minor damage to superficial blood vessels can lead to the accumulation of subarachnoid blood, subarachnoid hemorrhage (SAH), with resultant headache, agitation, and delirium.

Cerebral contusions or lacerations produce more serious injuries to brain tissue; seizures, reduced alertness, and focal neurologic signs are present directly after trauma. These lesions are usually located in regions of brain adjacent to bony prominences at the skull base, that is, basal frontal lobe and temporal lobe. Contusions are associated with considerable brain swelling. If the patient survives the acute episode, the long-term prognosis is good. Corticosteroids and reduced fluid intake may help control the brain swelling.

In contrast to concussion, subarachnoid hemorrhage, and contusion, the clinical signs of epidural hematoma usually develop hours after the injury in relation to the rapid accumulation of arterial or venous blood that compresses the dura, elevating intracranial pressure. All elderly patients with a history of significant head trauma should be observed carefully for the first 72 hours after the trauma. In some circumstances this may be possible outside the hospital.

Frequently overlooked in patients with head trauma is the possibility of associated damage to osseous and ligamentous structures in the neck that may lead to delayed spinal cord damage. The patient with serious head trauma should have his or her neck immobilized while being transported to the x-ray room. Films of the neck and cranioverterbral junction should be obtained in addition to a skull plate.

In the weeks or months following trauma, surveillance for the development of a subdural hematoma should be maintained. Most often, however, there is no available history of preceding head trauma in patients with subdural hematoma. Trauma is forgotten or mental state abnormalities limit the patient's recall and reporting of the traumatic event. The hematoma evolves gradually and raises intracranial pressure. Headache is prominent, frequently nocturnal, and may lateralize to the side of the clot. Increased intracranial pressure leads to altered consciousness, with drowsiness and lethargy as early signs. Focal neurologic signs are present but are usually "soft" and involve multiple modalities, reflecting the wide area of pressure produced by the superficial clot. Slight aphasia, mild weakness or drift of the outstretched arm, and slight sensory or visual neglect are more common than severe hemiplegia or dense hemianopsia. Radionucleotide brain scan, EEG, and CT scanning are all effective diagnostic procedures available on an outpatient basis to substantiate the diagnosis of subdural hematoma.

Skull fractures are commonly associated with tears in the dura and leakage of cerebrospinal fluid. Subsequent indolent or recurrent aggressive meningitis can ensue. Clear fluid with a high sugar content draining from the nose or ears should be evaluated carefully in anticipation of serious infection.

Meningoencephalitis and Encephalopathy

Inflammatory diseases of the brain or its coverings are less common in the geriatric population. Immunity to the viral pathogens that most commonly involve the brain (infectious hepatitis, infectious mononucleosis, enterovirus, cytomegalovirus) has usually developed by adulthood and remains effective except in the immunocompromised host.

One disease that does remain a problem in later life, however, is herpes simplex encephalitis. The disorder may develop in any season, as opposed to arbovirus and enterovirus infections, which are usually warm-weather problems. Confusion, poor memory, drowsiness, and seizures are early symptoms of herpes simplex encephalitis. Fever and systemic symptoms are often absent or minor in the elderly. Herpes frequently affects the limbic cortex, especially orbital, frontal, and temporal lobes. The resultant clinical findings include severe memory loss, with inability to make new memories; increased interest in food and sexual activity; and aphasia. The inflammatory changes frequently are asymmetrical and may produce a focal temporal lobe "mass" detectable on EEG, CT scan, or arteriography. The cerebrospinal fluid contains some red blood cells and a modest leukocytic reaction. Enthusiasm for a new therapy (adenine arabinoside) [28] has made the diagnosis of this disorder more important.

Bacterial endocarditis, a difficult diagnosis in some elderly patients, may present as a confusional state with cells in the cerebrospinal fluid, presumably due to infected meningeal emboli. Tumor may metastasize to the meninges, producing a sheet of spreading cells just as it does in the regions of the pleural or peritoneal surfaces.

Meningeal tumor leads to headache, confusion, and disturbance of cranial nerve and spinal root structures. Widely spaced, localized regions of root pain and sensory, motor, and reflex loss result. A careful cytologic search for neoplastic cells is important in elderly patients with an unexplained spinal fluid pleocytosis.

Any disturbance in general body metabolism may have profound effects on the brain, especially in the elderly patient with less reserve of brain tissue.

The brain provides the alert clinician with a readily available "litmus paper"; the least departure from a physiologic milieu interieur may be reflected early in disordered cerebral function. Usually a metabolic confusional state is characterized by: (1) altered level of alertness, drowsiness, agitation, or stupor; (2) reduced attention span, with frequent drifting from one topic to another, and inability to persevere with a task; (3) generalized decrease in all intellectual functions, especially writing and arithmetic capability; and (4) asterixis. In many encephalopathies multiple factors interrelate with each other, rather than there being a single isolated factor. Frequently the actual quantitative number measurement of one substance (e.g., sodium) will not differ from normal enough to explain dysfunction in a younger patient. However, when combined with slight fever, slight decreased ventilation, and medicines in an elderly patient with little cerebral reserve tissue, the additive effects may be responsible for serious alterations in brain function. In addition, the brain takes longer to equilibrate than serum. An older patient may take months to become fully normal after severe hyponatremia, despite the fact that the serum sodium may have returned to normal in 24 hours.

Table 5-2 presents the most common etiologies of metabolic encephalopathy. One should first consider situations within the body metabolism that lead to too little or too much of a factor. The most common deficiency in this era of frequent diuretic use is hyponatremia. Altered behavior may develop slowly, with stupor eventually intervening. Hypothermia, which is especially important in northern regions in the winter, may go undetected if temperature is recorded carelessly or if a nonreadable temperature is dismissed by an aide as meaning a faulty instrument or patient noncompliance. Vitamin B_{12} deficiency can produce demyelinative changes in cerebral white matter and optic nerves in addition to the more widely recognized spinal cord lesion. Paranoia, behavioral change, and poor memory may accompany the spastic ataxic gait, hyperreflexia, and reduced vibration sense in the lower extremities seen in the subacute combined degeneration that accompanies anemia.

Endogenous "intoxications" are also very common. Hypercalcemia produces drowsiness, lethargy, and difficulty in concentrating, as well as depressed reflexes and hypotonic muscles [29]. Hypoventilation, with carbon dioxide retention, is frequently not obvious and may be responsible for nocturnal confusion in patients with chronic lung disease who hypoventilate when asleep. Hyperviscosity states (e.g., Waldenstrom's macroglobulinemia) leads to sludging in blood vessels and resultant confusion, seizures, and retinopathy.

Exogenous intoxication is often difficult to diagnose since the toxin may be used surreptitiously or be unknown to the patient. Sleeping pills, especially barbiturates, are frequently abused or misused. The patient may, when awakened at night by restlessness, take additional pills, forgetting that he had already taken one or two. Depression with suicidal feelings may lead to

Table 5-2. Most Common Etiologies of Metabolic Encephalopathy

Common endogenous deficiencies
  Glucose
  Sodium
  Calcium
  Thyroxine
  Cortisol
  Temperature (hypothermia)
  Vitamin B_{12}

Common endogenous "intoxications" (too much of these factors)
  Liver failure
  Kidney failure
  Pulmonary failure
  Calcium
  Thyroxine
  Glucose
  Viscosity (e.g., Waldenstrom's macroglobulinemia)
  Sodium
  Cortisol

Exogenous intoxications
  Drugs
  Carbon monoxide
  Heavy metals
  Alcohol

Miscellaneous causes
  Cardiac encephalopathy
  "Fractured hip" syndrome

intentional drug overdose in the elderly, some of whom may not have shared their despair with others for fear of intervention by their loved ones. A continuous lidocaine drip, so frequently used in intensive care areas, can lead to a confusion and coma that mimic brain stem stroke when the mechanical control of the infusion fails, emptying a large bolus into the circulation. Atropine derivatives used as eye drops for glaucoma or orally for gastrointestinal disorders may cause agitation, delirium, and tachycardia.

Alcohol abuse is not limited to youth; lonely elderly patients frequently turn to drink for solace and hide this from their friends and associates. Unexplained burning feet, peripheral neuropathy, shakiness, or a seizure 24 to 48 hours after hospitalization for an acute illness should make the physician alert to the possibility of alcohol or barbiturate abuse. Bromism is still occasionally seen as a result of the chronic use of remedies now unknown to youths.

Unpredicted swings in blood levels of drugs (e.g., Dilantin) can produce intermittent confusional states that might go undiagnosed without blood measurements. When confronted with an elderly patient showing altered behavior the physician should first consider toxic effects of medicines and compulsively acquire data concerning the patient's drug use. Because this form of confusional state is easily remedied by changing or stopping medicines, it is critical that it be recognized for what it is.

Nondrug intoxications are uncommon. Headache, confusion, and sleepiness secondary to carbon monoxide intoxication should be considered if the patient feels better when he or she leaves the responsible environment. Heavy metal intoxication is usually related to occupational exposure but occasionally arsenic, thallium, mercury, or lead exposure can be a result of environmental conditions. Ataxia, peripheral neuropathy, loss of hair, dry nails and skin, and confusion are clues to heavy metal intoxication. Blood levels of metals can be checked in most toxicology labs.

Two encephalopathies common in geriatric patients deserve emphasis. Confusion, agitation, and altered mental state is especially common in older patients hospitalized and immobilized with broken bones, especially hip fractures, although the pathophysiology of this problem has not been fully clarified. Confusion leads to moving about, falling, and an inability to cooperate with medical and nursing caretakers. These factors clearly contribute to the high mortality seen in patients with fractured hips. The presence of pain and blood loss, a strange environment, restraint in bed in a fixed position, sensory deprivation (these patients frequently have subnormal vision and hearing), analgesics, and sedatives may all be contributing factors. Alterations in calcium from unrecognized systemic disease may have contributed to bone disorders leading to fracture; head trauma also may have occurred at the time of the fall. These patients require intensive medical and nursing supervision, but, alas, they are frequently placed in traction on wards in which the doctor or nurse/patient ratio is low. Maximization of sensory stimuli, minimization of medicines, early ambulation, and quick return to familiar surroundings can be lifesaving in the older patient with a broken hip.

Patients with congestive heart failure frequently pass through a period of apathy, reduced interest in the environment, confusion, and even incontinence. These symptoms may develop at a time when heart failure, edema, and dyspnea seem to be improving. Mental changes are usually temporary but may worry the physician and family sufficiently to lead to uncomfortable and sometimes invasive diagnostic procedures. Reduced cardiac output, hypoventilation, elevated venous and intracranial pressure, volume depletion, and possible toxic effects of cardiac or diuretic drugs are all possible contributing factors to the apathy. The syndrome usually clears in the days to weeks following treatment of heart failure. The brain takes a while to equilibrate after rapid fluid changes.

Parkinsonism

The age distribution of Parkinson's disease has not changed within the past century and it remains primarily a disease of the geriatric age group. The establishment by George Cotzias and coworkers that the drug L-dopa ameliorates symptoms and signs of parkinsonism has led to an awakening of interest in basal ganglia disease and an explosion of literature concerning the biochemistry, physiology, and treatment of Parkinson's disease. The availability of effective treatment has increased the importance of accurate diagnosis.

Parkinson's disease may begin slowly, and early symptoms may be vague (e.g., lack of initiative, difficulty initiating movement, slight drag of a foot, less facility using a hand, slowness of thought with reduced attention span). Many such patients do not have a prominent or characteristic tremor. The diagnosis is based on the total picture of the patient as the physician watches him enter the consulting room, speak, adjust himself on the examining table, and move about the room. The telltale signs of Parkinson's disease are noticeable as one greets a sufferer from a distance (remember, Parkinson himself lived in an era that preceded formal examination). In fact, it may be difficult to substantiate the reason for the patient's disability strictly on formal motor, sensory, or reflex testing alone. Expressionless face; decreased frequency of blinking; en bloc movement of the trunk and limbs; diminished arm swing; stooped posture; hesitation in initiating gait; soft voice, which trails off in volume and articulation; seborrhea; faint, variable finger tremor; slight drool at the corner of the mouth; and difficulty manipulating the body on and off the examining table—all are characteristic early features.

More recently physicians have become aware that the abnormality may not be limited to the motor system. Intellectual dysfunction is quite common and frequently takes the form of fixity of thought and difficulty learning or using new ideas. Sensory dysfunction, including pain, may be a prominent symptom [30]. Shoulder or thigh pain may be the presenting symptom of Parkinson's disease. Often the patient has been seen by several orthopedic surgeons and rheumatologists before the correct diagnosis is considered. A frozen shoulder due to decreased movement, or involvement of brain structures subserving sensation are likely explanations. Bladder and bowel dysfunction and decreased potency are common concomitants of the parkinsonian state. Increased frequency of urination, dribbling of urine, and obstipation are almost always present.

The disease progresses inexorably despite L-dopa treatment. L-dopa improves symptoms but *does not* stop disease progression. In addition, experience indicates that the longer a patient uses L-dopa, the more likely it is that side effects will develop and the less effective the drug becomes. For these reasons, one should not begin all patients with parkinsonism on L-dopa as soon as the diagnosis is suspected or made. Many patients with minor symptoms can be treated effectively with physical conditioning or therapy. It is absolutely essential that the patient maintain full activity and that he or she be encouraged to remain physically active and to exercise frequently. In the pre-L-dopa era, it was clear that vigorous physical activity could ameliorate even severe symptoms and signs. The patient and his family must be continually reminded of the need to increase activity, even when L-dopa is used. Other less effective drugs such as amantadine, diphenhydramine (Benadryl), or trihexyphenidyl (Artane) can be used early in the illness. When L-dopa is begun (alone or with a dopa decarboxylase inhibitor) one should not push the drug to toxicity but should seek amelioration of symptoms at the lowest possible dose.

Side effects from L-dopa are common. Nausea, stomach upset, and postural hypotension are usually managed by beginning the medicine slowly and varying its relation to meals. The cardiac side effects of L-dopa (arrythmia, increased ischemia, and congestive heart failure) are less prevalent when L-dopa is combined with a dopa decarboxylase inhibitor, which makes less drug available to the heart and peripheral blood vessels. With time, patients notice a wearing off effect, that is, as the time comes for the next dose, L-dopa's antiparkinsonian effect wanes. This can be improved by increasing the frequency of dosage. Sudden onset of muscular rigidity, or "on-off" effects, refers to a sudden loss of drug effectiveness. The variability and unpredictability of effect are extremely disconcerting to some patients with this problem. Increasing the frequency of dose and dissolving the pill in water or plain soda water may help the absorption of L-dopa and partially diminish the variability of the drug effect. In some patients it is helpful to stop the medicine for a few days, the so-called "drug holiday." Patients taking L-dopa on a long-term basis will frequently have periods of confusion and agitation. In my experience, this is often coincident with an intercurrent illness, such as infection, minor trauma, or congestive heart failure. Stopping the L-dopa for days or weeks often leads to a return to the prior mental state.

Hallucinating people or objects is common and is also dose-related. Dyskinesia—disturbing writhing or wiggling of limbs or mouth—may develop as the dose increases and may limit the amount of L-dopa that can be given. Recent realization of the side effects and limitations of L-dopa has stimulated the search for other effective agents, especially for that group of patients whose response to L-dopa is suboptimal.

Normal pressure hydrocephalus, discussed later in this chapter, and progressive supranuclear palsy are less common conditions frequently confused with parkinsonism. Limited voluntary vertical and, later, horizontal gaze is the earliest finding in progressive supranuclear palsy (PSP), but dementia and parkinsonian stiffness and gait abnormalities soon occur. This disorder responds less well to L-dopa but there is recent interest in methysergide treatment for it [31].

Spinal Cord Disease

When one considers the total number of patients with neurologic illness, disease of the spinal cord is relatively uncommon. Spinal cord disorders are especially important to diagnose, however, because of the potential, when untreated, for severe permanent disability and the remediable nature of some forms of myelopathy due to extradural compression. Despite its importance, extradural spinal compression is seldom diagnosed accurately when patients with this disorder are seen in a nursing home or the general medical wards of a hospital.

CERVICAL SPONDYLOSIS
Degenerative changes in the cervical spine, cervical spondylosis [32], are almost an inevitable accompaniment of aging. Spur formation, arthritic overgrowth, and disk degeneration all may lead to compression of nerve roots and spinal cord. There are two distinct clinical syndromes encountered: (1) the "lateral" or nerve root syndrome, and (2) "spondylitic myelopathy," the medial or spinal cord syndrome.

Lateral Root Syndrome
In the lateral root syndrome the nerve root is compressed during its course through the neural foramina. The cardinal symptom is root pain, usually in the shoulder, arm, or radial border of the hand. Pain is sharp and knife-like and is increased by neck movement. Movement of the limbs does not usually produce pain, in contrast to the situation in patients with bursitis, acute arthritis of the shoulder or elbow, or periarticular rheumatism, in all of which limb movement greatly increases the pain. Paresthesias along the same nerve root clinch the neurogenic nature of the symptoms. Root pain is usually accompanied by stiffness and neck pain. Examination reveals motor weakness, and atrophy if the disorder is chronic. Fifth cervical (C_5) root encroachment leads to weakness of deltoid and spinati muscles; C_6, the biceps; and C_7, the triceps and wrist extensors. In a C_5 or C_6 root lesion, the biceps reflex may be lost, and at C_7 the triceps reflex is absent. Sensory loss is frequently minimal; when present it conforms to standard dermatomal distribution. Nerve root compression due to spondylitic spurs frequently responds to conservative measures (e.g., cervical collar or traction). Surgery is seldom required unless disabling weakness or unremitting pain fails to respond to conservative treatment.

Spondylitic Myelopathy
In spondylitic myelopathy the cord itself is compressed by bony spurs or ridges. Spinal cord dysfunction usually develops gradually and is referable to compression of lateral and posterior columns. Stiffness and spasticity of the legs, clumsy gait, and tingling of the feet are the initial complaints. Hand atrophy and paresthesia and sphincter disturbances develop later. The syndrome is usually gradually progressive but acute decompensation may accompany trauma, even of minor degree. There may be a history of coexistent nerve root compression affecting the upper limbs. Films of the cervical spine,

especially the lateral view, are quite helpful in the evaluation of patients with myelopathy. The measurement from the most posterior aspect of the body of the vertebrae (or spur) to the anterior aspect of the spine conforms to the width of the dural sac. When this measurement is greater than 13 mm, cord compression due to bony encroachment is unlikely; when it is less than 10 mm, cord compression is very likely (Fig. 5-1).

Treatment of myelopathy includes immobilization in a cervical collar for 24 hours a day. If signs continue to progress or the myelopathy is severe, a decompressive laminectomy is warranted. The operation can be done without opening the dura mater. Advanced age is never an absolute contraindication to surgery, since the alternative is often severe disability, with loss of

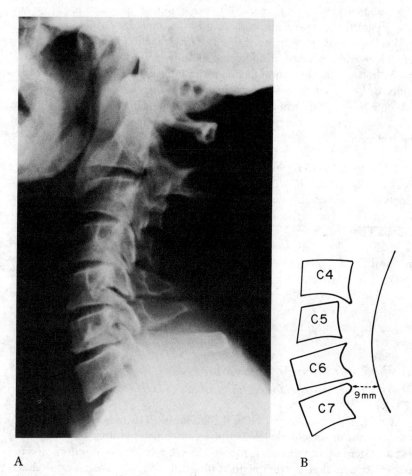

A   B

Figure 5-1. (A) Lateral view of the cervical spine. Multiple posterior spurs or osteophytes narrow the spinal canal. (B) Diagram shows the measurements of the diameter of the dural sac, in this case 9 mm.

mobility and frequently a bed or wheelchair existence with all of the associated risks to physical and psychologic well-being. In some personally observed patients in the eighth or ninth decade, decompressive laminectomy for spondylitic myelopathy has been associated with considerable improvement in gait, allowing continuing mobility.

LUMBAR SPONDYLOSIS—THE SPINAL STENOSIS SYNDROME
The spinal stenosis syndrome [33] has only recently been recognized and is quite common in the elderly. Narrowing of the sagittal plane of the lumbar spinal canal due to enlarged apophyseal joints, shortened pedicles, thickened ligamenta flava, and posterior protrusion of intervertebral disks causes chronic compression of lower spinal roots. The predominant symptom is pain, usually of a paresthetic nature and radiating to the buttocks and lower extremities. Weakness may accompany the sensory dysfunction. The symptoms are intermittent and characteristically are strikingly related to activity and position. Walking, standing immobile, or leaning backward will precipitate the symptoms. Often when the patient is examined in the supine position the neurologic findings are minimal. X-ray examination reveals a small lumbar canal. If surgery is contemplated, extensive decompression of the lumbar canal is needed.

EXTRADURAL TUMOR OR INFECTION
WITH CORD COMPRESSION
Patients with metastatic carcinoma, lymphoma, plasmacytoma, or abscess may come to the physician because of the development of spinal cord compression. This syndrome is usually associated with local bone pain or tenderness at the level of compression and, often, root pain or paresthesia at the same level. If the compression is not treated, paralysis may become complete and irreversible. Any patient with known tumor who develops numbness or weakness in the legs, sphincter abnormalities, or severe back pain should be evaluated carefully for spinal cord compression. The condition should be called to the attention of a neurologist or neurosurgeon as an emergency.

Miscellaneous Neurologic Symptoms or Conditions
of Importance to the Geriatrician
DIZZINESS
Dizziness [34], an abnormal sense of motion, is an extremely common, protean symptom in the elderly. When unaccompanied by other serious central nervous system dysfunction, it is most often not a symptom of serious disease. The geriatrician should attempt to distinguish five separate types of dizziness, each representing a separate pathogenesis and mode of evaluation.

Lightheadedness Secondary to Depression or Loss of Self-confidence
The dizziness in this condition is generally described in vague terms—"I

can't feel my head"—or "my head feels vacant, empty"—or "I am woozy." The feeling is nearly constant throughout the day and may last weeks to months. It is commonly associated with a feeling that there is a band about the head and scalp tightness or sensitivity. The dizziness is improved by activity and is usually worse when sitting quietly. Inertia or disability is usually attributed to the dizziness. The abnormal sensation of dizziness is due to loss of proprioception from the tight neck muscles, one of the receptors that yields constant information regarding the position of the head vis-à-vis the body. Antidepressants alone or with muscle-relaxing agents will often provide symptomatic relief.

Postural Lightheadedness Secondary to Altered Vascular Reflexes

A lightheaded, faint feeling occurs when the patient assumes the upright position or stands in one place for awhile. The lightheadedness is often associated with sweating and slight nausea and a sense of being about to pass out. It is relieved by lying down. Hyponatremia secondary to diuretics; aortic stenosis; Addison's disease; peripheral neuropathy, especially diabetic; or drugs are common causes that need to be considered. The cause is usually extracerebral.

Multisensory Organ Deprivation

The sense of awareness of the position of the head in space is derived from a composite input from the eyes, peripheral labyrinthian system within the inner ear, and peripheral proprioceptors in the feet and joints. In the elderly, changes in all of these receptors are quite common and have an additive effect. Cataracts and glaucoma, aging changes in the end organs of the ear, cervical spondylitis, and slight neuropathy are common causes of end organ dysfunction. The resultant sensation of dizziness is usually present only when the patient is walking or moving and is not present when he or she is supine or seated. There is a feeling of insecurity of gait and motion. Treatment consists of an attempt to improve any of the receptor regions (e.g., removal of cataracts, vitamins for a neuropathy, and so on).

Spinning Vertigo of Labyrinthian Origin

Most peripheral vestibular disorders are not life-threatening, not subject to anatomic definition in life (e.g., x-ray), and rarely subject to postmortem examination. As a result we know very little about the causes of labyrinthian vertigo, an extremely common affliction. When dizziness is related to labyrinth dysfunction, patients usually describe turning, whirling, or spinning of the room or themselves. Sweating, nausea, and vomiting frequently result. If the patient turns or moves, the vertigo is worsened; he or she prefers to remain very still, usually holding tight to an object for fear of falling. The vertigo is usually brief (lasting seconds to minutes to hours) but may be recurrent, especially when the patient first rises in the morning or turns in bed at night. Reputed etiologies include viral illness, allergy, Meniere's disease, and drug reactions. The condition is quite common after sudden fluid shifts (e.g., fluid given intravenously after operation in the hospital) and may be more common in the elderly.

Dizziness that is brief, recurrent, accentuated by movement, and unassociated with other important neurologic symptoms is rarely of serious etiology (e.g., brain tumor or vascular disease). This is especially true if the disorder is chronic (that is, lasting longer than three months) or associated with signs of peripheral hearing loss or tinnitus. Treatment is symptomatic; dimenhydrinate (Dramamine) is effective as are other antivertiginous agents. Extensive neurologic evaluation is generally not warranted.

Dizziness of Central Nervous System Origin
The dizziness accompanying brain disease is usually not described as true spinning but a wavering, oscillating feeling [35]. The central regions for interpretation of vestibular data, brain stem and temporal lobes, are packed with other important structures; nearly all important lesions affecting these regions will produce accompanying symptoms. Dysarthria, double vision, facial numbness, and weakness or numbness of the limbs on one side of the body are frequent symptoms. Nystagmus is present in patients with central dizziness and may be quite prominent, even if subjective dizziness is slight. Contrary to common belief, dizziness unaccompanied by other symptoms or signs is not commonly due to vascular disease. Some patients with vertebral or basilar occlusive disease have spells of dizziness. In most cases there are other attacks of a different nature, and headache may be present between spells in patients with vascular disease of the posterior circulation. With cerebrovascular disease, a stroke usually develops within days to six weeks. Patients with chronic, unaccompanied dizziness should *not* be treated with anticoagulants. In the patient in whom diagnosis is uncertain, angiography can help to clarify the nature of the symptoms [16] and is safer than the empiric use of warfarin.

NORMAL PRESSURE HYDROCEPHALUS
The important observations of Adams and associates [36] reawakened interest in the subject of normal pressure hydrocephalus (NPH). These authors described patients, usually older than 60 years, who have no known accompanying brain pathology other than the hydrocephalus. Thus it was possible to attribute the patient's clinical picture solely to the dilated ventricular system. Formerly, in patients with hydrocephalus due to tumor or congenital malformations, it was not possible to differentiate the symptom component due to tumor from that due to hydrocephalus.

When the ventricles enlarge in a mature or aged adult, the expansion is primarily frontal. Regions surrounding the frontal horns carry fibers from the leg region and from regions principally concerned with voluntary control of the bladder. In addition, many higher functions are controlled frontally. The clinical picture usually includes a triad of dysfunction: (1) abulia, referring to a diminished quantity and speed of behavior; (2) gait abnormalities; and (3) poor bladder control. In abulia there is less spontaneous speech or interaction; when spoken to, there is often a long latency period before a reply is forthcoming. Replies, when made, are brief, and the patient does not persevere with the task at hand. The patient, in this situation, can be viewed as a sputtering car with poor spark plugs—it has no zip to get started, and sputters out quickly, requiring frequent prodding to get moving. Despite the diminished performance, intellectual function (e.g., speech function, memory, computing capability) may be surprisingly preserved. With gait abnormalities, steps are usually slow and of small amplitude. The patient has difficulty starting, and then shuffles very slowly. This abnormality is frequently accompanied by extensor plantar reflexes. With poor bladder control the patient knows when he or she must void but seems unable to inhibit bladder emptying.

Hydrocephalus is now readily diagnosed on CT scan. In some patients a tumor, especially in the posterior fossa or in regions near the third ventricle, will produce hydrocephalus by distorting the ventricular system, as will prior scarring of the arachnoid regions that drain spinal fluid due to blood (trauma, subarachnoid hemorrhage from aneurysm, or vascular malformation) or prior infection. In the idiopathic form (NPH), symptoms usually develop gradually over months, and the syndrome is fully developed within a year. In vascular dementia with hydrocephalus (see p. 66), symptoms usually evolve more slowly, the history is punctuated by definite strokes, and there are findings of asymmetrical brain disease. It usually takes years to evolve, and gait and sphincter disturbances appear quite late.

Unfortunately, none of the tests for NPH have proved definitive or predictive of relief of symptoms by surgery. Temporary drainage of cerebrospinal fluid (by repeated lumbar punctures or lumbar drain) is a therapeutic test of some help; if the patient improves, a shunt is likely to be effective. Acetazolamide (Diamox) can decrease the production rate of cerebrospinal fluid and is of occasional therapeutic benefit. In most patients with a compatible clinical picture and CT or PEG evidence of hydrocephalus without prominent cerebral atrophy, the surgical placement of a shunting device should be considered. Infection of the shunt, subdural hematoma, and other complications have unfortunately proved common; thus, shunting should only be undertaken after the patient has been extensively evaluated and the untreated clinical course becomes apparent. There are patients with miraculous recoveries after shunting; alas, they are all too rare.

PERNICIOUS ANEMIA

Pernicious anemia is a treatable disorder with a variable clinical picture. The earliest neurologic symptoms are usually tingling in the hands and toes associated with an unsteady gait. On examination, the findings may include:

nystagmus; pallor of the optic disk, with slight reduction in visual acuity; increased deep tendon reflex in the upper limbs; diminished vibration sense in the lower extremities, often extending to the thoracic region; positive Romberg sign; and extensor plantar reflexes. Occasionally there is a distal symmetrical "stocking" distribution of touch, pin, and position loss in the legs. In some patients, careful sensory examination will reveal a level of pin loss across the chest in thoracic dermatones. These signs are due to pathology in the peripheral nerves and the lateral and posterior columns of the thoracic spinal cord. In some patients, there is also some involvement of cerebral white matter, producing irritability, paranoia, or loss of the usual inhibitions.

Some, but not all, patients with the neurologic dysfunction of pernicious anemia have an associated glossitis, with a history of sore tongue and a red, beefy, or glazed smooth tongue on examination. Anemia is usually present. In the absence of significant anemia, a careful examination of the peripheral blood smear almost always reveals hypersegmented polymorphonuclear leukocytes, and prominent anisocytosis and poikilocytosis with microovalocytes. Vitamin B_{12} levels in the blood are *not* absolutely reliable. In a patient with typical neurologic findings but a normal B_{12} level, more intense evaluation, including gastric acid and a Schilling test, or empirical treatment with B_{12} is in order (see Chap. 7).

TRANSIENT GLOBAL AMNESIA

A curious but common syndrome in the elderly usually called transient global amnesia (TGA) consists of an isolated temporary episode of memory loss [37]. The disorder can be baffling and frightening to physicians unfamiliar with it. The onset is usually sudden. The patient looks bewildered and begins to ask questions concerning his whereabouts or what he is doing. Often the queries reveal a lack of knowledge of recent events in the patient's own life; for example, a grandmother asked her daughter where grandson Jon was. Jon had left on a European trip months before, and since his departure the grandmother had corresponded with him regularly. Often questions are repeated, despite the fact that an answer was supplied. The patient may inquire repeatedly as to the time or his whereabouts less than one minute after a reply to the same question. During the episode the patient speaks normally and fully comprehends spoken speech, reads and writes normally, and can do complex arithmetic computations. There are no abnormalities of visual, motor, sensory, or reflex examination. The defect is solely in memory function. The patient cannot lay down new, lasting memory traces. In addition, there is a variable period of retrograde amnesia—the patient usually cannot recall events of recent days, months, and sometimes years before the episode, but can recall more accurately details from childhood. Generally the disorder is self-limited and lasts only hours (always less than 24 hours). Onset is often after a sudden change in temperature (e.g., a hot bath or shower or immersion in cold water). Just as suddenly, recall seems to turn on, and the period of retrograde amnesia gradually shrinks. The patient never regains recall of the period during which he or she was amnestic. Etiology is not certain, but most observers believe that typical TGA is a benign phenomenon. It usually does not recur.

Some have hypothesized an epileptic mechanism for TGA. In patients with seizures, however, memory loss is usually brief and follows loss of consciousness. Patients with temporal lobe epilepsy (memory is primarily a temporal lobe phenomenon) do not have episodes of TGA and patients with TGA may have normal EEGs and usually do not have seizures. Occlusive vascular disease is also not a likely explanation. Posterior cerebral artery occlusion can produce a stroke with associated memory loss, usually accompanied by visual or sensory abnormalities, but the memory loss is usually more persistent and the patient does not repeatedly query others. Patients with known vertebrobasilar stroke do not give a history of TGA and patients with TGA do not subsequently develop posterior circulation strokes. TGA is more likely an unusual migraine variant [38].

DROP ATTACKS

Some elderly patients give a history of suddenly falling to the ground without a preceding indication of being in any way unwell and without losing consciousness. They are then able to pick themselves up relatively quickly without noticing any obvious aftereffect. These events are usually referred to as "drop attacks." Although some authorities consider drop attacks to be indicative of vascular disease of the vertebrobasilar circulation, this is certainly not a uniform finding.

Physiologically, a drop attack simply means a sudden alteration in the motor systems controlling tone in the lower extremities. The extrapyramidal motor system that controls posture and tone consists of a multitude of nuclear structures and pathways within the cerebral hemispheres, brain stem, cerebellum, and spinal cord. The differential diagnosis of drop attacks includes the following.

1. Parkinsonism or other extrapyramidal disorders. Sudden jerks or giving way of limbs can be due to variability of tone seen in some parkinsonians.
2. Seizures. Akinetic seizures can be brief and may be associated with loss of tone. Usually there is a short period of lapse of consciousness.
3. Cervical spine disease (spondylitis or atlantoaxial dislocation or subluxation). Neck movement can produce a sudden change in spinal cord function in some patients with chronic spinal compression or unstable bony structures, due, for example, to rheumatoid disease of the cervical spine.
4. Hydrocephalus. In this circumstance, falling is due to involvement of frontal regions that control motor function in the legs; the falling is associated with an abnormality of gait.
5. Bruns' ataxia of gait. This term refers to a common syndrome of gait dis-

turbance in elderly patients with frontal lobe atrophy. The patient walks with small short steps and has great difficulty initiating motion. The feet may "stick" to the ground and the patient will suddenly fall.

6. A flexion reflex not related to important clinical disease. In many patients, dropping may simply be a manifestation of a heightened flexion reflex. When one steps on a rock, or without warning has the foot pinched or scraped, there is a reflex withdrawal of the lower extremity with sudden flexion of the thigh, leg, and ankle. If one were erect this would make the lower extremity bend; this may be enough in the elderly to precipitate sudden dropping to the ground.

7. Vertebrobasilar insufficiency. This diagnosis should not be made unless there are other spells indicative of transient brain stem or posterior cerebral artery dysfunction (see p. 61). Anticoagulants should *not* be given to patients whose only symptom is drop spells; instead the patient should be evaluated with respect to the differential diagnostic possibilities just mentioned.

MYOPATHY IN THE ELDERLY

The presence of muscle weakness is difficult to assess in some elderly patients who seem unable to perform a particular motor act on command or exert power against the resistance of an examiner. Frequently this is due to an inability to conceive of and integrate the act (an apraxia) rather than being related to intrinsic muscle disease. A myopathic origin of weakness should only be diagnosed in the presence of symptoms and signs of symmetrical weakness of both the upper and lower extremities, especially involving the pelvic and pectoral girdles and proximal limbs. Difficulty arising from a chair or from a stooped posture, inability to ascend steps, waddling gait, inability to lift objects onto a shelf above, or to manipulate clothing fasteners behind the upper back are all symptoms frequently described by patients with a myopathy. Most myopathies in the elderly are due to systemic, metabolic, or immune disturbances and are not due to primary disease of muscle fiber such as muscular dystrophy. The contractile process of muscle is a finely tuned mechanism easily disturbed by many metabolic abnormalities. Endocrinopathies (e.g., hypothyroidism or hyperthyroidism, Addison's disease, Cushing's syndrome, hypopituitarism, hypoparathyroidism or hyperparathyroidism) may present as muscle weakness. Electrolyte abnormalities, especially relating to potassium and calcium, can produce severe muscle weakness. Hypokalemia, and malabsorption with hypocalcemia and osteomalacia are common examples. In some patients with systemic cancer, there is a remote, poorly understood disturbance of muscle function. Sometimes this is associated with inflammatory changes in muscle (polymyositis), but in other cases only loss of muscle fiber is appreciated on muscle biopsy. In some cases, the myopathy of carcinoma is reversed with steroids or removal of the primary tumor. Other metabolic myopathies are usually reversible if the abnormality is corrected. The polymyalgia rheumatica syndrome is usually characterized by muscle and limb pain and sensitivity to touch, but not by true muscle weakness (see Chap. 16).

References

1. Adams, R. D. Pathological Reactions of the Skeletal Muscle Fibre in Man in Disorders of Voluntary Muscle. In J. Walton (Ed.), *Disorders of Voluntary Muscle* (3rd ed.). London: Churchill Livingstone, 1974.
2. Dorfman, L., and Bosley, T. Age-related changes in peripheral and central nerve conduction in man. *Neurology* 29:38, 1979.
3. Jervis, G. Senile Dementia in Pathology of the Nervous System. In J. Minckler (Ed.), *Pathology of the Nervous System.* New York: McGraw-Hill, 1971. Vol. II.
4. Brody, H. Aging of the Vertebrate Brain. In M. Rockstein and M. L. Sussman (Eds.), *Development and Aging in the Nervous System.* New York: Academic Press, 1973.
5. Lassen, N., Feinberg, I., and Lane, M. Bilateral studies of cerebral oxygen uptake in young and aging normal subjects and in patients with organic dementia. *J. Clin. Invest.* 39:491, 1960.
6. Naritome, H., et al. Effect of advancing age on regional residual blood flow. *Arch. Neurol.* 36:410, 1979.
7. Kety, S. Human cerebral blood flow and oxygen consumption as related to aging. *J. Chronic Dis.* 3:478, 1956.
8. Caplan, L. R. Lacunar infarction; a neglected concept. *Geriatrics* 21:71, 1976.
9. Mohr, J., et al. The Harvard Cooperative Stroke Registry: a prospective registry. *Neurology* 28:754, 1978.
10. Fisher, C. M., and Curry, H. Pure motor hemiplegia of vascular origin. *Arch. Neurol.* 13:30, 1965.
11. Fisher, C. M. Ataxic hemiparesis: a pathologic study. *Arch. Neurol.* 35:126, 1978.
12. Fisher, C. M. A lacunar stroke: the dysarthria—clumsy hand syndrome. *Neurology* 17:614, 1967.
13. Fisher, C. M. Migrainous accompaniments versus arteriosclerotic ischemia. *Trans. Am. Neurol. Assoc.* 93:211, 1968.
14. Fisher, C. M. Facial pulses in internal carotid artery occlusion. *Neurology* 20:476, 1970.
15. Caplan, L. The frontal artery sign—a bedside indicator of internal carotid occlusive disease. *N. Engl. J. Med.* 288:1008, 1973.
16. Caplan, L., and Rosenbaum, A. The role of cerebral angiography in vertebrobasilar occlusive disease. *J. Neurol. Neurosurg. Psychiatry* 38:601, 1975.
17. Faught, E., Trader, S., and Hanna, G. Cerebral complications of angiography for transient ischemia and stroke: prediction of risk. *Neurology* 29:4, 1979.
18. Fisher, C. M. Transient migrainous accompaniments of late onset. *Stroke* 10:96, 1979.

19. Fisher, C. M., and Pearlman, A. The nonsudden onset of cerebral embolism. *Neurology* 17:1025, 1967.
20. Hinton, R., et al. Influence of etiology of atrial fibrillation on incidence of systemic embolism. *Am. J. Cardiol.* 40:509, 1977.
21. Wolf, P., et al. Epidemiologic assessment of chronic atrial fibrillation and risk of stroke: the Framingham Study. *Neurology* 28:973, 1978.
22. Fisher, C. M. Stroke with atrial fibrillation. *Stroke* 9:96, 1978.
23. Barnett, H. J., et al. Cerebral ischemic events occurring in patients with prolapsing mitral valve. *Arch. Neurol.* 33:777, 1976.
24. Duncan, A., Caplan, L., and Rumbaugh, C. Aneurysms: a source of cerebral emboli. *Neurology* 29:592, 1978.
25. Caplan, L., and Mohr, J. Intracerebral hemorrhage: an update. *Geriatrics* 33:42, 1978.
26. Caplan, L. R. Intracerebral Hemorrhage. In H. R. Tyler and D. Dawson, (Eds.), *Current Neurology*. Boston: Houghton Mifflin, 1979. Vol. II.
27. Caplan, L. R., and Schoene, W. Subcortical arteriosclerotic encephalopathy (Binswanger disease); clinical features. *Neurology* 28:1206, 1978.
28. Whitley, R., et al. Adenine arabinoside therapy of biopsy-proved herpes simplex encephalitis. *N. Engl. J. Med.* 297:289, 1977.
29. Schwartz, T., and Hedges, R. N. Hypercalcemia and hypocalcemia. *D. M.* December, 1960, p. 1.
30. Snider, S., et al. Primary sensory symptoms in parkinsonism. *Neurology* 26:423, 1976.
31. Rafal, R., Gummow, L., and Grimm, R. Treatment of progressive supranuclear palsy with methysergide with neuropsychological improvement in five patients. *Neurology* 27:351, 1977.
32. Brain, R., and Wilkinson, M. *Cervical Spondylosis*. Philadelphia: Saunders, 1967.
33. Wilson, C. Significance of the small lumbar spinal canal: cauda equina compression syndrome due to spondylosis. *J. Neurosurg.* 31:499, 1969.
34. Drachman, D., and Hart, C. An approach to the dizzy patient. *Neurology* 22:323, 1972.
35. Fisher, C. M. Vertigo in cerebrovascular disease. *Arch. Otolaryngol.* 85:529, 1967.
36. Adams, R., et al. Symptomatic occult hydrocephalus with normal cerebrospinal fluid pressure. *N. Engl. J. Med.* 273:117, 1965.
37. Fisher, C. M., and Adams, R. D. Transient global amnesia. *Acta Neurol. Scand.* 40 (Suppl. 9): 1, 1964.
38. Caplan, L., Chedru, F., and Lhermitte, F. Transient global amnesia and migraine. *Neurology* 28:387, 1978.

6. Psychiatric Aspects of Aging

Benjamin Liptzin

Recent years have seen an upsurge of interest in psychology and psychiatry in relation to late life. In part this reflects the increasing numbers of elderly persons and the large public expenditures for their health and welfare that have been discussed elsewhere in this book. In addition, it reflects the outstanding contributions of a number of pioneers in the field. As psychiatrists and other mental health professionals have dipped their toes in the water of geriatric problems, they have been compelled to discard their stereotypes of the elderly as senile, unsuitable for psychotherapy, and not interested in psychiatric care. While the upsurge in clinical interest has not yet been matched by a similarly large increase in our knowledge base, this chapter will summarize the currently available information on the normal psychology of aging and on psychopathology in the elderly. Those areas of the research literature that are of clinical relevance will be highlighted. The reader interested in more detail should refer to one of the more extensive reviews listed at the end of this chapter.

Normal Psychology of Aging
INTELLIGENCE
Studies of intelligence in the elderly are dependent on the concept of intelligence adopted by the investigator as well as the particular instruments used to measure various aspects of intelligence. The most widely used instrument in the United States for measuring intelligence is the Wechsler Adult Intelligence Scale. Wechsler's cross-sectional studies showed the highest level of "mental ability" at age 24 with a decline after age 30 that continued into old age. He suggested that verbal performance holds up well but that performance on tests that require perceptual motor skills decline with increasing age. Longitudinal studies of the same persons over time have shown no changes or minimal decline from ages 62 to 72 and from 74 to 86, suggesting that the earlier findings of age differences in intelligence from cross-sectional studies may reflect cohort differences in variables such as amount of education, recency of education, occupation, and familiarity with tests. Healthy subjects perform significantly better than ill subjects on intellectual tests. In summary, many intellectual functions show little or no decline in individuals past age 60, although there may be a decline in perceptual motor skills, particularly on timed tasks.

LEARNING AND MEMORY
A substantial body of experimental psychology research has accumulated in the last 20 years on age-related changes in learning and memory. There are decrements in performance on many experimental learning tasks with increasing age, some of which may be due to speed of presentation or to moti-

vational factors. Older subjects may develop more anxiety in fast-paced test situations, with fear of failure leading to fewer responses and withdrawal from the testing situation. Current research is focusing on factors that may improve learning in the elderly, such as slowing the rate of presentation or the expected speed of response, or developing strategies for learning. In contrast to the saying "you can't teach an old dog new tricks," learning can occur even at advanced ages. A better understanding of how learning occurs at advanced ages may improve the ability of older persons to adapt to new work or living conditions such as learning to use the thermostat or stove in a new apartment.

Experimental studies of memory employ a variety of tasks that measure specific aspects of memory function, including short-term and long-term memory. Older subjects have more difficulty than younger subjects on short-term memory tasks when asked to divide their attention or to reorganize the material presented. Memory for remote events is also impaired in the elderly compared to younger subjects, but recall and recognition of past events remains quite high. The clinician must consider approaches that will assist normal older persons with minimal or mild difficulties. Moderate or severe memory difficulties reflect pathologic changes in the brain and not normal aging. This distinction is important since persons with mild forgetfulness may function better if reassured that such mild changes do not indicate senility in the sense of progressive dementia.

ADAPTATION AND COPING

Problem-solving ability still exists in older people, despite decreases in memory and in performance on visuoperceptual tasks with advancing age. A clinician dealing with an older individual should keep in clear focus the person's ability to adapt and consider ways to sustain or supplement that coping.

Studies of late adulthood by developmental psychologists have suggested that older persons, like younger, have differing capacities for coping with life stresses and for coming to terms with their changing life situations. The aging individual plays an active role in adapting to the biologic and social changes that occur over time as well as in finding ways to achieve greater life satisfaction.

Various theorists and empirical investigators have discussed the normative crises associated with the changes of late adulthood. These changes begin with menopause in women and extend through grandparenthood, retirement, widowhood, and expectation of one's own death. From a clinical perspective, the idea of normative crises suggests that most persons make successful adaptations to expectable life transitions. This challenges some conventional wisdom, but it is supported by research findings. A review of the epidemiology of depression found no increase in depression for menopausal women. Studies of morbidity and mortality in the year following bereavement found that there was an increase for younger widows but not for older widows for whom widowhood is more expectable. Unsuccessful adaptations to life transitions may require professional help in the elderly just as they may in the young.

Epidemiology of Mental Disorders in the Elderly

Regrettably little systematic descriptive epidemiologic data exists on mental disorders in the elderly. A study of the prevalence of mental disorders in the aged population of Newcastle upon Tyne estimated the total prevalence rate for psychiatric disorders as 263 per 1,000 persons aged 65 years and over. The number of elderly with severe organic brain syndromes was 56 per 1,000 persons. Less than 7 percent of the total cases represented institutionalized persons and even for the persons with psychoses, less than 12 percent of the total were institutionalized. Chronological age was the only demographic variable that was clearly related to the organic mental syndromes. For persons with functional disorders such as depression, complaints of loneliness were independent of the number of daily contacts.

SUICIDE

Epidemiologic studies consistently show that elderly men have the highest rates of suicide, with the rate increasing with each decade. For women the highest rate occurs around age 50, with a gradual decline thereafter. The elderly account for about 11 percent of the population, but 25 percent of the suicides. A number of studies have attempted to elucidate the reasons for the high suicide rate among the elderly, especially for men. Depression, which might be a factor, has been found to be more common among younger than older persons. Furthermore, the rate of suicide attempts is much higher in young persons than in the elderly but with fewer successful attempts and, thus, a lower suicide rate. One major difference is that elderly men tend to use more lethal methods (e.g., firearms, hanging, drowning) in their suicide attempts and are therefore more likely to be successful.

Utilization of Health and Mental Health Services

For many years it was believed that the elderly had a higher prevalence of mental disorders than younger persons because of their higher rate of being admitted to and remaining residents of state and county mental hospitals, which were the major sources of psychiatric care. By the mid-1960s, states began to restrict systematically admissions of older persons to state mental hospitals; by 1975 many fewer elderly were treated in these hospitals. In 1975, less than 1 percent of the population 65 years and over were admitted to inpatient services of state and county mental hospitals, private psychiatric hospitals, general hospital psychiatric inpatient units, community mental health centers, and outpatient psychiatric services. Individuals 65 and over accounted for only 4.8 percent of admissions to this group of psychiatric services and for less than 2 percent of the patients seen in private psychiatrists' offices.

This change in utilization patterns has led to the assertion that the elderly are underserved by specialized mental health programs. However, many elderly persons with mental disorders receive some general health services. A recent study found that over one-fourth of elderly outpatients at a medical clinic met the criteria for having a major depressive disorder. Almost two-thirds of these were not recognized as being depressed by their physicians. Furthermore, as the number of mentally ill elderly in state mental hospitals has dwindled, the number in nursing homes has increased dramatically and now far exceeds the number who receive specialized mental health services. Elderly persons with mental disorders who are in nursing homes or who visit nonpsychiatric physicians usually have little contact with a mental health specialist. It is essential, therefore, that nonpsychiatric physicians effectively recognize and treat psychiatric disorders in their elderly patients.

Psychiatric Assessment of the Older Patient

A careful assessment is the first step in understanding the emotional, psychologic, behavioral, or cognitive difficulties presented by an older patient. Furthermore, ongoing assessment is essential for validating initial impressions or evaluating therapeutic interventions. The psychiatric signs and symptoms presented by an older patient must be considered in relation to factors influencing their presentation or treatment, including medical illnesses and the medications used to treat them; neurologic disorders, especially those that produce cognitive deficits; sensory limitations, especially decreased vision or hearing; and the psychosocial support system available to the older person.

HISTORY-TAKING

Most often an elderly person is referred for psychiatric assessment by someone else—a family member, neighbor, friend, police, or staff of the person's residence. It is essential that history-taking include their observations and concerns as well as those of the identified patient. The first step is to elicit the "chief complaint." While a psychiatric assessment should be part of any complete medical assessment, the symptoms that may flag a psychiatric problem include weight loss, crying, suicidal thoughts, apathy, confusion, assaultiveness, agitation, hypochondriasis, memory difficulty, and paranoid ideas. Several clinical examples illustrate the importance of eliciting a specific complaint and not jumping to the conclusion that the presenting problem is "depression" or "senility."

A woman was referred for inpatient treatment of "depression" so severe that she could not get out of bed. When seen she was inappropriately cheerful. A careful history uncovered a complaint of absent smell that was confirmed by computed tomographic (CT) scan to be due to a large olfactory meningioma. Removal of the tumor completely cured her inability to get out of bed.

A woman was referred for psychiatric consultation because of "depression" evidenced by loss of appetite. A careful history elicited no other symptoms of depression, but it did reveal that the loss of appetite was secondary to food tasting bad and that this complaint began soon after the patient began taking a new antiarthritis drug. When the drug was stopped, the patient's appetite returned to normal.

An elderly woman was referred for an apparent organic brain syndrome characterized by memory complaint and incontinence. A careful history indicated that the memory complaint was out of proportion to the actual impairment. For example, she complained that she couldn't even remember her doctor's name, but it was something like Liptzin, which she then proceeded to spell perfectly. (Kahn and associates have suggested that such a memory complaint is more often a sign of depression than of dementia.) Appropriate treatment for depression led to improvements in her memory and incontinence.

The second step in history-taking is to explore the development of the presenting problem. Was it a gradual process over months or years or did the problem appear abruptly? (Sometimes the family may date the onset of cognitive difficulties to retirement or death of a spouse, when in fact there were signs of slippage even earlier.) What other findings accompanied the current problem? In trying to answer the question "why these particular symptoms and why now?" it is imperative to explore any recent changes in medication and in the patient's life situation, including family relationships. A relatively short history of confusion is unlikely to be due to a dementing process but rather to an acute confusional state or, in some cases, to depression.

The next step is to explore the patient's past psychiatric and medical history. Has the person previously had problems similar to the current ones? If yes, how were they diagnosed and treated? How successful was the treatment? A previous history of very similar problems suggests an affective disorder, since both depression and mania tend to be recurrent disorders while organic brain syndromes tend to be progressive. This clue is very important since the presence of any cognitive symptoms in an elderly patient often leads to a diagnosis of organic brain syndrome and therapeutic nihilism. Two case examples will illustrate the problem.

An 85-year-old woman was a patient in a state mental hospital where she rarely spoke and was tied in a chair all day because of contractures that had developed as a result of inactivity. The diagnosis on her record (and the one the staff accepted) was "chronic organic brain syndrome." Her chart, however, described numerous episodes of severe depression that had been treated successfully with electroconvulsive therapy until she turned 80 and was felt to be too old for further treatments. A trial of antidepressants uncovered an alert woman who was able to detail to her son the goings and comings of staff in the previous five years. Regrettably her contractures were not as reversible as her chronic brain syndrome.

A 78-year-old woman who appeared forgetful, hostile, and paranoid was thought to have early dementia. Past history revealed clear-cut depressive episodes that had previously responded to a combination of antidepressant and antipsychotic medication. When medication was restarted she became more active and cheerful, and was able to remember her favorite baseball team's games in great detail.

A careful medication history will often reveal the iatrogenic cause of acute confusional states or depression. While many medications can cause or aggravate confusion in an elderly person, the most common offenders are psychotropic drugs, including antidepressants and antipsychotic drugs that have anticholinergic side effects, and hypnotics and antianxiety drugs that cause central nervous system depression. Alcohol ingestion, alone or together with the above drugs, can also produce a confusional state. Cimetidine is a widely prescribed drug for ulcers that is reported to produce confusion as a side effect in the elderly. Reserpine is well known as a cause of depression, but it is still prescribed despite the availability of numerous other antihypertensive medications.

A person's family and social history is vital since a change in family relationships may either precipitate or signal a psychologic disturbance. Understanding the individual's cultural background and lifelong personality is a precondition to therapeutic planning. Furthermore, understanding changes in the individual's support system may explain why the problem is emerging or being referred now.

MENTAL STATUS EXAMINATION

Evaluation of mental status begins from the first contact, whether by telephone or in person with the identified patient or with the person referring the patient. The first observations on seeing a patient involve appearance, including dress and grooming. This is followed quickly by behavioral observations of alertness, activity level, and reaction to the interviewer.

After the initial observations it is important to evaluate the person's cognitive functioning. This begins with how the person relates the history of his or her problem. Is the story logical, coherent in proper temporal sequence, and in sufficient detail to make sense? Whether or not the person gives a coherent history, some questions formally to assess cognitive functioning are essential. These usually include questions of orientation, memory, and general information.

The next areas to consider are mood and affect, with the former the subjective state of the individual and the latter a state inferred by the listener. Any person who appears to be significantly depressed should be asked about thoughts of suicide. "Do you ever think you just can't go on anymore?" "Have you ever thought you would be better off dead?" "Have you ever tried to harm yourself?" The presence of serious suicidal intentions requires the clinician to take protective steps that may include hospitalization. One indicator of seriousness is whether the person has any future plans for trips, activities, or projects. Someone who is not planning anything for next week is more at risk than someone who is looking forward to a grandchild's wedding in six months.

Judgment, thinking, and perceptions are the last areas to be covered in the mental status examination. A person's judgment may be affected either by cognitive deficit or by a functional psychosis. For example, someone may go out for a walk in winter without a coat because he can't remember what time of year it is or because he thinks he is the Messiah and needs no coat. Or a person may not eat because he forgets or can't cook or because he believes the food is poisoned or because he has no appetite. It is important to assess whether the person understands his situation or not and whether he does anything dangerous. Delusions are false beliefs that are fixed and not changed by arguments or facts. Paranoid delusions may be either persecutory or sexual in nature. Decreased vision and hearing may also lead to heightened vigilance and on occasion to frank paranoid delusions. Perceptual disturbances include illusions, which are misperceptions of stimuli, or hallucinations, which are perceptions without external stimuli.

PHYSICAL ASSESSMENT

To complete the data base for a psychiatric assessment it is necessary to have the results of a complete physical examination, with particular attention to the neurologic examination as well as routine laboratory studies (see the discussion in Chap. 7 on treatable dementias). In addition to finding physical factors that may produce psychologic symptoms directly, a thorough physical assessment has four other purposes. First, it may identify treatable conditions, such as hearing loss, decreased vision, and decreased mobility, all or any of which may lead to social isolation and hence aggravate psychologic symptoms. Second, it may uncover areas of concern that the patient might otherwise not have expressed. Third, it reinforces the point that psychologic and physical problems are closely related and allows the psychiatrist or other mental health specialists to benefit from the generally positive feelings that patients have toward physicians. Finally, knowledge of the patient's physical condition is an obvious precondition to treatment with any psychotropic medication.

Common Psychiatric Problems
COGNITIVE DEFICIT

The evaluation of cognitive symptoms (disorientation, poor memory, and concentration) is a task often faced by health care providers who work with the elderly. Cognitive functioning should be assessed even in persons with a straightforward focal medical symptom such as shortness of breath. Poor memory can interfere with the patient's ability to comply with a medication regimen, particularly in a person living alone with no outside supports.

Mild forgetfulness is common in older patients, but significant memory problems, especially if fairly recent in onset, should be evaluated and not dismissed because of the person's age. Chapter 7 provides a more complete discussion of dementia and acute confusional states. The latter are often treatable, and the physician should always consider the possibility of treatable conditions. Patients with known senile dementia often develop confusional states from common conditions such as fever, infection, trauma, surgery, heart failure, or medications, including alcohol. Cognitive functioning will return to baseline after the acute condition clears. Cognitive symptoms may also be a sign of depression, as discussed in the next section.

DEPRESSION

The diagnosis of a typical depression does not present much challenge. Few physicians would miss the diagnosis of a patient with complaints of sadness, crying, decreased energy, decreased appetite, weight loss, decreased libido, early morning awakening, and thoughts of suicide. Severe depression may be associated with characteristic delusions: (1) somatic delusions of cancer, brain tumor, or the body viscera rotting. These are much stronger and fixed than occasional hypochondriacal preoccupations that are fairly common as people get older and develop various illnesses. (2) Delusions of poverty, the feeling that one has no money to eat or pay for other necessities of life. When confronted with a large bank balance the person will respond, "Banks make mistakes." Again this is far beyond normal concerns about living on a reduced and often fixed income that is eroded by inflation. (3) Delusions of guilt that one has committed some terrible sin and deserves to be punished for the terrible deed. To the outsider the transgression appears to be non-existent or of little consequence, but the person believes otherwise and is terrified. The delusion may have a core of reality as the person reminisces about the successes and failures in his life.

Older depressed persons are less likely than younger persons to report feeling depressed, but they are more likely to voice physical symptoms and complaints and to be irritable or suspicious. Most importantly, depression may present with signs and symptoms that mimic dementia, including apathy, decreased cognitive ability, memory complaint, loss of self-care skills, incontinence, confusion, and agitation. Since depression is a reversible illness, while dementia is not, the physician is better off overtreating for depression if there is any suspicion that depression is contributing to the older person's problems.

MANIA

Since mania is considerably rarer than depression, most physicians are unfamiliar with the typical picture of elated mood, hyperactivity, decreased sleep, and flight of ideas. Atypical features of mania in the elderly are a tendency toward confusion at the outset, more pronounced paranoid features, the presence of mixed depression and elation, and more labile affect. It is highly unusual for mania to first present after age 65, and a previous history of depression is generally found. Treatment with antidepressants may also precipitate manic attacks.

PARANOID THINKING AND BEHAVIOR

As noted previously, paranoid thinking may be associated with depression or mania in the elderly. It may also be a defensive response to changes in the individual or in his or her environment. For example, a patient who is becoming more forgetful may develop the idea that someone is stealing from her rather than accept that she can't remember where she left her purse. Or a patient who has some hearing deficit may believe people are talking about him rather than admit to needing a hearing aid. On the other hand, a certain degree of suspiciousness may be appropriate in an elderly person whose apartment has been robbed or whose purse has been stolen on the street.

HYPOCHONDRIASIS

Excessive preoccupation with and complaining about physical problems may be a sign of depression. It may also be an exaggeration of a normal response to increasing physical disabilities and limitations. Somatic complaints may also be the only acceptable avenue of asking for attention from relatives, friends, or neighbors, although it may also reflect a lifelong personality pattern.

SCHIZOPHRENIA

Persons with paranoid illnesses that come on late in life are sometimes thought of as having a variant of schizophrenia. Generally these patients do not have the personality disintegration associated with the usual adolescent or early adult onset schizophrenia. For many persons, schizophrenia is a chronic illness, and state mental hospitals used to be filled with persons who were institutionalized when young and never recovered. Currently many of these persons have been reinstitutionalized "in the community" in nursing homes.

ALCOHOLISM

Alcoholism is a serious behavioral disturbance that has numerous medical complications that shorten life if the drinking begins early in life and is of large quantities. However, alcoholism is still quite prevalent in the older population for several reasons. As work and family expectations are reduced by retirement, children growing up, and widowhood, some of the pressures to control drinking are reduced. Alcohol may be used to fill bored and lonely hours. Even in small amounts, alcohol can precipitate severe confusion in older persons with mild cognitive impairment, and it may take weeks of abstinence for such confusion to clear completely.

Treatment Approaches
ENVIRONMENTAL CHANGE
Appropriate changes in the physical or social environment of the individual may either lead to improvements in function or compensation for functional deficits. Physical changes may compensate for decreased hearing, vision, or mobility and allow the person to carry on previous activities. Examples of social changes include increased social contact in or outside the house, and provision of supportive services such as homemakers or meals on wheels.

PSYCHOTHERAPY
The full range of individual and group psychotherapies can be of use to older persons. Traditional psychoanalysts had avoided older patients because it was assumed they were too rigid and that an extensive investment in personality change was not practical with so few years of life remaining. In recent years, however, some psychoanalysts have provided evidence that insight therapy can be quite useful to some older persons. For most patients supportive therapy is more appropriate. This includes techniques of listening, empathizing, and providing advice or reassurance in the context of a concerned professional relationship. Psychotherapy can be carried out even with patients who have some cognitive deficit, since such patients can often talk openly about the losses they have experienced as well as take pride in the accomplishments of their lifetime.

PSYCHOTROPIC MEDICATION
Chapters 4 and 8 provide a more complete description of the use of psychotropic drugs in the elderly. Despite some special problems that make the elderly more sensitive to these drugs and more prone to suffer from side effects, these agents can be enormously helpful in treating psychiatric disorders in the elderly.

FAMILY INTERVENTION
Often when an older relative presents with a psychiatric problem, it precipitates a crisis in the patient's family. Attention to the family's needs will not only improve their ability to cope but also allow them to be more helpful to their relative.

COMMUNITY GEROPSYCHIATRY
Because of the nature of psychiatric disorders in the elderly, a community psychiatry approach has many benefits. First, since few elderly persons are seen in specialized mental health programs, this approach emphasizes consultation and education for other health and social service practitioners and agencies. Consultation and education may change attitudes, increase awareness of mental problems in the elderly, provide assistance in managing difficult cases, and help to identify cases that require specialized treatment.

Second, it emphasizes the need for an interdisciplinary team of psychiatrists, nurses, social workers, clinical psychologists, occupational therapists, and other mental health personnel. Each discipline brings unique skills and insights to the care of older persons with psychiatric disorders. Third, it emphasizes outreach and case-finding, including home visits when needed, with the goal of preventing psychiatric disability. Fourth, it attempts to provide a comprehensive range of clinical services in institutional and noninstitutional settings. Fifth, it is concerned about services being available, accessible, and acceptable to patients. Finally, it attempts to take an organized view of the problems in a given community and match resources to the areas with the highest needs.

While much of this rhetoric is not yet a reality in most communities, community mental health centers are beginning to pay more attention to the elderly as required by law. Furthermore, most of the emphases noted should be part of any mental health services for the elderly.

Suggested Reading

Berezin, M. A., and Cath, S. H. (Eds.). *Geriatric Psychiatry: Grief, Loss, and Emotional Disorders in the Aging Process.* New York: International Universities Press, 1965.

Birren, J. E., and Schaie, K. W. *Handbook of the Psychology of Aging.* New York: Van Nostrand Reinhold, 1977.

Blazer, D., and Williams, C. Epidemiology of dysphoria and depression in an elderly population. *Am. J. Psych.* 137:439, 1980.

Busse, E. W., and Pfeiffer, E. *Mental Illness in Later Life.* Washington, D.C.: American Psychiatric Association, 1973.

Busse, E. W., and Pfeiffer, E. (Eds.) *Behavior and Adaptation in Late Life* (2nd ed.). Boston: Little, Brown, 1977.

Glasscote, R., Gudiman, J. E., and Miles, D. *Creative Mental Health Services for the Elderly.* Washington, D.C.: Joint Information Service, 1977.

Group for the Advancement of Psychiatry. *The Aged and Community Mental Health—A Guide to Program Development.* GAP Report No. 81. New York: GAP, 1971.

Kahn, R. L., et al. Memory complaint and impairment in the aged: the effect of depression and altered brain function. *Arch. Gen. Psychiatry* 32:1569, 1975.

Kaplan, O. J. (Ed.). *Psychopathology of Aging.* New York: Academic Press, 1979.

Kay, D. W. K., Beamish, P., and Roth, M. Old age mental disorders in Newcastle upon Tyne. I: A study of prevalence. *Br. J. Psychiatry* 110:146, 1964.

Levin, S., Kahana, R. J. (Eds.). *Psychodynamic Studies on Aging: Creativity, Reminiscing and Dying.* New York: International Universities Press, 1967.

Levinson, D. J. *The Seasons of a Man's Life.* New York: Alfred A. Knopf, 1978.

Neugarten, B. L. Time, age, and the life cycle. *Am. J. Psychiatry* 136:887, 1979.

Post, F. *The Clinical Psychiatry of Late Life.* Oxford, England: Pergamon Press, 1965.

Steury, S., and Blank, M. L.   *Readings in Psychotherapy with Older People.* DHEW Publication No. (ADM)77-409. Rockville, MD.: Department of Health, Education, and Welfare, 1977.

Wells, C. E.   Pseudodementia. *Am. J. Psych.* 136:895, 1979.

Zinberg, N. E., and Kaufman, I. (Eds.).   *Normal Psychology of the Aging Process* (rev. ed.). New York: International Universities Press, 1978.

7. Dementia

Richard W. Besdine

Human brain function is precious and unique, and deranged intellect is feared more than death by most people. Ironically, many health professionals are loath to confront the frightening specter of brain impairment. The elderly have the highest prevalance of cognitive impairment, and even when mentally firm, they are burdened by less enthusiastic and careful health care compared with younger patients [1–3]. Thus, opportunity for identification of reversible causes of intellectual loss is lessened in the very population that needs investigation most.

Impaired intellectual function is an abnormal state. Although it has been widely assumed that normal aging carries with it an inevitable and important decline in intelligence, the American Psychological Association (APA) has taken a strong contrary position. As early as 1973 [4], the APA suggested that data purporting to correlate intellectual loss with aging were collected using methodology known to be faulty for gerontologic study. Intelligence tests designed for young individuals were applied in cross-sectional investigations to young and old subjects. The different life experiences of nutrition, infection, education, psychosocial milieu, and so on were neglected—the cohort effect—and observed differences were attributed to age alone. The artifact and invalidity introduced by the cohort effect has been well documented in research in gerontology (see Chap. 27), yet the pernicious, false myth of cognitive loss with normal aging persists in both scientific and lay communities.

Normal aging does not include depression, paranoia, confusion, or dementia. The frequency of cognitive impairment does increase sharply with age, however, affecting 10 percent of all people over 65, and 30 percent of those over 80 [5,6]. Among the over one million American nursing-home dwellers, 50 to 75 percent suffer from cognitive impairment. Conservative estimates identify three million Americans over 65 years old afflicted with cognitive impairment, and two-thirds of them live in the community. The most modest estimates of the cost, both in dollars and in human energy, are great. The quality of the lives of the afflicted and their families is heavily compromised. If all the financial and human cost were inevitable, it would be an unfortunate but necessary reality. Recognition of the fact that retrieval of certain individuals from the diagnostic wastebasket of "senility" is possible by the identification of a specific treatable disease makes the cost intolerable.

Cognitive Impairment as a Treatable Disorder
CATEGORIES
Because much is yet to be learned through research about cognitive impairment in the elderly, the nomenclature is controversial and confusing. Terms

in common use will be employed and clarified. Organic mental disorders (DSM-III*) include all intellectual impairment. Two categories of syndromes can occur as subdivisions of the organic mental disorders: the global and the focal syndromes. The first include delirium and dementia—both disturbances of all facets of intellectual function. The second include disturbances only of single or a few intellectual functions. The global syndromes of delirium and dementia are the common intellectual deficits provoked by reversible illness in the elderly. Older terms for delirium and dementia are acute and chronic organic brain syndrome, respectively. Delirium and dementia have recently been redefined operationally and can serve as useful descriptions of the common manifestations of brain failure in the elderly [7].

Although often regarded as a diagnosis, cognitive impairment is a symptom or syndrome. It has been called senile dementia, senility, hardening of the arteries, and many other names; but whatever intellectual impairment is called, it is not a disease or a diagnosis. It is a symptom when the patient or the family complains, or it is a syndrome when a number of characteristic features are described together. This syndrome, as any other, has its own differential diagnosis, including reversible and irreversible diseases. The potential causes must be sifted and evaluated to identify the one afflicting each impaired individual patient. An incorrect historical assumption has persisted that dementia syndromes are irreversible and hopeless, and that only delirious states are reversible and curable; but, geriatric studies have shown that curable diseases can provoke a classic dementia syndrome that is reversible when the disease is treated [8]. The crucial point is that the dementia syndrome in older individuals is often a nonspecific response to many medical illnesses occurring in the absence of primary neuronal degeneration [9].

EPIDEMIOLOGY
There are as yet no good studies identifying the prevalence and cause of reversible cognitive impairment in elderly Americans. Cumulative inferential data from small samples and the European literature suggest that 10 to 25 percent of all people over 65 with cognitive impairment have an underlying, unrecognized treatable disease [10–12]. The prospect of there being 300,000 impaired people in the United States today who might have been restored to useful life by appropriate evaluation and treatment urges further study and intervention.

PRESENTATION OF DEMENTIA
Dementia develops slowly, generally has been present for several months when detected, is progressive, and has an uncertain time of onset. It can

* From *Diagnostic and Statistical Manual* of the American Psychiatric Association.

best be detected by mental status examination (MSE). Many simple tests have been popularized, but learning and using one test regularly is a clinical necessity [13–15]. Whatever MSE is used, certain functions should be evaluated, including social adjustment, reasoning, orientation, memory, arithmetical ability, judgment, and emotional state.

Social Adjustment

Social adjustment is disordered early in the patient with dementia. Previous relationships with friends, family, and work associates deteriorate and antisocial or regressive behavior is common.

Reasoning Ability

Reasoning ability declines and the attention span shortens. The patient often gets lost in the performance of simple tasks requiring more than one step. Learning failure may surface by inability to remember new information such as names, addresses, or room numbers, or it may only become apparent in a new situation requiring flexibility and adaptability.

Orientation

Orientation becomes increasingly disturbed as dementia progresses. Time orientation usually fails first, most often in the order of date first, then day, month, year, and, finally, season. Place becomes progressively misidentified, and patients often think they are at home in unfamiliar environments. People are similarly misidentified. First, people in the immediate environment are confused with one another, then with past acquaintances; strangers may become relatives; and finally no one is familiar. Loss of self-identification rarely occurs.

Memory

Memory is the most easily measured cognitive function. In clinical examination, memory is divided into recent and remote. Although recent memory is more disturbed in dementia, both are impaired. A useful distinction can be made between benign forgetfulness and dementia. In the former, details of an event can be temporarily forgotten; in the latter, entire events may be irretrievably lost. The afflicted patient, particularly if previously intelligent, verbal, and socially adept, may improvise—more accurately, confabulate—to cover memory deficit. Responses of the patient must be checked against reality, so that the examiner is not fooled by a demented but facile patient.

Mental Arithmetic

When mental arithmetic fails, simple calculations can no longer be performed. Here, previous employment and education must be considered in formulating expectations.

Judgment

Judgment is a complex intellectual function that is usually disturbed. Failing judgment is often the precipitating event in the institutionalization of a long-demented old person. Confusion, poor memory, and inability to learn can often be managed for an indefinite period in the community; however, poor judgment provokes potentially dangerous acts by the old person that cannot be monitored at home. The family is then driven to seek placement for an elderly relative.

Emotional State

The person's emotional state is usually disturbed. The previous personality changes or becomes exaggerated. Although dementia is an organic deficit, there is usually an emotional reaction to the perceived loss of intellectual function. Anxiety and depression commonly follow awareness of failing memory. Progressive dementia produces a paradoxical easing of distress. As insight and awareness fade and disappear, there may be a false impression of improvement due to lessened anxiety.

Deficits in brain function can usually be detected by careful interview combined with formal mental status examination. In doubtful or confusing situations, psychological testing can be valuable in uncovering dementia [16].

PRESENTATION OF DELIRIUM

Delirium, unlike dementia, develops abruptly, has generally been present only for hours or a few days, may not progress, and has an easily identifiable time of onset. Restlessness, diminished attention span, decrease in amount and quality of sleep with day-night reversal, fluctuating alertness, memory deficits, and perception defects with hallucinations are all common.

Frequently, in aged patients delirium is superimposed on preexisting dementia, sharply reducing the delirium's turmoil. When these patients are thus doubly afflicted, they appear to have the abrupt onset of a new dementia or the sudden dramatic worsening of an established one. In either instance, the superimposed attenuated delirium may be overlooked and its cause untreated.

Evaluation of Cognitively Impaired Patients

Thorough evaluation of the cognitively impaired elderly patient is as essential as the workup of the patient with unexplained fever, chest pain, or any other important symptom complex. Although few patients would accept the diagnosis of "chest pain of early middle age" from their physician to explain substernal distress, most health consumers and many professionals are satisfied with no investigation of mental decline in the elderly and accept a label of "senility," or "hardening of the arteries," or "old age." Different presenting syndromes suggest different specific diagnostic evaluations, but often distinction between dementia and delirium or determination of whether both are present cannot be made, especially when history is scanty or unavailable. In these instances, comprehensive diagnostic screening is necessary to uncover the underlying cause of the impairment [17,18].

MEDICAL

Evaluating cognitively impaired elderly patients requires careful sequencing of diagnostic tests to avoid iatrogenic harm. When diagnosis and treatment of a potentially reversible syndrome are easy and harmless to the patient, however, they should be pursued vigorously. As complete a history as possible, including identification of recent environmental events and losses relevant to mental health, should be taken of every cognitively impaired patient. A comprehensive physical examination, including rectal, genital, neurologic, and mental status examination should be performed. A complete blood count; measurement of sedimentation rate; study of stool for occult blood; thyroid tests, measurements of electrolytes, blood urea nitrogen, calcium, and phosphorus; urinalysis and culture; serum B_{12} measurement; tests of liver function and blood sugar; syphilis serology; chest x-ray; and ECG should all be performed routinely. If initial screening tests are uninformative, additional diagnostic studies specifically aimed at each of the many causes of cognitive impairment must be undertaken. Further tests should be done proceeding from the least invasive first, in stages, as directed by any clinical or preceding laboratory data that suggest possible etiology. Studies undertaken may include checking blood levels of toxins or therapeutic drugs, plain or contrast x-rays, lumbar puncture, tuberculin skin test, measurement of blood gases, blood culture, EEG, diagnostic ultrasound, and radioisotopic brain scanning and CT scans. These and other indicated studies must be employed in sequence, with results analyzed carefully before proceeding with additional investigation. Because of the patient's limited ability to cooperate, pursuit of medical diagnosis in the presence of mental impairment must often rely disproportionately on laboratory and radiologic tests to find a reversible cause of the impairment [17]. If comprehensive laboratory and radiographic screening are not undertaken in elderly, cognitively impaired patients, medical disease presenting as mental impairment will remain undiagnosed and the patient will be irretrievably lost.

PSYCHIATRIC

Psychiatric evaluation of the patient with the dementia syndrome can be vital, since depressive illness in the elderly may masquerade as dementia

[19]. The term *pseudodementia* has been coined to describe elderly depressed patients who present with a dementia syndrome [18]. Depression in old age commonly includes vegetative signs of sleep, bowel, and eating disturbance; somatic complaints; anxiety and agitation; withdrawal and apathy; and psychomotor retardation [20]. Often missing are the guilt, self-pity, and low self-esteem that are prominent in younger depressed patients. Occult depression should be considered in the evaluation of all elderly demented patients. Useful points for differentiating depression from organic dementia include, in the depressed patient, a history or family history of prior depression, recent provocative loss, no progression of an apparent severe dementia, extensive complaints by the patient of memory loss that is found to be less severe on formal testing, and a rapid onset [21]. A therapeutic trial of antidepressant drugs has been recommended for apparently demented elderly patients in whom no etiology for the dementia has been found [20].

COMPUTED TOMOGRAPHY
Computed tomography of the head (CT scan) is a recent valuable addition to the evaluation of elderly patients with cognitive impairment [22]. CT scanning can reliably detect subdural and epidural hematoma, tumor, intracerebral hemorrhage, brain abscess, subdural empyema, hydrocephalus, and nonhemorrhagic stroke. In addition to focal lesions, the CT scan delivers information about ventricular size and width of cortical sulci. Unfortunately, these measurements have been used in attempts to identify brain shrinkage as the cause of clinical dementia. Currently there is insufficient evidence to conclude that ventricular enlargement and sulcal widening correlate with Alzheimer's disease or any other cause of the dementia syndrome [23].

The CT scan is useful in either establishing the diagnosis of one of the focal intracranial diseases previously enumerated or ruling them out and prompting other diagnostic studies. The CT scan cannot verify or exclude Alzheimer's disease, a clinical and pathologic diagnosis. Timing of CT scanning in the evaluation of cognitively impaired patients will vary, depending upon the clinical presentation and neurologic examination. When focal intracranial pathology is suspected, the CT scan should be done very early. When global dysfunction without focal signs is present, CT scanning should be a secondary or tertiary study in patients for whom there is persistent diagnostic uncertainty.

Causes of Cognitive Impairment
Many individual causes of cognitive impairment in the elderly are reversible, although a majority of cases are irreversible. Reversible causes are defined as diseases with specific treatments that, when applied, allow the return of previous intellectual function. Irreversible causes are brain diseases that

have no known specific treatment. Irreversible does not mean hopeless, however, and there is substantial literature documenting successful techniques for making patients with irreversible brain disease more comfortable and more manageable [24]. Reversible causes are the crucial focus. If reversible causes of cognitive impairment are untreated, they result either in death or in the eventual establishment of fixed dementia. Because most causes of delirium are reversible, a common misconception is that the causes of dementia are irreversible. More and more specific illnesses are now being extracted from the diagnostic wastebasket of "senility," leaving fewer old people requiring custodial care.

Reversible Dementia

It is particularly important to identify reversible causes of dementia promptly. If untreated, these diseases often allow survival, but the dementia becomes fixed and irreversible, even if the underlying disorder is eventually discovered and treated. Furthermore, untreated, these diseases usually result in costly institutionalization and shorten life span. Accordingly, it is urgent to evaluate the patient with newly discovered dementia, in spite of the apparent adynamic nature of the disorder. Those syndromes due to reversible diseases are sometimes called secondary dementias, to emphasize that the primary disease process is outside the brain itself and exerting a secondary detrimental effect on the brain.

Delirium is a very common nonspecific manifestation of systemic illness in the elderly. The aged brain is exquisitely sensitive to pathophysiologic changes caused by a host of physical illnesses, and early in the development of such illnesses the delicate function of the brain is easily disturbed [25,26]. Most deliria in the elderly are provoked by reversible disease. A danger is that the delirium, superimposed on dementia and less dramatic than pure delirium, will be missed.

Conditions most likely to produce global organic mental disorders in the elderly, in decreasing order of frequency, are listed in Table 7-1. Also noted is whether dementia or delirium, or both can be expected.

Irreversible Dementia

When reversible causes of dementia in the elderly are enumerated, few irreversible disorders are left behind, but these remaining diseases still account for the majority of cases of cognitive loss in old age. The irreversible disorders producing cognitive impairment are often grouped as primary dementias, emphasizing that the pathology exists in the neurons serving cognition itself. It seems certain that senile dementia of the Alzheimer type (SDAT) is the most common disorder requiring nursing home care in America. SDAT is responsible for 60 to 70 percent of the irreversible

Table 7-1. Reversible Causes of Organic Mental Disorders in the Elderly

Causes	Dementia	Delirium	Either or Both
Therapeutic drug intoxication			X
Depression	X		
Metabolic factors			
Azotemia/renal failure (dehydration, diuretics, obstruction, hypokalemia)			X
Hyponatremia (diuretics, excess ADH, salt wasting, intravenous fluids)			X
Hypernatremia (dehydration, intravenous saline)		X	
Volume depletion (diuretics, bleeding, inadequate fluids)			X
Acid-base disturbance		X	
Hypoglycemia, insulin, oral hypoglycemics, starvation)			X
Hyperglycemia (diabetic ketoacidosis or hyperosmolar coma)		X	
Hepatic failure			X
Hypothyroidism	X		
Hyperthyroidism (especially apathetic)	X		
Hypercalcemia			X
Cushing's syndrome	X		
Hypopituitarism	X		
Infection and/or fever			
Viral respiratory or gastrointestinal		X	
Bacterial			
Pneumonia		X	
Pyelonephritis		X	
Cholecystitis		X	
Diverticulitis		X	
Tuberculosis (TB)			X
Endocarditis			X
Cardiovascular			
Acute myocardial infarction		X	
Congestive heart failure			X
Arrhythmia			X
Vascular occlusion		X	
Pulmonary embolus		X	
Brain disorders			
Vascular insufficiency			
Transient ischemia		X	
Stroke			X
Trauma			
Subdural hematoma			X
Concussion/contusion		X	
Intracerebral hemorrhage		X	
Epidural hematoma		X	

Table 7-1 (continued)

Causes	Dementia	Delirium	Either or Both
Infection			
Acute meningitis (pyogenic, viral)		X	
Chronic meningitis (TB, fungal)			X
Neurosyphilis	X		
Subdural empyema			X
Brain abscess			X
Tumors			
Metastatic to brain			X
Primary in brain			X
Pain			
Fecal impaction			X
Urinary retention		X	
Fracture		X	
Surgical abdomen		X	
Sensory deprivation states such as blindness or deafness	X		
Hospitalization			
Anesthesia or surgery			X
Environmental change and isolation			X
Alcohol toxicities			
Lifelong alcoholism	X		
Alcoholism new in old age			X
Decreased tolerance with age, producing increasing intoxication	X		
Acute hallucinosis		X	
Delirium tremens		X	
Anemia			X
Tumor: systemic effects of nonmetastatic malignancy			X
Chronic lung disease with hypoxia or hypercapnia			X
Deficiency states such as vitamin B_{12}, folic acid, or niacin	X		
Normal pressure hydrocephalus	X		
Accidental hypothermia		X	
Chemical intoxications			
Heavy metals such as arsenic, lead, or mercury			X
Consciousness-altering agents			X
Carbon monoxide			X

Source: From National Institute on Aging Task Force. Senility reconsidered: treatment possibilities for mental impairment in the elderly. *J.A.M.A.* 244:259, 1980. Copyright 1980, American Medical Association.

dementias. Multiinfarct dementia accounts for 15 to 25 percent, and 10 to 20 percent of cases show mixed pathology. The remaining causes include exceedingly rare but important and, in some instances, well-known diseases (see p. 110).

ALZHEIMER'S DISEASE
Pathology and Definition

In 1906, at a meeting of the Southwest German Society of Alienists, Alois Alzheimer recounted unique neuronal degenerative changes seen in the brain of a 51-year-old woman who suffered rapid and devastating cognitive decline that terminated in death after two years [27]. During the next 50 years, the characteristic pathology of Alzheimer's disease (AD) was described, including: (1) the original neurofibrillary tangles identified by Alzheimer, now thought to be paired helical protein filaments of synaptic origin but antigenically related to neurotubules; (2) the characteristic "senile" or neuritic plaque now known to contain amyloid and probably representing neuronal degeneration; (3) cytoplasmic neuronal granulovacuolar degeneration; (4) loss of dendritic spines; and (5) Hirano bodies, found extraneuronally and probably not central to the pathology of AD. The characteristic lesions predominate in the neocortex and especially the hippocampus, and although plaques appear and increase modestly with normal brain aging, sharp quantitative distinctions are made easily between the Alzheimer brain and the normal brain.

For the half-century following Alzheimer's original description, AD was defined as a rare, presenile (patients younger than 60 years of age) cause of dementia unrelated to the senile dementias of aging. However, a series of painstaking and meticulous clinicopathologic studies [9,28,29] has convinced most investigators that the most common forms of senile dementia and of AD share a specific identical pathology. Accordingly, a single name of AD is given to both; the age-defined variety in the elderly is called senile dementia of the Alzheimer type (SDAT), with AD applied to patients under age 65. Though classic teaching describes brain atrophy with cortical shrinkage and ventricular dilatation, current data do not corroborate any such gross anatomic differences between SDAT and normal brains [30].

Diagnosis

The antemortem diagnosis of SDAT is made solely on clinical grounds, using comprehensive laboratory evaluation to exclude reversible causes of the dementia syndrome. Among the irreversible dementias, the only other common cause that must be distinguished from SDAT is multiinfarct dementia (see p. 110), the clinical behavior of which should be distinctive in its pure form. The dementia of SDAT is of gradual and retrospectively uncertain onset, progresses slowly and linearly, shows few focal or lateralizing neurologic signs or symptoms, and is generally found in a setting of emotional blandness. Very rarely, compelling financial or personal reasons bring families or patients to request diagnostic brain biopsy to identify SDAT.

Epidemiology

The epidemiology of SDAT is poorly understood. Virtually all data come from institutionalized populations, providing a highly skewed view of the disorder. For this reason, a major initiative of the National Institute on Aging is to study the prevalence, incidence, and course of SDAT early in its appearance in community-dwelling elderly. Currently available information indicates greater risk among women, but, given the greater longevity of women and the greater likelihood that women will be institutionalized (men are far more likely to have living spouses at home to care for them), the female preponderance may be artifactual. SDAT leads to premature death in most victims, not due to the neuronal degeneration itself, but usually to some complication of the intellectual loss. Recent survival figures, when studied in patients given optimal custodial medical care, show improvement, although longevity is still reduced sharply for SDAT sufferers [31].

Possible Causes

A definitive etiology for SDAT has not been identified. Current research is pursuing several possibilities. SDAT is a primary neuronal degeneration, and recent reliable reports show reduced regional brain blood flow measured in the hippocampus of victims as secondary to the neuronal atrophy rather than etiologic.

Aluminum poisoning. Aluminum has been associated with SDAT through several lines of suggestive evidence. First, it causes "dialysis dementia" when blood levels rise inadvertently because of high aluminum levels in dialysis fluid. Second, aluminum salts injected into experimental animals produce neurofibrillary tangles, although these aluminum tangles differ from those in SDAT patients and no plaques appear in the animals. Third, total aluminum in the brains of patients dying with SDAT is 10 to 30 times that of appropriate controls. Finally, Perl and Brody [32] have localized aluminum accumulation in SDAT brains to the nuclei of the very neurons with tangles. Current majority opinion, however, sees aluminum accumulation as a marker of neuronal damage rather than the cause. Aluminum is one of the half-dozen most common elements in the earth's crust and its ubiquity could explain passive accumulation in injured neurons. Formal statements have come from several sources, reassuring the public that aluminum cookware is safe.

Viral. A viral etiology has been suspected for SDAT since the documentation that several other degenerative neurologic diseases, such as kuru and Creutzfeldt-Jakob disease, are transmitted by slow viruses. However, direct corroborating evidence of this hypothesis is scanty, limited currently to the observation of paired helical filaments in human fetal cortical neurons exposed in vitro to Alzheimer brain homogenates [33].

Genetic. Multiple studies suggest a genetic or hereditary influence on the appearance of SDAT [34]. A classic Swedish study found a five-fold greater risk among first-degree relatives of institutionalized SDAT victims [35]. Chromosomal defects appear more often in females with SDAT, and certain HLA types are more prevalent in SDAT patients. Down's syndrome and lymphoproliferative disorders are more common in relatives of SDAT victims, and most Down's patients living into their thirties show intellectual decline and postmortem brain changes identical with AD. Most recently, Cohen and Eisdorfer [36] have found that SDAT patients were born significantly later during their mothers' childbearing years than unaffected siblings or controls [36].

Neurotransmitter deficiency. Whatever the initiating lesion, there is accumulating, convincing evidence that defects in cholinergic synaptic transmission accompany the failure of brain cognitive function. Choline acetyltransferase (CAT), the enzyme allowing the final step of intraneuronal synthesis of the cholinergic synaptic transmitter acetylcholine (ACH); ACH itself; and acetylcholine esterase (ACE), the enzyme degrading ACH, are all decreased in SDAT brains [37]. These cholinergic system deteriorations correlate with clinical and pathologic evidence of SDAT. The greatest declines were measured in the specific areas most afflicted with plaques and tangles, the neocortex and hippocampus, and the plaques and tangles show high concentrations of ACE, indicating their cholinergic origins [38]. There is general agreement that the neuronal degeneration of SDAT selects cholinergic cells, and their functional decline and disappearance produce the clinical deficit of SDAT. The therapeutic implications of neurotransmitter chemistry in SDAT are discussed on page 109.

Treatment

In managing patients with SDAT or any other irreversible dementia, numerous strategies and approaches are properly recommended to maximize cognitive function, and some will be discussed here. The present discussion is limited to treatment specifically preserving or restoring lost intellectual function in SDAT patients. A major problem in many studies has been the failure to apply clinical distinctions within groups of demented subjects to separate SDAT from multiinfarct patients when evaluating therapeutic interventions. Strong recommendations now exist for defining treatment groups when evaluating any therapeutic strategy [39].

Drugs. Excluding the judicious use of psychoactive agents for the affective or behavioral complications of SDAT, there are encouraging data concerning the use of specific drugs to treat the dementia itself [40].

Hydergine is a commercial preparation of three dihydrogenated ergot alkaloids with direct neuronal biochemical effects unrelated to cerebral blood flow. A dozen studies reviewed in 1976 showed modest but significant improvement in numerous parameters, most often depression, during three months' treatment, but methodological problems existed in many [40]. More recent double-blind studies verified improvement, and one in Germany documented long-term quantitative intellectual improvement compared with decline in the placebo group [41]. European studies documenting efficacy use 4.5 to 8 mg per day for at least several months, compared with the American FDA-approved dose of 3 mg per day maximum, usually given only for weeks to a month or two. It seems likely that hydergine produces long-term intellectual improvement in SDAT, but future studies must clarify dose, duration, evaluation, and patient selection problems in existing data.

Cerebral vasodilators, Gerovital-H3, hyperbaric oxygen, and *psychostimulants* have all been evaluated in demented elderly individuals and are of no value [40].

Nootropics, a new group of agents, and certain *neuropeptides* have shown promise, largely in experimental animals, although discussion of their early clinical trials is beyond the scope of this chapter.

Neurotransmitter-enhancing therapy. Not surprisingly, neurotransmitter-enhancing therapy has been tried, largely because of implications from the observations concerning cholinergic decline in SDAT [42]. Since cholinergic afferent neurons to the hippocampus and levels of ACE, CAT, and ACH are all diminished, and since the postsynaptic muscarinic cholinergic receptor activity is unimpaired, it is logical to try to increase ACH or to prevent its degradation, or both. Because exogenous ACH is degraded rapidly and cannot enter the brain, preventing degradation of ACH was attempted. Physostigmine, an inhibitor of ACE, has shown some memory-enhancing effects, but they are brief and side effects are substantial. Although direct administration of the deficient synthetic enzyme CAT makes theoretical sense, no practical approaches have been found along this line.

Another approach is suggested by the treatment of parkinsonism with L-dopa, whereby precursor of the deficient dopamine is given and gets into the brain to be made into more dopamine and treat the disease. Since ACH is synthesized by CAT, using choline and acetyl-coenzyme A, the analogous strategy was to feed choline precursor to SDAT patients and increase ACH brain levels. Although choline chloride increases blood and brain choline levels, phosphatidyl choline (lecithin) was found to produce greater increases, and also increased ACH in brain and cerebrospinal fluid. Thus trials have been undertaken in which phosphatidyl choline (lecithin) has been administered to SDAT patients. Preliminary results are mixed, with occasional patients showing sharp improvement, but to date no statistically significant data have been produced [42]. One important caveat about lecithin concerns the peculiarity of FDA nomenclature that also allows phosphatidyl serine to be called lecithin. The lecithin health food stores sell is predominantly phosphatidyl serine, which is of no conceivable benefit in the treatment or prevention of SDAT.

MULTIINFARCT DEMENTIA

As already mentioned, in addition to SDAT, the other common irreversible cause of dementia in the elderly is multiinfarct dementia (MID); together they account for 99 percent of cases. MID is more common in men and tends to begin at a younger age than SDAT. Brought to prominence by Hachinski and coworkers [43], MID is the result of repeated strokes; post-mortem examination shows multiple areas of infarcted, softened brain. A threshold phenomenon has been demonstrated, showing that dementia correlates with more than 50 ml of infarcted brain tissue. Most patients have antecedent hypertension or diabetes, and numerous characteristics of MID have been assembled to differentiate it clinically from SDAT [44], including: (1) rapid onset, (2) stepwise fluctuating mental decline, (3) associated atherosclerotic pathology elsewhere in the body, (4) focal or laterilizing signs or symptoms, (5) diabetes or hypertension, (6) male sex, (7) marked emotional lability, and (8) pseudobulbar palsy. Nonetheless, certain patients show clinical features of both, and the brains of such patients often show features of both SDAT and MID at postmortem. Treatment of MID is limited primarily to prevention by detecting and controlling antecedent diabetes and hypertension. The recent decline in stroke morbidity and mortality should lessen the future prevalence of MID.

RARE IRREVERSIBLE DEMENTIAS

Rare irreversible dementias account for only one to two percent of cases, but the following five disorders are described for completeness of differential diagnosis and because of the need to distinguish them from SDAT when considering treatment.

Creutzfeldt-Jakob Disease

Creutzfeldt-Jakob disease (CJD) is a rare cause of the dementia syndrome generally occurring in middle-aged patients, although with considerable variation in presenting age. In addition to dementia, cerebellar ataxia, myoclonic jerks, and seizures are common. Progression to death is rapid, usually within a year or two of diagnosis, although a variant of the disease occurs in which survival is six months or less. The brain shows spongiform degeneration (CJD is categorized as one of the spongiform encephalopathies). Senile plaques are found in CJD, but the abnormal filaments and thickened neurites of SDAT are absent. CJD has come to prominence in spite of its rarity because it is the first North American dementia known to be caused by a slow virus, one that has been transmitted from human material to higher apes and other experimental animals.

Reports of accidental contagion, combined with the heartiness of the virus, have provoked discussion of precautions needed in dealing with afflicted patients [45]. Recommendations include careful handling of and avoidance of exposure to central nervous system tissue, cerebrospinal fluid, and blood of victims. Skin contact requires only washing, but inoculation should be guarded against carefully. Postmortem central nervous system specimens should be regarded as infectious. Patient isolation is not recommended. Although transmitted by a slow virus that is related to the agents of kuru and scrapie, an autosomally dominant mechanism of heritability has been documented as well, possibly suggesting an underlying genetic predisposition to infection with the virus. Documenting the viral etiology and transmission of CJD does not imply or confirm viral cause of SDAT.

Dementia Pugilistica

The punchdrunk syndrome, dementia pugilistica, is a dementia afflicting boxers, usually well after cessation of prizefighting. A latent period of 10 years or more has been documented. Although it is assumed that repeated brain trauma initiates this reversible dementia, the brain pathology is not dominated by evidence of injury, but rather by the appearance at postmortem examination of typical SDAT neurofibrillary tangles. SDAT plaques, however, are not found with increased frequency.

Pick Disease

Pick disease (PD) is an exceedingly rare degenerative brain disease with a clinical presentation indistinguishable from AD. The definitive Swedish study suggests autosomal dominance, with high penetrance as the mode of inheritance. Pathologically there is atrophy of frontal and temporal lobes bilaterally, distinguishing PD grossly from SDAT. Microscopically there are no similarities in spite of the congruence of clinical presentation. PD brains lack plaques or tangles. Instead one sees a characteristic Pick body or cell—a neuron with a large silver-staining cytoplasmic inclusion—as well as neuronal loss, gliosis, and Hirano bodies.

Parkinson's Disease

Parkinson's disease is said to have an associated dementia, but it is argued that parkinsonism and SDAT, two diseases commonly found in the elderly, coincide frequently enough to account for the component of dementia. Plaques do seem to be more common in postencephalitic parkinsonism. The Guam parkinsonism-dementia complex is a clearer situation, in which the frequent and familial occurrence of parkinsonism and dementia is well documented on the island of Guam. The brains of these patients show classic SDAT neurofibrillary tangles as well as granulovacuolar degeneration, but no plaques. The relevance of the Guam syndrome to classic idiopathic parkinsonism is uncertain.

Huntington's Disease

Beginning in early middle age, Huntington's disease presents with a variety of nonspecific cognitive and behavioral abnormalities that progress to severe dementia over the 10- to 20-year survival of afflicted individuals. However, the hallmark of Huntington's disease is the onset of involuntary choreiform movements, usually appearing a year or two after onset of the disease. Half the offspring of patients are afflicted, indicating autosomal-dominant inheritance with complete penetrance. Neuropathology shows neuronal loss, especially in the cerebral cortex.

General Principles of Treatment

The physician interacting with cognitively impaired patients has three responsibilities. First, comprehensive diagnostic evaluation must be carried out. Second, a prognosis should be clearly provided for the family and, when suitable, for the patient. Third, treatment of any reversible disease should be carried out thoughtfully. Specifics of treatment of each reversible cause of dementia are largely within the boundaries of the appropriate medical or surgical or psychiatric discipline and are discussed in relevant chapters elsewhere in this book. But even when the diagnosis of an irreversible cause of cognitive impairment is made, responsibility for involvement with family and patient continues. Irreversible does not mean hopeless. Whether the impairment remains fixed or worsens, dementia exists on a continuum of highly variable severity. After appropriate evaluation of the patient's deficits, a prosthetic supportive environment to compensate for losses and emphasize remaining function can be constructed that will make demands on the impaired brain commensurate with its capacities. When new diseases surface in elderly individuals who have cognitive impairment of any cause, sharp decline in intellect can be anticipated. Recovery to previous functional levels demands optimum and prompt treatment of the complicating problem.

References

1. Cyrus-Lutz, C., and Gaitz, C. Psychiatrists' attitudes towards the aged and aging. *Gerontologist* 12:163, 1972.
2. Miller, D., et al. Physicians' attitudes towards the ill aged and nursing homes. *J. Am. Geriatr. Soc.* 24:498, 1976.
3. Spence, D., and Feigenbaum, E. Medical students' attitudes towards the geriatric patient. *J. Gerontol.* 16:976, 1968.
4. Eisdorfer, C., and Lawton, M. P. (Eds.). *The Psychology of Adult Development and Aging.* Washington, D.C.: American Psychological Association Task Force, 1973.
5. Gilmore, A. J. J. Community Surveys and Mental Health. In W. F. Anderson and T. G. Judge (Eds.), *Geriatric Medicine.* New York: Academic Press, 1974.

6. Gruenberg, E. M. Epidemiology of Senile Dementia. In B. S. Schoenberg (Ed.), *Advances in Neurology*. New York: Raven Press, 1978.
7. Lipowski, Z. J. Organic brain syndromes: A reformulation. *Compr. Psychiatry* 19:309, 1978.
8. National Institute on Aging Task Force. Senility reconsidered: Treatment possibilities for mental impairment in the elderly. *J.A.M.A.* 244:259, 1980.
9. Besdine, R. W. Geriatric medicine: An overview. *Annu. Rev. Gerontol. Geriatr.* 1:135, 1980.
10. Marsden, C. D., and Harrison, M. J. G. Outcome of investigation in patients with presenile dementia. *Br. Med. J.* 2:249, 1972.
11. Pfeiffer, E. Psychopathology and Social Pathology. In J. E. Birren and K. W. Schaie (Eds.). *Handbook of the Psychology of Aging*. New York: Van Nostrand Reinhold, 1977.
12. Tomlinson, B. E., Blessed, G., and Roth, M. Observations on the brains of demented old people. *J. Neurol. Sci.* 11:205, 1970.
13. Copeland, J. R. M., et al. A semi-structured clinical interview for the assessment of diagnosis and mental state in the elderly: The geriatric mental status schedule. *Psychol. Med.* 6:439, 1976.
14. Jacobs, J. W., et al. Screening for organic mental syndromes in the medically ill. *Ann. Intern. Med.* 86:40, 1977.
15. Kahn, R. L., Goldfarb, A. I., et al. Brief objective measures for the determination of mental status in the aged. *Am. J. Psychiatry* 3:326, 1960.
16. Wells, C. E., and Buchanan, D. C. The Clinical Use of Psychological Testing in Evaluation for Dementia. In C. E. Wells (Ed.), *Dementia* (2nd ed.). Philadelphia: Davis, 1977.
17. Kampmeier, R. H. Diagnosis and treatment of physical disease in the mentally ill. *Ann. Intern. Med.* 86:637, 1977.
18. Robinson, R. A. Differential diagnosis and assessment in brain failure. *Age Ageing* (Suppl.) 6:42, 1977.
19. Goldfarb, A. I. Masked Depression in the Elderly. In S. Lesse (Ed.), *Masked Depression*. New York: Jason Aronson, 1974.
20. Busse, E. W., and Pfeiffer, E. *Mental Illness in Later Life*. Washington, D.C.: American Psychiatric Association, 1973.
21. Wells, C. E. Pseudodementia. *Am. J. Psychiatry* 136:895, 1979.
22. Caird, F. Computerized tomography (EMI scan). In Brain Failure in Old Age. *Age Ageing* (Suppl.) 6:50, 1977.
23. Ford, C. V., and Winter, J. Computerized axial tomograms and dementia in elderly patients. *J. Gerontol.* 36:164, 1981.
24. Lawton, M. P. Psychosocial and Environmental Approaches to the Care of Senile Dementia Patients. In J. O. Cole and J. E. Barrett (Eds.), *Psychopathology in the Aged*. New York: Raven Press, 1980.
25. Libow, L. S. Pseudo-senility: Acute and reversible organic brain syndromes. *J. Am. Geriatr. Soc.* 21:112, 1973.
26. Engel, G. L., and Romano, J. Delirium, a syndrome of cerebral insufficiency. *J. Chronic Dis.* 9:260, 1959.
27. Alzheimer, A. Ueber eine eigenartige Erkrankung der Hirnrinde. *Col. Nervenheilk Psychiat.* 18:177, 1907. Referenced in C. E. Wells (Ed.), *Dementia* (2nd ed.). Philadelphia: Davis, 1977.

28. Blessed, G., Tomlinson, B. E., and Roth, M.   The association between quantitative measures of dementia and of senile change in the cerebral grey matter of elderly subjects. *Br. J. Psychiatry* 114:797, 1968.
29. Terry, R., and Wisniewski, H. M.   Ultrastructure of senile dementia and of experimental analogs. In C. M. Gaitz (Ed.), *Aging and the Brain*. New York: Plenum Press, 1972.
30. Terry, R.   Discussion in J. O. Cole and J. Barrett (Eds.). *Psychopathology in the Aged*. New York: Raven Press, 1980.
31. Gruenberg, E. M., and Hagnell, O.   The failure of success. *Milbank Mem. Fund Q.* 55:3, 1977.
32. Perl, D. P., and Brody, A. R.   Alzheimer's disease: X-ray spectrometric evidence of aluminum accumulation in neurofibrillary tangle-bearing neurons. *Science* 208:297, 1980.
33. DeBoni, U., and Crapper, D. R.   Paired helical filaments of the Alzheimer type in cultured neurons. *Nature* 271:566, 1978.
34. Jarvick, L. F.   Genetic Factors and Chromosomal Aberrations in Alzheimer's Disease, Senile Dementia, and Related Disorders. In R. Katzman et al. (Eds.), *Alzheimer's Disease: Senile Dementia and Related Disorders*. New York: Raven Press, 1978.
35. Larson, T., Sjogren, T., and Jacobson, G.   Senile dementia: A clinical, sociomedical, and genetic study. *Acta Psychiatr. Scand.* 39(Suppl. 167):1, 1963.
36. Cohen, D., and Eisdorfer, C.   White House Conference on Alzheimer's Disease. Washington, D.C., January 1980.
37. Davies, P., and Malmey, A. J. F.   Selective loss of central cholinergic neurons in Alzheimer's disease. *Lancet* 2:1403, 1976.
38. Perry, E. K.   The cholinergic system in old age and Alzheimer's disease. *Age Ageing* 9:1, 1980.
39. Isaacs, B.   The evaluation of drugs in Alzheimer's disease. *Age Ageing* 8:1, 1979.
40. Reisberg, B., Ferris, S. H., and Gershon, S.   Pharmacotherapy of Senile Dementia. In J. O. Cole and J. E. Barrett (Eds.), *Psychopathology in the Aged*. New York: Raven Press, 1980.
41. Kugler, J., et al. Long-term treatment of the symptoms of senile cerebral insufficiency: A prospective study of hydergine. *Dtsch. Med. Wochenschr.* 103: 456, 1978.
42. Growdon, J. H., and Corkin, S.   Neurochemical Approaches to the Treatment of Senile Dementia. In J. O. Cole and J. E. Barrett (Eds.), *Psychopathology in the Aged*. New York: Raven Press, 1980.
43. Hachinski, V., Lassen, M. A., and Marshall, J.   Multi-infarct dementia. *Lancet* 2:207, 1974.
44. Hachinski, V., et al.   Cerebral blood flow in dementia. *Arch. Neurol.* 32:632, 1975.
45. Gajdusek, D. C., et al.   Precautions in medical care of, and in handling materials from, patients with transmissible virus dementia. *N. Engl. J. Med.* 297: 1253, 1977.

8. Management of Psychiatric Problems

Carl Salzman

Americans 65 years and older receive 22 percent of all drug prescriptions. Nearly two-thirds use drugs on a regular basis, averaging 5 to 12 medications every day and more than 13 prescriptions per year [1]. Fewer than five percent of this group abstain from all drug use.

Psychotropic drug use also increases significantly with age and tends to be associated with long term use [2]. Thirty-six percent of noninstitutionalized people over 60 use a medically prescribed drug at least once, and 9 percent use such drugs regularly. One-third of elderly patients hospitalized for treatment of medical or surgical illness in a general hospital received at least one psychotropic drug [3]. The incidence of psychotropic drug prescription to institutionalized elderly patients has been reported to vary between 7 and 92 percent. Approximately one-half of the elderly users of psychotropic drugs report that they could not perform regular daily activities without using a drug. The incidence of polypharmacy also increases with age, and the elderly are inclined to take psychotropic drugs in combination with other medical and psychotropic drugs [4,5].

The conditions for which psychotropic drugs are prescribed to older patients may be placed into five general categories on the basis of clinical use. This categorization stresses target symptoms rather than official diagnostic classifications, since disturbances for which psychotropic drugs are prescribed often overlap such categories. Furthermore, in many instances, a clear diagnosis is not possible, and the clinician is forced to treat manifest pathologic symptoms.

1. *Disordered behavior.* This category includes agitation, wandering, and assaultiveness. Patients who have disordered psychotic thinking (schizophrenic, paranoid, or manic) or who are demented or acutely delirious are also included.

2. *Depression.* This category includes serious depressive affect regardless of etiology. Agitation due to depression is included in this category.

3. *Anxiety.* There is considerable overlap between the treatment of subjective anxiety and objective agitation. Drugs used for disorders in this category are used only for the mild to moderate states of subjective anxiety.

4. *Memory disturbances.* Memory changes in old age may have a variety of causes. The drugs discussed for use in this category of disorders are prescribed to patients whose memory failure is idiopathic and not secondary to another treatable illness.

5. *Sleep disorders.* Like the memory disorder, this category of sleep disturbance excludes disorders of sleep secondary to other treatable illness.

Treatment of Disordered, Agitated Behavior and Psychotic Thinking

INDICATIONS FOR NEUROLEPTIC AGENTS

Behavioral disorders and psychotic thinking may accompany a psychosis that began in earlier years and has continued into late life. Both schizophrenia and affective psychosis of early adulthood can persist into later years and can occur in patients who may additionally develop organic central nervous system (CNS) disorders. Late-onset psychoses such as "late paraphrenia," while less common, may also be associated with behavioral disorders. Agitation, assaultiveness, and wandering may appear as behavioral concomitants of psychosis or of organic brain disease, such as senile dementia and arteriosclerosis. Behavior disorders may also be the only presenting sign of physical illness and pain, or may accompany toxic deliria from medications that alter CNS arousal levels or CNS cholinergic function.

Specific treatment of these various disorders depends on the etiology of the symptoms. Although neuroleptic drugs may improve logical thinking, decrease loose associations and ideas of reference, and diminish delusions and hallucinations, the geriatric clinician more commonly employs neuroleptics to control agitation, wandering, belligerence, and assaultiveness, as well as to assist in nighttime sleep or daytime sedation.

CLINICAL PHARMACOLOGY OF NEUROLEPTICS

Neuroleptics theoretically share the altered bioavailability of other orally absorbed, lipid-soluble drugs so that age-related changes in gastric pH, intestinal surface area, and gastrointestinal mobility may delay the absorption and the onset of clinical activity. Neuroleptics possess anticholinergic activity and thus may also delay their own absorption. Age-related decreases in plasma proteins may lead to higher proportions of unbound neuroleptic, thereby predisposing the older patient to increased toxicity. Since neuroleptics are highly lipid-soluble, and since body fat increases with age as lean body mass decreases, the volume of distribution may increase with age. Too, since neuroleptics are metabolized in the liver, bioavailability of oral forms is influenced by first-pass hepatic extraction, which may change with age. Metabolism of some neuroleptics by demethylation may also be altered by age-related decreases in hepatic enzyme activity.

Neuroleptic drugs are thought to decrease psychotic symptoms by central dopaminergic blockade. The mechanism of their antiagitation effect remains unexplained. All neuroleptics share antiagitation properties as well as the ability to control psychosis, and if milligram equivalency is considered, then all neuroleptic drugs are equally effective. Neuroleptic drugs, however, differ in side-effect production. Selection of the appropriate neuroleptic for each elderly patient thus depends more on knowledge of differential toxicity than on differential clinical efficacy. Certain neuroleptic side effects that can be particularly hazardous for older people are correlated in part with affinity for the dopamine receptor site. These are: sedation, orthostatic hypotension, and extrapyramidal symptoms. As the drug's receptor site affinity increases, milligram potency increases, and the number of milligrams necessary for clinical effect decreases. Sedation and orthostatic hypotension decrease and extrapyramidal symptoms increase as the milligram potency increases. Table 8-1 lists these relative side effects of neuroleptic drugs.

Sedation

Sedation is a side effect that may sometimes be used for therapeutic purposes. For the elderly patient who has trouble falling asleep, neuroleptics with sedative side effects are excellent inducers of sleep. Sedating neuroleptics may also be used to quiet the agitated patient during the day. More commonly, however, sedation is an unwanted side effect for the elderly patient. Daytime sedation due to a neuroleptic may cause or aggravate nighttime insomnia and may increase confusion and disorientation in the elderly patient with dementia. These symptoms may be worse in the evening (sundowning syndrome), and in extreme cases, may include visual hallucinosis. As disorientation and confusion increase, the elderly patient typically becomes more agitated. A frequent medical response is to increase the sedating neuroleptic, which will only further aggravate the symptoms. Sedation and its consequences are also likely when sedating neuroleptics are combined with other sedating drugs. Elderly patients in a general hospital survey often received sedating neuroleptics, such as chlorpromazine or thioridazine in combination with narcotics, analgesics, and hypnotics.

Orthostatic Hypotension

Orthostatic hypotension is a consequence of neuroleptic blockade of central vasoregulatory centers as well as peripheral alpha-adrenergic blockade. Dizziness may be quite uncomfortable for the older person who is already somewhat unsteady. In the elderly patient, sudden decreases in blood pressure may also precipitate falls with secondary fracture, strokes, or even heart attacks. Orthostatic hypotensive episodes may occur at night when the older person awakens to urinate. Patients taking low milligram potency neuroleptics should be advised to arise slowly from the recumbent position. Supportive stockings may be used, but drugs that elevate blood pressure, such as amphetamines, may aggravate psychosis and agitation and should be avoided. Epinephrine will lower blood pressure further due to beta-adrenergic activity and should be avoided. Since sedation and orthostatic hypotension are inversely correlated with milligram potency, selection of a sedating neuroleptic for clinical purposes entails an increased risk of a drop in blood pressure and thus is probably unwise for the elderly patient. Use of drugs such as chlorpromazine, chlorprothixene, and thioridazine should be restricted to those situations in which sedation is clinically necessary, or when other neuroleptic drugs cannot be used.

Table 8-1. Representative Neuroleptic Drugs for the Elderly Patient and Their Side Effects

Generic Name	Trade Name	Approximate Geriatric Dose Range (mg/day)	Relative Incidence of Side Effects		
			Sedation	Hypotension	Extrapyramidal Symptoms
Chlorpromazine	Thorazine Chlor-PZ	10–300	Marked	Marked	Moderate
Thioridazine	Mellaril	10–300	Marked	Marked	Mild–moderate
Acetophenazine	Tindal	10–60	Mild	Mild	Moderate
Trifluoperazine	Stelazine	4–20	Mild	Mild	Marked
Thiothixene	Navane				
Haloperidol	Haldol	0.25–6	Minimal	Minimal	Very marked

Extrapyramidal Symptoms
The elderly are increasingly susceptible to the production of extrapyramidal symptoms (EPS) by neuroleptics [6]. In fact, extrapyramidal symptoms develop in as many as 50 percent of all patients between ages 60 and 80 who receive neuroleptics. Those with brain damage or dementia or endogenously reduced dopaminergic transmission (i.e., from Parkinson's disease) may be even more sensitive.

Extrapyramidal symptoms due to neuroleptic drugs include acute dystonia, akathisia, and parkinsonism. Acute dystonic reactions are likely with rapid increases in neuroleptic dosage. The "Pisa syndrome" refers to a drug-induced dystonic reaction in geriatric patients in which the trunk is flexed to one side. Akathisia may be confused with agitation, prompting an increased neuroleptic dosage rather than a decrease. Parkinsonism is the most common drug-induced extrapyramidal symptom in old age; the peak incidence is in the eighth decade.

A fourth form of neuroleptic-related extrapyramidal symptoms that is sometimes noted in the elderly is akinesia. The patient appears anergic, mute, and often immobile. Although the facial expression is blank, it may sometimes appear sad, and akinetic patients sometimes speak of feeling sad or depressed. Akinesia is more commonly produced by high-potency neuroleptics. Because this side effect sometimes resembles retarded depression, the clinician is sometimes misled into considering antidepressant treatment for an affective illness. The addition of other drugs or electroconvulsive therapy (ECT) only produces more side effects and further confuses the clinical picture. Akinesia is best treated by reducing the neuroleptic dose, or switching to a lower potency drug that produces a lower incidence of extrapyramidal symptoms.

CLINICAL PRESCRIPTION OF NEUROLEPTIC DRUGS
Clinicians who wish to prescribe a neuroleptic drug to an older patient face a difficult choice. If they wish to avoid extrapyramidal symptoms, they must select a relatively low-potency neuroleptic and risk sedation and hypotension. If sedation and/or hypotension must be avoided, a high-potency drug must be selected and the development of extrapyramidal symptoms is likely.

Table 8-1 suggests that middle-range neuroleptics, those that are neither extremely high nor low potency, may be the best choice for the agitated, psychotic elderly patient. On these theoretical grounds, a drug such as acetophenazine would be the best compromise among neuroleptics. Acetophenazine is, in fact, a well-tolerated and useful drug for the older patient.

In actual practice, however, a broad range of neuroleptics has been used successfully with older patients, with doses adjusted to minimize side effects. Thioridazine and haloperidol have been prescribed extensively for elderly psychiatric patients [7] and are the most commonly prescribed neuroleptic drugs for elderly medical patients in a general hospital [3]. Haloperidol and thioridazine have been compared with each other in geriatric patient populations [8]. The drugs are clinically equivalent, although haloperidol was associated with greater improvement in alertness and social functioning. Thioridazine produced more depression, but haloperidol produced more extrapyramidal symptoms. Trifluroperazine and thiothixene, which are high-potency neuroleptics of approximately equal milligram strength, have been found to resemble haloperidol in improving alertness but cause fewer extrapyramidal symptoms [9]. Newer neuroleptics such as molindone and loxitane can be expected to share properties with other neuroleptics of equivalent milligram potency. Studies of their effect in older patients have not been reported, however.

Dose
The net result of the age-related alterations in absorption, binding, metabolism, volume of distribution, half-life, and excretion of neuroleptics, as well as increased receptor sensitivity, is a need for reduced doses in the elderly. Exact dosages for each drug cannot be recommended. Starting doses should be low, particularly for the very frail, very old patient (e.g., 0.25 mg of haloperidol), and increments should be equally small. In general, an average daily dose of neuroleptic is 75 to 100 mg per day of chlorpromazine equivalents and it is seldom necessary to exceed 300 mg per day [10].

Treatment of EPS and Anticholinergic Drug Toxicity
Most extrapyramidal symptoms are best treated by dose reduction or a change to low-potency neuroleptics. As already noted, however, central cholinergic blockade accomplished by using anticholinergic drugs can help restore a dopamine-acetylcholine balance. Anticholinergic drugs such as trihexyphenyl, beperiden, benztropine, and so on, are useful in reducing the severity of extrapyramidal symptoms and, in some cases, preventing their onset. They are particularly useful with high-potency neuroleptics such as haloperidol. These drugs, however, produce anticholinergic side effects of their own.

Tardive Dyskinesia
Tardive dyskinesia, a movement disorder involving the mouth, limbs, and trunk, has been associated with prolonged high-dose neuroleptic drug treatment. The prevalence of tardive dyskinesia in elderly recipients of neuroleptics is 20 times greater than in geriatric patients who receive little or no drug therapy. Its symptoms include smacking, puckering movements of the lips, fly-catching movements or cheeking of the tongue (bon-bon sign), rabbit-like "snouting," and rhythmic, rolling choreiform movements of the arms, trunk, and big toe. It is disfiguring and uncomfortable. For the elderly patient, it adds a gross movement disorder to an already progressively decreasing motor coordination and tremor. The mouth movements cause great

embarrassment and tend to foster social isolation, already a problem for many older people. In addition, mouth movements make eating and drinking difficult and wearing dentures nearly impossible. Older patients, particularly women, seem to be increasingly susceptible to tardive dyskinesia.

The best treatment is prevention by using as little neuroleptic for as brief a time as possible. If tardive dyskinesia is observed near to its onset, drug discontinuance may reverse the symptoms. There is currently no treatment for prolonged severe tardive dyskinesia.

Treatment of Depression

Loss, grief, and sadness are inevitable experiences of late life and do not necessarily imply a clinical depression. Clinical depression, however, is a severe affective disturbance that affects nearly one million older Americans and is the most common psychologic disorder of advanced age [11,12].

The development of depressive symptoms may be insidious, with no clear precipitant. Progressive social isolation, somatic complaints (particularly of gastrointestinal disturbance), and irritability may signal an impending depression. Deterioration of cognitive functions—with memory loss, confusion, and disorientation—may accompany or aggravate the mood disturbance. Agitation or retardation, early morning insomnia, and severe anorexia are hallmarks of severe depression in all ages. Extended loss of sleep and weight in older people, however, may be life-threatening. Severely depressed elderly patients, especially white men, may be high suicide risks.

Treatment of the depressed older patient includes a variety of psychotherapeutic, environmental, and behavioral approaches as well as somatic therapies. The latter include electroconvulsive therapy (ECT), as well as chemical antidepressants.

ELECTROCONVULSIVE THERAPY

Electroconvulsive therapy, which should be employed when the depression is life-threatening, has been found useful and safe for older patients [13] if appropriate precautions and medical evaluation are employed. It may be more beneficial than chemical antidepressants if the depression is accompanied by somatic delusions. Memory loss and confusion following ECT are correlated with the number and frequency of treatments and with electrode placement. Elderly patients should receive unilateral treatment to the nondominant temporal hemisphere. Treatment should be given on alternate days, if clinically possible. Most older patients will show a response after three to six treatments. An occasional older patient may require more treatments, particularly if he or she has had many previous ECT treatments. If the older patient has had well-documented prior episodes of depression, low-dose maintenance medication should be prescribed following the ECT response. This medication may be a tricyclic antidepressant (see below) or lithium carbonate (see p. 127). Table 8-2 summarizes potential problems with ECT in treatment of the elderly [14].

MONOAMINE OXIDASE INHIBITORS

It has been determined that monoamine oxidase (MAO) levels increase in platelets and the brain with aging. If this increase in MAO is responsible for a decrease in catecholamine synaptic neurotransmission in the elderly, then inhibition of MAO may have special therapeutic benefit [15]. Recent studies have found MAO inhibitors, phenelzine, and tranylcypromine to be successful in the treatment of the depressed older patient [16,17]. Monoamine oxidase inhibitors have not been advocated for the treatment of most depressed older patients, however, because of potential toxicity. The production of a hypertensive crisis resulting from the combination of a MAO inhibitor and pressor amines in foods or other drugs may be particularly hazardous in an elderly individual with fragile, arteriosclerotic cerebral blood vessels.

TRICYCLIC ANTIDEPRESSANTS

Tricyclic antidepressants are the primary chemical treatment of depression in all age groups. Since serious depression is common in older people, it is not surprising that these drugs are prescribed increasingly often to the elderly. At least 10 percent of elderly patients hospitalized for medical illness receive tricyclic antidepressants.

Clinical Pharmacology

Tricyclic antidepressants available for current use are listed in Table 8-3 along with their distinguishing characteristics. Under the control of hepatic microsomal enzymes, the tertiary tricyclics, imipramine and amitriptyline, undergo N-demethylation to active desmethyl metabolites. Steady state plasma levels of imipramine, amitriptyline, and nortriptyline are increased with age, whereas levels of desipramine are not increased [18]. This suggests decreased N-demethylation, which has also been found with benzodiazepine metabolism. The metabolites desipramine and nortriptyline, as well as their parent compounds, bind extensively to plasma proteins. Reduced plasma proteins, which sometimes occur with advanced age, may predispose the elderly to tricyclic antidepressant toxicity (see section on benzodiazepines). Older patients are also inclined to have long plasma disappearance half-lives of imipramine and of amitriptyline, but not of nortriptyline or desmethylimipramine. Age-related decreases in hepatic metabolism may account for the increased toxicity of these compounds in older patients. The 2-hydroxy metabolites of imipramine and desipramine, however, have been shown to produce cardiotoxicity in dogs. This potential cardiotoxic metabolite and the prolonged elimination of half-life tricyclics might explain, in part, the increased cardiotoxic sensitivity of the elderly to tricyclic compounds.

Table 8-2. Potential Problems with Electroconvulsive Therapy in Treatment of the Elderly

Problem	Treatment
Acute organic brain syndrome	Use unilateral treatment to the nondominant hemisphere
	Use fewer treatments than for younger adults; 2 to 6 treatments will usually suffice
	Space treatments to avoid compounding of the confusion occurring after each treatment; use at least an alternate-day treatment schedule
Cardiac arrhythmias	Obtain a pretreatment ECG, and then follow cardiac rhythm during treatment with cardiac monitor or ECG
	Use of pretreatment atropine may protect patient against poststimulus arrhythmias; may need higher doses of atropine in elderly patients
	In patients with recent history of infarctions and arrhythmias, pretreatment with lidocaine may be indicated; a cardiologist or internist should attend the treatment of elderly patients with serious cardiac pathology; hyperoxygenate just prior to treatment
Augmentation of hypertension	Consider elimination of or reduction in dose of pretreatment atropine
	Pretreatment with 5 mg of diazepam may protect against large increase in blood pressure
Increased susceptibility to fractures	Requires careful determination of adequate dose of succinylcholine to achieve complete muscle relaxation
Prolonged sleep	May require lower dose of barbiturate anesthesia
Prolonged apnea	Serum pseudocholinesterase may be reduced or absent due to hydrolysis by another medication, such as echothiophate treatment for glaucoma

Source: From Salzman, C., van der Kolk, B., and Shader, R. I. Psychopharmacology and the Geriatric Patient. In R. I. Shader (Ed.), *Manual of Psychiatric Therapeutics.* Boston: Little, Brown, 1975.

Table 8-3. Tricyclic Antidepressants*

Generic Name		Trade Name	Sedation	Hypotension	Anticholinergic Side Effects	Cardiac Irritability
Tertiary Amine	Secondary Amine					
Imipramine		Tofranil, Immavate, Antipress, Janimine, Presamine, SK-Pramine	Mild	Moderate	Moderate	Moderate
	Desmethylimipramine	Norpramin, Pertofrane	Mild	Mild	Mild	Mild
Doxepin		Sinequan, Adapin	Moderate	Moderate	Strong	Mild
	Desmethyldoxepin	—	—	—	—	—
Amitriptyline		Elavil, Amitril, Endep	Strong	Moderate	Strong	Strong
	Nortriptyline	Aventyl, Pamelor	Mild	Mild	Moderate	Mild
	Protriptyline	Vivactil	Mild	Mild	Strong	Mild

*Two additional antidepressants are available: amoxapine (Asendin) and maprotiline (Ludiomil). They are effective in elderly patients, but comparative side-effect data with the above antidepressants are lacking.

Choice of Tricyclic Antidepressants

For clinical purposes one may assume that for any individual elderly patient all tricyclic antidepressants are equally efficacious. Selection of an antidepressant, like a neuroleptic, is based on differential side effect production rather than differential clinical efficacy. Table 8-3 gives an outline of the approximate tendency for side effect production, which may assist the clinician.

Orthostatic hypotension and cardiac irritability are the most serious potential side effects of tricyclic antidepressants for older patients. Patients with irregular cardiac rhythm or bundle branch block may develop varying degrees of heart block from tricyclic antidepressants. Ventricular arrythmias may also occur, particularly ventricular premature depolarizations; and ventricular tachycardias and ventricular fibrillation may be seen. In the elderly patient with preexisting heart disease, therefore, tricyclic antidepressants may present significant hazard.

As indicated in Table 8-3, the secondary (demethylated) amines—desipramine and nortriptyline and doxepin—are less cardiotoxic than the primary, tertiary amines—imipramine and amitriptyline—although these differences have been observed primarily in nongeriatric patient populations.

Anticholinergic toxicity is also a serious potential consequence of tricyclic antidepressant use in the elderly. At low doses, peripheral anticholinergic side effects resemble those of the neuroleptic drugs: dry mouth, constipation, urinary retention, blurred vision, and aggravation of glaucoma. Dry mouth and constipation, which are also symptoms of depression in the elderly, are the most uncomfortable side effects and may aggravate the depression or lead to poor drug compliance. The dry mouth may lead to a loss of porcelain dental fillings or poor fitting dentures. With higher tricyclic doses, a central anticholinergic toxic syndrome becomes more likely. Symptoms are like those found with use of high-dose neuroleptics: disorientation, confusion, memory loss, a sensation of bugs crawling on the skin. In extreme cases, there are visual hallucinations, confusion in identification of familiar faces, and restlessness leading to agitation.

Physostigmine has been advocated for the treatment of the central anticholinergic syndrome, but this drug has its own potential toxicity. Physostigmine has been associated with symptoms of cholinergic excess such as heart block, seizures, increased salivary secretions, and bronchoconstriction. There has been little or no experience with physostigmine in the elderly, and it should be used with caution.

Sedation is also a potentially unwanted consequence of tricyclic administration. Amitriptyline and doxepin are the tricyclics with the strongest sedative effects; they have been used to quiet the agitated, depressed, elderly patient as well as to accelerate sleep induction. Increased sedation in the elderly patient, however, is more often a troubling side effect. As noted previously, increased sedation in the elderly that is produced by sedating psychotropic drugs (or a combination of such drugs) may lead to disorientation, confusion, and agitation, particularly in the evening and at night (sundowning syndrome). Sedative drugs commonly cause daytime sleeping, which is one of the most frequent causes of nighttime insomnia in the elderly. For these reasons, tricyclic antidepressants with sedative effect should be used with caution and limited, when possible, to the more agitated or sleepless, depressed elderly patient.

Tricyclic antidepressants of the imipramine series tend to be less sedating. For the withdrawn, apathetic elderly patient who does not have a dementia, methylphenidate has been recommended as an activating drug with low toxicity [19].

On the basis of differential side effect production, desipramine, nortriptyline, and doxepin are the tricyclic antidepressants with lowest relative toxicity and are probably the best tolerated by the older person. Desipramine or nortriptyline should be used if the patient has a depression characterized by anergia, apathy, psychomotor retardation, or hypersomnia. Desipramine is probably the tricyclic of choice for the older person who is known to be very sensitive to anticholinergic side effects, or who has physical disabilities, such as glaucoma or prostatic disease, that would be exacerbated by anticholinergic side effects. Similarly, if the patient is taking other medications with anticholinergic effects, desipramine should be the tricyclic used first. For patients who are agitated, have insomnia, or who have cardiovascular disease, doxepin may be considered as a tricyclic of first choice. Doxepin is well tolerated and effective in older patients [20]. Tertiary amines, imipramine and amitriptyline, probably should not be first choice tricyclics for the elderly. Protriptyline should be avoided because of its long half-life.

Dose

Older patients have exhibited higher plasma levels of some tricyclics than have younger adults. In prescribing tricyclics to the elderly, it is prudent to start with low doses. A safe starting dose is 10 mg, one to three times a day. Response is often noted at doses between 50 and 150 mg per day since steady state tricyclic levels are achieved later in older patients. Clinical effect may not appear for 10 to 21 days. Prescribing physicians should obtain pretreatment ECGs on all elderly patients and repeat the ECG periodically during the course of treatment. Blood pressure, taken with the patient seated and standing, should be obtained before treatment is initiated and repeated before each increased dosage or as indicated clinically.

Anticholinergic side effects, particularly dry mouth and constipation, challenge the physician's ingenuity and may lead to discontinuance of the tricyclic by the patient. Petroleum jelly applied to the junction of gums and teeth at night may reduce bad taste in the morning. Hard candies are sometimes helpful. A peripheral cholinergic agonist such as bethanachol is sometimes helpful in reducing these symptoms. Dosage reduction of the tricyclic, or an alternative antidepressant treatment such as ECT or monoamine oxidase inhibitors, may be necessary.

LITHIUM

Late-onset mania without preexisting manic-depressive illness has not yet been reported. Most older patients who receive lithium, therefore, either have preexisting bipolar illness or have developed a late-life depression. In either case, lithium should be used as a prophylaxis against symptom recurrence rather than as a specific treatment.

Lithium is excreted almost entirely through the kidney and thus elimination half-life is prolonged (36–48 hours) in older patients [21]. Sodium-depleting diuretics, often taken by the elderly, may result in further lithium retention [22], leading to higher intracellular lithium levels and an increased likelihood of toxicity.

The elderly are more susceptible than younger patients to lithium side effects. These side effects may be confused with other common symptoms of older patients. Gastrointestinal symptoms such as nausea and vomiting, which are early signs of lithium intoxication, may also accompany numerous medical diseases as well as be a symptom of depression in the elderly [23]. Neuromuscular irritability may develop at relatively low doses in the elderly [24] and may be confused with idiopathic tremor of old age, or tremor secondary to other medications such as neuroleptics. Confusion may commonly occur with lithium in the elderly, even at relatively low blood levels. This side effect may be mistaken for confusion due to progressive dementia or many other diseases. Lithium-induced hypothyroidism may also mimic depression or dementia in the elderly [25].

Lithium should be used with caution in the elderly, and its use should be restricted to prophylaxis of well-documented, recurrent affective illness. Dosages should be reduced and blood levels monitored carefully. Cardiac and renal function should be checked regularly, and inquiry into polypharmacy should be routine. Guidelines and procedures to follow for lithium prescription in older patients are as follows:

1. Careful medical history and physical examination
2. History of concomitant drug use
3. ECG
4. Check of thyroid status
5. Urinalysis, electrolytes, BUN, creatinine clearance measurements
6. Daily doses of 150 to 900 mg per day; blood levels at 0.4 to 0.8 mEq/L

Treatment of Anxiety

Anxiety about failing health and personal loss are common in the elderly. Feelings of uselessness, the experience of physical and intellectual decline, and loss of loved ones or peer support systems may also aggravate pre-existing anxiety conditions. Anxiety may be experienced as cognitive apprehension, agitation, or as somatic symptoms with hypochondriacal components. Antianxiety agents are prescribed to approximately 11 percent of the population. Benzodiazepines have virtually replaced all other forms of chemical antianxiety treatment. For example, one-third of elderly patients hospitalized for medical illness were taking a benzodiazepine antianxiety drug, and diazepam was the most commonly prescribed of all psychotropic drugs. Benzodiazepines have also been found useful in the behavioral management of patients with chronic organic brain syndrome [26]. For the very severely agitated patient, however, a neuroleptic such as thioridazine has been shown to be superior to diazepam [27].

CLINICAL PHARMACOLOGY OF BENZODIAZEPINES

The biotransformation of benzodiazepines changes with age. Absorption of chlordiazepoxide is delayed in the elderly [28], although the clinical significance of this delay is uncertain. Decreases in stomach acid due to age or to magnesium-aluminum hydroxide antacid therapy have also been shown to substantially delay this acid hydrolysis and onset of clinical activity.

Intramuscular absorption of chlordiazepoxide and diazepam is slower and less regular than after oral administration and cannot be relied upon to reliably circumvent oral absorption problems when rapid administration of benzodiazepines is necessary. Since chlordiazepoxide and diazepam bind extensively to plasma albumin, elderly persons with decreased albumin levels may be at risk for increased levels of unbound drug and thus increased adverse reactions.

Hepatic metabolism of long-acting benzodiazepines such as diazepam or chlordiazepoxide to active metabolites may be delayed, elimination half-life is considerably prolonged for diazepam and chlordiazepoxide, and the plasma clearance of diazepam may be reduced in elderly women [29]. Benzodiazepines with active metabolites and long half-lives may take even longer to reach clinically useful steady state blood levels and may accumulate more in the older than in the younger patient. Short-acting benzodiazepines that do not undergo biotransformation to active metabolites, such as oxazepam and lorazepam [30], do not undergo age-related alterations in metabolism.

The benzodiazepine-metabolizing capacities of the elderly patient may be further reduced by disease or by other medications that inhibit the biotransformation of these drugs, thus extending the period of potential toxicity. The clinical consequences of altered benzodiazepine pharmacology in the elderly may be unwanted sedation or impaired motor coordination as well as apathy and reversible confusion, disorientation, and dysarthria. The increasing sensitivity of the elderly to these effects may be a result of increased receptor sensitivity [31]. In one survey, benzodiazepine-induced drowsiness was almost twice as high in patients over the age of 70 years as it was in those aged 40 years or less.

All benzodiazepines interact with drugs that depress the CNS, further reducing arousal levels. The clinical consequences of this interaction may be unwanted sedation, aggravated sundowning or disorientation, confusion, and its attendant increased agitation. The combined prescribing of benzodiazepines with other depressant drugs is common in the elderly, particularly old patients in a general hospital. In one review, diazepam was the most frequently prescribed psychotropic drug, and it was frequently combined with narcotics and analgesics as well as other sedatives and psychotropic drugs with sedative action. Thus it was not uncommon for an elderly general hospital recipient to receive several CNS depressant drugs simultaneously.

CHOICE OF BENZODIAZEPINE

Benzodiazepine derivatives share equivalent antianxiety properties when differences in milligram potency are taken into account. Thus, selection of an appropriate benzodiazepine should be based on the pharmacokinetic profile of each specific drug. Relevant clinical prescribing information is surveyed in Table 8-4.

Long-acting benzodiazepines, such as diazepam, that have active metabolites may be selected when a single daily dose is preferred. However, since the long-acting benzodiazepines are likely to predispose the elderly patient to toxicity, alternate-day dosage may be required. Short-acting benzo-

Table 8-4. Antianxiety Benzodiazepines

Generic Name	Trade Name	Presence of Active Metabolites	Approximate Geriatric Dose Range (mg/day)
Long-acting			
Chlordiazepoxide	Librium A-Pexide SK-Lygen	Yes	5–40
Diazepam	Valium	Yes	2–20
Chlorazepate	Tranxene	Yes	7.5–30
Prazepam	Centrax	Yes	10–30
Halazepam	Paxipam	Yes	20–60
Short-acting			
Lorazepam	Ativan	No	0.5–4
Oxazepam	Serax	No	10–40
Alprazolam	Xanax	No	0.25–1

diazepines without active metabolites, such as oxazepam or lorazepam, allow for more flexibility in dosage scheduling and are the preferred antianxiety drugs for the elderly.

DOSE
Benzodiazepine dosage should be adjusted according to the clinical requirements of the patient's symptoms and the production of side effects. As with other psychotherapeutic drugs, dosages of approximately one-third to one-half of that prescribed for younger adults (e.g., 5–10 mg of oxazepam) three or four times a day may be sufficient for an antianxiety effect without producing excessive sedation. Dosage increments should be based on elimination half-life data of the chosen benzodiazepine.

Treatment of Memory and Cognitive Disorders

The quest for memory-enhancing drugs, the "holy grail" of geriatric research, seems to constantly provide potentially exciting new compounds. Unfortunately, no treatments have been found clinically efficacious for the older patient with severe memory disturbance or with irreversible neuronal loss and structural or cerebrovascular pathology. Most research efforts, therefore, are being directed toward the treatment of mild to moderate memory loss in the older person without demonstrable neuropathology.

Many, but not all, older people experience mild forgetfulness. Memory loss serious enough to impair function may be a symptom of treatable illness such as depression [32], or a symptom of an acute brain syndrome due to toxicity, trauma, disorders of metabolism, or reduced sensory input (e.g., the sundowning syndrome). Treatment of the underlying disorder may bring about a surprising restoration of memory function. Successful treatment of depression with ECT, for example, has been noted to be accompanied by clinical improvement in memory and concentration.

The target population for pharmacotherapy of memory disorders can be characterized as older people with gradually worsening memory problems. They cannot remember the previous day's activities, tend to repeat themselves, occasionally get lost or confused, and have difficulty concentrating. These older people are usually aware of their disorder, but try to deny it or hide it with excuses or jokes. Their mood may be labile or secondarily depressed. There is little decrease in self-care, or in ability to act in a socially appropriate manner. Work is usually impossible, however, and retirement has become necessary.

The psychomotor stimulants were among the earliest drugs to be used for the treatment of cognitive impairment of the elderly. Only methylphenidate has proved useful in contemporary clinical practice. It has not been associated with improvement of memory function per se, however, but only for the treatment of apathy, withdrawal, and depression. The chief advantage of methylphenidate is the relative lack of side effects. The optimum dose is 30 mg per day or less [33].

Hydergine, a dihydrogenated ergot alkaloid, is widely used for mild to moderate memory disorder. Its mechanism of action, however, is unknown. Originally it was thought to dilate central blood vessels and increase blood flow and brain oxygen consumption. Recently, research suggests a direct metabolic effect on central receptor sites. Clinical studies of hydergine have been generally positive but not strikingly so. Long-term studies indicate that adequate doses of hydergine may exert modest improvement in cognitive function as well as some elevation of mood [34]. It remains uncertain, nevertheless, whether hydergine is a drug that should be regularly prescribed for mild to moderate memory and cognitive disorders of the elderly. The recommended daily dose is 3 to 6 mg taken orally.

Exciting new research into reduced cognitive functioning in older age is focused on the role of central neurotransmitters and the potential use of neurotransmitter precursors. Acetylcholine may be involved in memory processes and is reduced in aging and in dementia. Choline precursors such as lecithin may prove of some value in memory disorders that are not secondary to pathologic or cerebrovascular change [35]. Recent observations have also demonstrated a reduction in serotonin in nonvascular dementia as well as in very old age. This has lead to speculation that serotonin precursors such as L-tryptophan, or the use of specific serotonin reuptake blockers may be helpful for the treatment of dementia without anatomic pathology [36].

There is relatively little that pharmacotherapy can do to reverse memory loss associated with aging. Treatable depression is, perhaps, the most common cause of reversible memory loss in the aged and should always be considered in the differential diagnosis. Social and family assistance as well as psychotherapy and peer support may be as effective and helpful to the older person as pharmacotherapy in coming to terms with his or her progressive disability.

Treatment of Sleep Disturbance

It sometimes seems as though nearly every aged person has trouble sleeping. Subjectively, older people commonly complain of difficulties in initiating or maintaining sleep and a lack of feeling refreshed on awakening. In patients in their 60s and 70s, the average time taken to fall asleep (sleep latency) normally increases by 10 minutes as compared to patients in their 30s. Objectively, the duration of stage 4 (deep sleep) declines in the elderly as does the total number of hours of nightly sleep. The basic 90-minute REM cycle remains in old age, although dream recall associated with REM sleep declines [37].

Mild difficulties in falling asleep are very common in the elderly. Anxiety about health and the future contribute to extended sleep latency. Daytime napping, particularly in the bored, unoccupied older person, is an often overlooked cause of sleep-onset insomnia. Early morning awakening, which is normally very common in advanced age, may also be secondary to depression, medical illness, drugs, or physical discomfort.

The clinician must be aware of these normal disturbances of sleep in the elderly, as well as the numerous causes of pathologic sleep problems. Diagnosis of the etiology of the sleep disturbance is important in order to avoid improper or excessive prescription of hypnotic medication. Helping the older person to remain awake and productive during the daytime, for example, is far superior to prescribing potentially toxic medications.

Sleep difficulties in older people are reflected in the widespread prescription of hypnotics to the elderly. Of the hypnotics prescribed in 1977 39 percent were for persons over the age of 60 years [38]. Flurazepam was the most commonly prescribed drug of all to elderly medical-surgical patients in a general hospital. In another survey of 2,542 patients in a variety of hospitals, 42.7 percent of the flurazepam recipients were 60 years of age or older.

Barbiturates have been used successfully for many years to treat sleep disorders of the elderly [39]. Barbiturates and nonbarbiturate hypnotics such as methaqualone, glutethimide, and methyprylon, when combined with other sedatives, may produce paradoxical excitement and disinhibition as well as additive CNS depression, hepatic enzyme induction, hypotension, and withdrawal seizures. Barbiturate and nonbarbiturate hypnotic use in the elderly, if necessary, should be limited to very short-term use in medically controlled settings.

Chloral hydrate, 250 to 1,000 mg given at bedtime, is a drug of proved effectiveness. Gastric irritation and paradoxical excitement are potential hazards in the elderly. Diphenhydramine given before sleep is also helpful to some older patients, although anticholinergic side effects may cause confusion (see the section on antidepressants), particularly if the patient is taking other drugs with anticholinergic properties. Sleep-onset insomnia that is secondary to psychosis or behavioral disorders may be quite responsive to sedating neuroleptics such as chlorpromazine, thioridazine, or chlorprothixene. Early morning awakening that is secondary to depression often responds to tricyclic antidepressant therapy. Amitriptyline is the most sedating of the tricyclic antidepressants, although its use in the elderly may produce other toxic consequences (see the section on antidepressants). ECT almost always restores sleep rapidly to the severely depressed older patient.

The hypnotic effect of most drugs is time-limited and rarely extends beyond two weeks. Withdrawal may be accompanied by rebound insomnia or REM rebound with disturbed sleep and dreams.

Recently, the benzodiazepines have become the most commonly prescribed sleep-inducing drugs. All benzodiazepines have been used at bedtime, although comparative hypnotic efficacy data are lacking. Nighttime benzodiazepines, however, may produce excessive daytime drowsiness in the elderly as well as reversible confusion, disorientation, dysarthria, apathy, and drowsiness. Flurazepam is the most widely prescribed benzodiazepine for sleep. In contrast to other hypnotics, flurazepam produces very little or no alteration in REM sleep and no REM rebound on withdrawal. Flurazepam, however, also produced unwanted daytime drowsiness in elderly recipients, and 20 percent of elderly nursing home residents who received flurazepam on a long-term basis developed ataxia, confusion, or hallucinations [40]. The variable toxicity associated with flurazepam appears to be dose-dependent, producing fewer unwanted adverse effects in 15-mg rather than 30-mg doses. Flurazepam also undergoes metabolism to an active metabolite with a long half-life of approximately four to five days (90–100 hours). As noted in the section on benzodiazepines, this metabolism may be altered and the half-life extended even further, thus leading to prolonged potential adverse reactions. Since there are scanty research data to confirm the clinical superiority of the higher flurazepam dose, the 15-mg dose is suggested for the older patient. Flurazepam use should be restricted to brief periods of treatment of pathologic sleep disorder rather than chronic use for the normal problems of sleep onset and maintenance of the elderly.

A short-acting benzodiazepine hypnotic, temazepam, has recently become available. The metabolism of this drug is less complex than that of flurazepam, and there is no accumulation. On the basis of this pharmacologic difference between the two drugs, the shorter-acting one should be more beneficial for elderly patients. To date, however, no controlled comparisons have been made between temazepam and flurazepam in this group.

References

1. Lamy, P. P., and Vestal, R. E. Drug prescribing for the elderly. *Hosp. Pract.* 11:111, 1976.
2. Friedel, R. O. Pharmacokinetics in the Geropsychiatric Patient. In M. A. Lipton, A. DiMascio, and K. F. Killam (Eds.), *Psychopharmacology: A Generation of Progress.* New York: Raven Press, 1978.
3. Salzman, C., and van der Kolk, B. A. Psychotropic drug prescriptions to elderly patients in a general hospital. *J. Am. Geriat. Soc.* 28:18, 1980.
4. Salzman, C., and van der Kolk, B. A. Psychotropic drugs and polypharmacy in elderly patients in a general hospital. *J. Geriat. Psychiatry* 12:167, 1979.
5. Salzman, C. Polypharmacy and drug-drug interactions in the elderly. In K. Nandy (Ed.), *Geriatric Psychopharmacology.* New York: Elsevier, 1979.
6. Salzman, C., Shader, R. I., and Pearlman, M. Psychopharmacology and the Elderly. In R. I. Shader and A. DiMascio (Eds.), *Psychotropic Drug Side Effects.* Baltimore: Williams & Wilkins, 1970.
7. Stotsky, B. A. Psychoactive Drugs for Geriatric Patients with Psychiatric Disorders. In S. Gershon and A. Raskin (Eds.), *Aging.* Vol. 2, *Genesis and Treatment of Psychologic Disorders in the Elderly.* New York: Raven Press, 1975.

8. Smith, G. R., Taylor, C. W., and Linkous, P.   Haloperidol versus thioridazine for the treatment of psychogeriatric patients: A double-blind clinical trial.
Psychosomatics 15:134, 1974.
9. Birkett, D. P., Hirschfield, W., and Simpson, G. M.   Thiothixene in the
treatment of diseases of the senium. *Curr. Ther. Res.* 14:775, 1972.
10. Fann, W. E., and Wheless, J. C.   Some Special Considerations for Psychopharmacology in the Elderly. In J. C. Schoolar and J. L. Clagharn (Eds.),
The Kinetics of Psychiatric Drugs. New York: Bruner/Mazel, 1979.
11. Salzman, C., and Shader, R. I.   Depression in the elderly: I. Relationship between depression, psychologic defense mechanisms and physical illness. *J. Am.
Geriatr. Soc.* 26:253, 1978.
12. Salzman, C., and Shader, R. I.   Depression in the elderly: II. Possible drug
etiologies: Differential diagnostic criteria. *J. Am. Geriatr. Soc.* 26:303, 1978.
13. Wilson, W. P., and Major, L. F.   Electroshock and the Aged Patient. In
C. Eisdorfer and W. E. Fann (Eds.), *Psychopharmacology and Aging.* New
York: Plenum Press, 1973.
14. Salzman, C., van der Kolk, B., and Shader, R. I.   Psychopharmacology and
the Geriatric Patient. In R. I. Shader (Ed.), *Manual of Psychiatric Therapeutics.* Boston: Little, Brown, 1975.
15. Salzman, C.   Update on geriatric psychopharmacology. *Geriatrics* 34:87,
1979.
16. Robinson, D. S.   Age-related Factors Affecting Antidepressant Drug Metabolism and Clinical Response. In K. Nandy (Ed.), *Geriatric Psychopharmacology.* New York: Elsevier, 1979.
17. Ashford, J. W., and Ford, D. V.   Use of MAO inhibitors in elderly patients.
Am. J. Psychiatry 136:1466, 1979.
18. Nies, A., et al.   Relationship between age and tricyclic antidepressant plasma
levels. *Am. J. Psychiatry* 134:790, 1977.
19. Kaplitz, S. E.   Withdrawn, apathetic geriatric patients responsive to methylphenidate. *J. Am. Geriatr. Soc.* 23:271, 1975.
20. Ananth, J. V., et al.   Doxepin in geriatric patients. *Curr. Ther. Res.* 25:133,
1979.
21. Davis, J. M., et al.   Clinical Problems in Treating the Aged with Psychotropic Drugs. In C. Eisdorfer and W. E. Fann (Eds.), *Psychopharmacology
and Aging.* New York: Plenum Press, 1973.
22. Israili, Z. H.   Age-related Change in Pharmacokinetics of Some Psychotropic
Drugs and Its Clinical Implications. In K. Nandy (Ed.), *Geriatric Psychopharmacology.* New York: Elsevier, 1979.
23. Salzman, C., and Shader, R. I.   Clinical Evaluation of Depression in the
Elderly. In A. Raskin and L. F. Jarvik (Eds.), *Psychiatric Symptoms and
Cognitive Loss in the Elderly.* New York: Halstead, 1979.
24. van der Velde, C. D.   Toxicity of lithium carbonate in the elderly patient.
Am. J. Psychiatry 127:1075, 1971.
25. Eisdorfer, C., and Raskin, M. A.   Endocrinologic Bases of Behavior in Aging.
In R. L. Sprott and B. E. Eleftheriou (Eds.), *Hormonal Correlates of Behavior.* Bar Harbor: Jackson Laboratory, 1975.
26. Kirven, L. E., and Montero, E. F.   Comparison of thioridazine and diazepam
on the control of non-psychiatric symptoms associated with senility: Double-
blind study. *J. Am. Geriatr. Soc.* 21:546, 1973.

27. Covington, J. S. Alleviating agitation, apprehension, and related symptoms in geriatric patients. *South. Med. J.* 68:719, 1975.
28. Shader, R. I., et al. Absorption and disposition of chlordiazepoxide in young and elderly male volunteers. *J. Clin. Pharmacol.* 17:709, 1977.
29. MacLeod, S. M., et al. Age and gender related differences in diazepam pharmacokinetics. *J. Clin. Pharmacol.* 19:15, 1979.
30. Kraus, J. W., et al. Effects of aging and liver disease on disposition of lorazepam. *Clin. Pharmacol. Ther.* 24:411, 1978.
31. Greenblatt, D. J., Allen, M. D., and Shader, R. I. Toxicity of high-dose flurazepam in the elderly. *Clin. Pharmacol. Ther.* 21:355, 1977.
32. Kahn, R. L., et al. Memory complaint and impairment in the aged. The effect of depression and altered brain function. *Arch. Gen. Psychiatry* 32:1569, 1975.
33. Salzman, C. Stimulants in the Elderly. In M. Raskin et al. (Eds.), *Age and the Pharmacology of Psychoactive Drugs.* New York: Elsevier, 1982.
34. Yesavage, J. A., et al. Vasodilators in senile dementias: a review of the literature. *Arch. Gen. Psychiatry* 36:220, 1979.
35. Cole, J. O. Cholinergic Agents in Senile Dementia. In K. Nandy (Ed.), *Geriatric Psychopharmacology.* New York: Elsevier, 1979.
36. Carlson, A. Data presented at the annual meeting of the American College of Neuropsychopharmacology. San Juan, Puerto Rico, December 11–14, 1979.
37. Kramer, M. Sleep and Aging. In K. Nandy (Ed.), *Geriatric Psychopharmacology.* New York: Elsevier, 1979.
38. Soloman, F., et al. Sleeping pills, insomnia and medical practice. *N. Engl. J. Med.* 300:803, 1979.
39. Raskin, M., and Eisdorfer, C. Psychopharmacology of the Aged. In L. L. Simpson (Ed.), *Drug Treatment of Mental Disorders.* New York: Raven Press, 1976.
40. Marttila, J. K., et al. Potential untoward effects of long-term use of flurazepam in geriatric patients. *J. Am. Pharmacol. Assoc.* 17:692, 1977.

9. Endocrine and Metabolic Systems

John W. Rowe
Richard W. Besdine

Gerontologists have long been fascinated with endocrine systems because of the clear-cut, clinically relevant alterations in homeostatic mechanisms that occur with advancing age, and because of the possibility that the aging process itself may be secondary to endocrine changes. The latter possibility is reinforced by similarities between some states of hormone deficiency, such as diabetes, myxedema, and hypocorticism, and the clinical concomitants of normal aging.

Hormone Receptors and Aging

Alterations with aging have been documented at almost all molecular sites involved in mediating hormone actions. These include receptors, adenylate cyclase, the nucleus, and the chromatin. Most studies so far have focused on hormone receptors. Over 100 hormone receptor systems have now been examined during the aging process. About 70 percent exhibit decreases in receptor concentration with advancing age, 25 percent do not appear to show a change, and about 5 percent show increased concentration. This pattern seems to be equally distributed between cell membrane and intracellular receptors. Except for two or three cases, all age changes are in apparent receptor concentration rather than binding infinity. Correlations between age changes in receptors and biologic responsiveness have been made in many instances. Some of these appear to be closely linked, while in other cases receptor changes may not necessarily be responsible for altered responsiveness [1].

Carbohydrate Metabolism and Diabetes Mellitus

It is well known that increasing age in otherwise healthy individuals with no clinical evidence or family history of diabetes is associated with a progressive decline in the capacity to dispose of carbohydrates. This age-related decline in carbohydrate metabolism is evident on either oral or intravenous glucose testing, is progressive throughout adult life, and is of sufficient proportions to confound the diagnosis of chemical diabetes in the elderly. Using standard criteria based on the two-hour postprandial blood glucose after a standard oral glucose challenge, at least one-half of normal subjects over age 70 years would be diagnosed as chemical diabetics [2]. Although the prevalence of diabetes does increase with age, it is very unlikely that it reaches this proportion, and many of these individuals are not diabetic.

PHYSIOLOGY

The impairment of carbohydrate tolerance with aging is characterized by a normal fasting glucose, a generally intact serum insulin response to increased plasma glucose, and a decrease in peripheral sensitivity to insulin. The relative contributions of normal aging and alterations in body composition with age to this insulin resistance remains uncertain. The approach to diagnosis of chemical diabetes in the elderly must take into account these physiologic changes. Individuals with elevated fasting blood glucose (greater than 140 mg/dl) are probably diabetic (Fig. 9-1). Almost any acute illness and many chronic illnesses, including pancreatic carcinoma, thyrotoxicosis, or any condition that leads to impaired carbohydrate intake will also result in abnormal carbohydrate metabolism.

Another major cause of impaired glucose tolerance in the elderly is the administration of one or more of the numerous medications known to result in hyperglycemia. Glucose tolerance testing should be performed with the patient in the basal state after receiving an adequate carbohydrate intake (at least 200 g of carbohydrate per day) for at least three days. In order to avoid the inappropriate or misleading overdiagnosis of chemical diabetes in the elderly, age-adjusted guidelines have been established for interpretation of the oral glucose tolerance test (see Fig. 9-1).

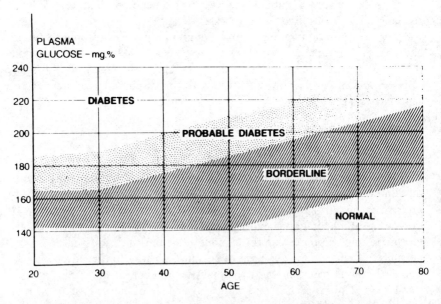

Figure 9-1. Diagnostic levels of plasma glucose for various ages two hours after glucose challenge.

DIABETES MELLITUS

The prevalence of symptomatic and asymptomatic diabetes mellitus substantially increases with age. It is estimated that at least 25 percent of all individuals over age 85 are diabetic. Reasons for this age-related increase include obesity, increased diagnostic screening for diabetes in the elderly, and longevity itself, since long life is associated with a normal decrease in carbohydrate tolerance, thus facilitating the expression of diabetes in an individual with a genetic predisposition.

There are several ways in which age plays an important role in the presentation of diabetes. Development of symptoms, especially polyuria and thirst secondary to hyperglycemia, is often delayed since the reduced glomerular filtration rate seen in the elderly reduces the salt and water losses normally associated with hyperglycemia and the resultant osmotic diuresis. Additionally, the renal threshold for spilling glucose into the urine increases with age, and thus glycosuria often does not appear until the plasma glucose reaches approximately 300 mg/dl. Frequently, neurologic abnormalities, either cranial or peripheral neuropathy, are the initial presenting symptom. Lack of a preexisting history of diabetes should never be taken as evidence against underlying diabetes as responsible for the development of a neurologic deficit. Thyrotoxicosis and pancreatic carcinoma should be carefully excluded in elderly individuals who have the rapid onset of impaired carbohydrate tolerance.

Uncontrolled Diabetes: Hyperosmolar Nonketotic Coma

The hallmark of acute, episodic, uncontrolled diabetes in the elderly is the syndrome of hyperosmolar nonketotic coma (HHNK) [3]. This is characterized by markedly elevated blood glucose levels near 700 mg/dl versus the level of approximately 300 mg/dl commonly seen in diabetic ketoacidosis. In HHNK, plasma osmolality may rise higher than 350 mOsm/kg (normal, 285–295 mOsm/kg), and marked extracellular fluid volume depletion and neurologic findings are prominent. Ketosis is absent and acidosis, when present, is mild in degree and associated with increased plasma levels of lactic acid. HHNK can be termed a geriatric syndrome since it is seen almost exclusively in individuals over age 65 years. Management differs in several important ways from that of uncontrolled diabetes in the younger adult, who generally presents with diabetic ketoacidosis.

Diagnosis of HHNK is often difficult since the patient may not have previously been known to be diabetic, and the prominent neurologic presentation may prompt the diagnosis of stroke or other acute neurologic event. Patients with HHNK generally present with marked depletion of extracellular fluid volume, which has been induced by an osmotic diuresis associated with a markedly elevated blood glucose level. Markedly depressed tissue turgor, lack of sweating, hypotension, and prerenal azotemia secondary to volume loss are not unusual.

Once the diagnosis is made, appropriate treatment includes administration of intravenous or subcutaneous insulin in small amounts and prompt repletion of the extracellular fluid volume. Patients with HHNK are often particularly sensitive to insulin and use of small doses (10–20 units of regular insulin initially) is indicated. Despite the hypertonic state, if hypotension or other evidence of marked volume depletion is present, therapy should be instituted with rapid intravenous infusions of isotonic saline solutions. This will have some effect of decreasing plasma osmolality, since, although the solution is isotonic, it will be significantly hypotonic compared to the patient's plasma. Once the patient is hemodynamically stable, infusions of one-half normal saline (0.45% NaCl) should be begun. Too rapid correction of the volume deficit may precipitate pulmonary edema, especially in elderly individuals with preexisting cardiac disease. In general, one-half of the deficit should be repleted within the first 24 hours of hospitalization. In order to avoid worsening of the neurologic status from too rapid correction of plasma osmolality, blood glucose should be brought to and maintained at approximately 200 to 250 mg/dl for approximately 24 hours while volume repletion is achieved [4].

A factor contributing to the hyperosmolality is that water loss is generally more substantial than salt losses. This may not be reflected in serum electrolytes, since hyperglycemia, by virtue of its osmotic effect on cells, will draw water from the intracellular space to the extracellular space, thus depressing the serum sodium concentration. As in the case of a younger patient with uncontrolled diabetes, a thorough evaluation, including history and physical examination, is important in order to determine the precipitating event, which is frequently an infection.

Patients with HHNK are generally stuporous or comatose upon admission and may, particularly in the very elderly or in those with preexisting central nervous system disease, recover to their previous neurologic state very slowly despite prompt correction of volume deficits and hyperosmolality. In some cases the patient's mental status will not clear for a week or more after correction of the metabolic abnormalities. In the absence of focal signs or evidence of worsening neurologic status, it is best to observe the patient rather than subject him or her to an arduous series of neurologic studies in order to detect the basis of the abnormal mental status. Following an episode of HHNK, some, but not all, patients will require insulin therapy.

Long-term Management of the Elderly Diabetic Patient
The chronic management of diabetes mellitus in elderly ambulatory patients follows the same general guidelines employed in younger adult diabetics. Since moderate levels of hyperglycemia may often be associated with complaints of weakness, lethargy, and decreased mental alertness, the therapy should be normalization, to whatever degree possible, of blood sugar levels. Many elderly patients with new onset of diabetes are obese, and dietary

management alone is effective in controlling blood glucose levels. Oral anti-diabetic agents may be employed, but one should avoid the use of particu-larly long-acting agents, such as chlorpropamide, that may induce late hypoglycemia. Additionally, elderly patients appear to be particularly sus-ceptible to the development of hyponatremia as a consequence of chlorpropa-mide administration.

Hypoglycemia may be particularly treacherous in the elderly since it will go undetected in many patients. This is related to the absence of peripheral symptoms (sweating, hunger, tachycardia, pallor), and lack of recognition or reporting of the symptoms by patients with mental failure. Hypogly-cemia may thus present solely as worsening of confusion. In patients on either oral antidiabetic agents or insulin, one must be vigilant in patient education and careful monitoring of medications at regular intervals in an attempt to avoid adverse drug effects.

Decreases in memory, vision, and motor coordination in the elderly de-crease the patient's capacity to reliably self-administer insulin. The simpler the regimen the more likely the patient is to follow it; one should avoid frequent changes in insulin dose and, whenever possible, manage patients with one dose of insulin daily. Careful attention to foot care is important in all diabetics but assumes even greater prominence in the elderly because of the effect of coincident vascular insufficiency in complicating foot infections and injuries.

Thyroid Gland

The function of the hypothalamic-hypophyseal-thyroid axis has long been the focus of intense interest to gerontologists. This interest is based not only on the clear age-related alteration in the presentation of certain thyroid diseases, but also in the possibility that the thyroid, with its central role in the regula-tion of many metabolic processes, somehow regulates the aging process itself. This area of research has been further stimulated by superficial similarities between the hypothyroid state and old age, such as hypercholesterolemia, increases in body fat, vulnerability to hypothermia, and decreases in auditory acuity. Despite the accumulation of much useful information, a clear view of the influence of age on all aspects of thyroid metabolism has not emerged and no strong support has accumulated for an important role of the thyroid gland in the aging process.

PHYSIOLOGY

Under normal conditions, the anterior pituitary plays a central role in the control of circulating levels of thyroid hormone through release of a peptide hormone–thyroid-stimulating hormone (TSH). TSH stimulates iodine up-take by the thyroid gland and the synthesis and ultimate release of thyroxine (T4) and, in lesser quantities, the more physiologically potent hormone triiodothronine (T3). At peripheral tissues thyroxine exerts an effect on target cells and also is converted to T3 so that the bulk of T3 available originates from peripheral monodeiodination of T4. TSH release is sensitive to two opposing regulatory factors. Thyroxine decreases pituitary TSH release; thyrotropic-releasing hormone (TRH), a tripeptide of hypothalamic origin, increases TSH release and depresses the pituitary response to T4. The net result is sensitive control of thyroid hormone production and release, whereby the free (not protein-bound) circulating level of thyroid hormone is maintained at a level sensed by the anterior pituitary gland as appropriate under the physiologic conditions operating at the time.

DIAGNOSIS OF THYROID DISEASE

The measurement of TSH by radioimmunoassay is an important diagnostic tool in clinical evaluation of the adequacy of thyroid hormone production; it frequently allows the diagnosis of subtle clinical abnormalities that are not readily apparent from measurement of the circulation thyroid hormones themselves. In cases of hypothyroidism resulting from failure at the level of the thyroid gland, TSH levels and the plasma TSH response to TRH are high. Conversely, in hyperthyroidism TSH levels are low and response to TRH is blunted.

The metabolic status of peripheral tissues sensitive to thyroid hormone remains the most direct measure of the adequacy and appropriateness of thyroid function for the entire organism. In this regard, starting about age 20 to 30 years, there is a gradual and significant decline in the basal metabolic rate (BMR) throughout the adult age range. This decline, however, parallels the loss in metabolizing tissues, lean body mass, so that the metabolic rate per unit of lean body mass appears to undergo no important change with age [5]. Studies of thyroid hormone kinetics indicate that a normal or slightly decreased circulation level of total and free thyroxine is maintained into healthy old age by a balanced reduction of as much as 50 percent in T4 production and degradation [6]. It is of special interest that the bulk of present evidence suggests that T3 levels fall with age [6]. Since T3 has also been found to be low in apparently euthyroid individuals with a variety of chronic illnesses or caloric deficiencies, the relationship between age itself and these other factors in the decline in T3 in the elderly remains uncertain. Plasma concentrations of thyroid-binding globulin (TBG), the proteins to which circulating thyroid hormones are bound, do not change with age.

Whether the apparent slight decline in T3 levels with age represents "hypothyroidism" in apparently normal elderly people is unclear. Evaluation of the hypothalamic-hypophyseal-thyroid axis with age indicates that basal and TRH-stimulated TSH secretion is either unchanged or slightly decreased in old age. Since even subtle hypothyroidism would be expected to result in a heightened secretion of TSH, these data are not consistent with the decrease in T3 values reported in some elderly. Likewise, the suggestion from the decreased pituitary response that thyroid hormone is present in excess cannot be supported by the data reviewed above on circulation thyroid hormones in the elderly. On a clinical level, the diagnostic procedures and interpretation of the results for the detection of abnormalities in thyroid function are not importantly influenced by age. The only exception to this general rule might be the slight decrease in T3 levels with age, which could be ambiguous in cases of borderline hypothyroidism. This does not assume major importance, however, since measurement of plasma T3 is often not a reliable index for the presence of mild hypothyroidism; measurement of thyroxine or TSH is more reliable.

THYROTOXICOSIS

The syndrome of thyrotoxicosis maintains in old age the importance that it holds in young adult life as a common treatable cause of morbidity, particularly in women. Age, however, has an important impact on the etiology, clinical presentation, and management of thyroid excess [7]. With regard to etiology, Graves' disease, with its diffusely enlarged thyroid gland and ophthalmopathy, is rarely seen in the elderly. With advancing age, multinodular goiter (Plummer's disease) plays an increasingly important role as the cause of clinically evident thyrotoxicosis.

Old age is accompanied by a decrease in the number and intensity of the symptoms of thyroid hormone excess so that the presentation is less striking and much less obvious to the physician. Not only is each individual symptom often less intense, but at the time of the diagnosis elderly patients often manifest only one prominent symptom, as opposed to young patients in whom a constellation of findings can easily be identified. The changes in the number and intensity of symptoms may be due, in part, to the decreased reserve of many organ systems, especially the cardiovascular system, in the elderly. Since metabolic demands increase proportionally to thyroid hormone levels, the decreased reserve may result in decompensation of one or another organ system, commonly the heart. Thus, elderly thyrotoxic patients, when brought to medical attention, are often seen with hormone levels lower than those that are tolerated well by younger patients. For this reason, thyrotoxicosis must be considered in all elderly patients with a new onset of atrial fibrillation, digitalis-resistant congestive heart failure, unexplained weight loss, or a new onset of hypertension.

The general decrease in intensity of the symptoms of excess thyroid hormone with advancing age, when extreme, results in a presentation that is primarily one of deactivation rather than activation. Such elderly patients, often said to have "apathetic thyrotoxicosis," present with a general syndrome of "failure-to-thrive," with weight loss, lethargy, and depression as common features. Although these patients do not appear to be suffering from thyroid excess as we think of it in the young, diagnosis and appropriate management of the thyroid hormone excess results in a gratifying return of the patients to their prior level of activity and well-being.

In addition to the changes in the severity and number of symptoms in old age, there is also, in many cases, an age-related change in a type of symptom present. The most striking change is the prevalence of goiter [7]. A palpably enlarged thyroid gland is the hallmark of thyrotoxicosis in young adults, and its absence makes the diagnosis of thyrotoxicosis unlikely. In old age, as many as 25 percent of patients with proved thyrotoxicosis will not have goiters, and in many patients no thyroid tissue can be palpated.

Nowhere is the change in the type of symptoms more evident than in the gastrointestinal tract. Anorexia is more common in the elderly than the increased appetite associated with hyperthyroidism in young adults. Diarrhea or hyperdefecation gives way to constipation, and often the triad of weight loss, anorexia, and constipation lead to a presumptive diagnosis of colonic malignancy. In many cases the diagnosis of hyperthyroidism is made only after a long and arduous search for malignancy.

Although the same treatment modalities are available for young and elderly patients, radioactive iodine is by far the most widely used in the older age group. Considerations that limit the usefulness of radioiodine in younger patients, including concern about genetic effects in future children and a wish to avoid late hypothyroidism, are essentially nonexistent in the elderly. When radioiodine is employed, a regimen of oral antithyroid drugs prior to and for several weeks after the administration of radioiodine often simplifies management by eliminating a postradioiodine period of excess hormone release.

HYPOTHYROIDISM

Primary hypothyroidism—failure at the level of the thyroid gland, with elevated TSH levels—appears more commonly in elderly individuals than in young adults. Although age has no important effect on the type or severity of the symptoms of hypothyroidism, recognition of the syndrome is made difficult in the elderly by the similarity of many of the symptoms and signs of thyroid deficiency to findings present in elderly individuals with normal thyroid function. These include dryness of skin, increase in weight, intolerance to cold, depression, lethargy, and apathy. Slow progression of hypothyroidism aggravates the diagnostic difficulty in chronically ill, gradually failing, elderly individuals. As is clear from the previous discussion of the influence of age on thyroid hormone levels, measurement of plasma thyroxine or TSH either under basal or stimulated conditions remains a sensitive and reliable test for the detection of hypothyroidism in the elderly. A slight decrease in T3 levels with age could conceivably be confused with mild thyroid hormone deficiency; however, this has not been found to be a reliable and sensitive test for the detection of mild hypothyroidism at any age. The decreased disposal of thyroxine with advancing age may result in a lowered daily requirement of thyroxine for elderly individuals to achieve a clinically euthyroid state. Generally, a starting daily dose of 50 μg of thyroxine is recommended, with close follow-up study and gradual increases in dose as dictated by the clinical picture and serum thyroid hormone level. Thyroid deficiency is often confounded by the presence of symptomatic ischemic heart disease. In this case the initial dose of thyroxine replacement should be low to avoid exacerbation of the heart disease. The resultant mild or moderate hypothyroidism may be managed by close follow-up and further cautious hormone replacement.

EVALUATION OF THYROID MASSES

The likelihood that a palpable thyroid nodule is benign increases with advancing age. In many cases, although only one nodule is evident on palpation, the gland is actually multinodular; this is particularly true in individuals with clinical evidence of hyperthyroidism. Despite the decreased likelihood of malignancy, a thyroid nodule that is very firm; rapidly growing; or encroaching on the laryngeal nerve, resulting in voice change, is highly suspicious for malignancy and deserves careful evaluation. Although thyroid cancers are less frequent with increasing age, those that do occur are more aggressive and carry a poor prognosis. The slow-growing papillary and somewhat more aggressive follicular carcinomas are rare in the elderly. Undifferentiated carcinomas, which grow rapidly and are apt to metastasize early in the course, take on increasing prominence after the sixth decade.

Adrenal Cortex

The major architectural change with age in the adrenal cortex is an increase in the presence of "benign cortical nodular hyperplasia" [8]. Autopsy studies indicate the presence of bilateral, multifocal nodules, varying in size from microscopic to macroscopic, in as many as two-thirds of elderly individuals. Even when quite large, these nodules are rarely associated with clinical or chemical evidence of glucocorticoid or mineralocorticoid excess.

CORTISOL

The production of cortisol, the major glucocorticoid, by the adrenal cortex is under the influence of the hypothalamic-hypophyseal axis. Corticotropin-releasing factor (CRF) of hypothalamic origin stimulates the release of adrenocorticotropic hormone (ACTH) from the anterior pituitary, which, in turn, stimulates the adrenocortical production of cortisol. Under normal conditions there is a nyctohemeral pattern of plasma cortisol, with a peak early in the morning and a stable low value throughout the remainder of the day. In response to stress, this pattern is abolished and plasma cortisol levels increase abruptly [9].

Basal plasma cortisol disposal rates decrease by 25 to 35 percent in healthy elderly individuals, presumably secondary to decreased hepatic metabolism of the hormone. This decreased disposal is matched by a 25- to 35-percent reduction in cortisol secretion rates [10]. This balancing of decreased disposal and secretion rates results in the maintenance of normal plasma levels in old age and suggests the presence of an intact negative feedback system by which cortisol secretion is down-regulated to compensate for the decreased disposal; thus, excess accumulation of cortisol in plasma is avoided.

Dynamic studies of glucocorticoid metabolism, including stimulation with ACTH and insulin-induced hypoglycemia, suppression with dexamethasone, and testing of the reserve capacity of the hypothalamic-hypophyseal axis (metyrapone), yield similar results in young and old subjects [11,12]. In addition, plasma cortisol response to surgery has been found to be intact in elderly individuals. Thus the occasional practice of "protecting" elderly individuals undergoing surgery with supplemental steroids would appear to be without justification in the absence of specific evidence of impaired adrenal reserve.

RENIN ALDOSTERONE

Aldosterone is produced by the zona glomerulosa of the adrenal cortex and is secreted in response to ACTH, elevations of plasma potassium, decreases in plasma sodium, and increases in circulation levels of angiotensin. Aldosterone is an important regulator of sodium reabsorption and potassium excretion in the distal nephron and plays a vital role in the maintenance of the volume and composition of the extracellular fluid. As with cortisol, the secretion rate of aldosterone is significantly lower in elderly individuals [13]; however, normal plasma levels are not maintained. Under basal conditions plasma aldosterone is approximately 30 percent lower in healthy individuals 70 to 80 years of age as compared to younger adults. In response to a low-sodium diet, aldosterone secretion increases three-fold in young subjects and doubles in the elderly [14]. The decreased aldosterone levels in old age do not appear to be related to any changes in plasma potassium or extracellular fluid volume; they are most likely related to the parallel reductions in renin that are found with advancing age. That the decrease in aldosterone does not represent absolute failure of the adrenal capacity to produce the hormone is suggested by the finding that plasma aldosterone levels after ACTH administration are the same in both young and old individuals.

These normal age-related changes in renin and aldosterone are important for several reasons. Since hypertensive individuals are often categorized into different physiologic groups depending upon their renin level, an elderly individual with normal renin for his age might be incorrectly categorized as a low-renin hypertensive if age-adjusted criteria are not utilized. Lower plasma aldosterone levels in the elderly may also predispose them to the development of hyperkalemia. The elderly are particularly vulnerable in this regard since glomerular filtration rate, a prime determinant of potassium disposal, is also impaired with age. This combination of physiologic impairments makes an elderly individual particularly susceptible to the development of hyperkalemia after the administration of potassium-sparing diuretics such as triamterene or spironolactone.

ADRENAL DISEASES

Neither the tests employed in the clinical evaluation of adrenal function nor the interpretation of the results are changed by age. Both adrenal hyperfunction (Cushing's disease and Cushing's syndrome) and hypofunction (Addison's disease) are primarily diseases of middle age and occur rarely in the elderly. Cases of hypercorticism in old age are easily overlooked since several of the clinical expressions of glucocorticoid excess—including weight gain, osteoporosis, carbohydrate intolerance, and hypertension—are each commonly seen in elderly individuals with normal adrenal function. Suspicion for Cushing's disease in the elderly must be high to avoid overlooking this treatable entity.

In elderly patients with adrenal insufficiency, miliary tuberculosis must be high on the list of possible causes. In addition, acute adrenal hemorrhage occurs in the elderly and may complicate the course of serious acute illness. In approaching the treatment of adrenal insufficiency, from whatever cause, the decreased disposal of cortisol with age should be taken into account. Frequently, normal plasma cortisol values can be obtained with a total dose of 25 mg daily; doses of 37.5 mg, or even in some cases 50 mg, per day may result in a development of mild hypercorticism if given for a long period of time.

Parathyroid
PHYSIOLOGY

Recognition of the importance of parathyroid hormone in the maintenance of calcium homeostasis and skeletal integrity has focused considerable interest on possible age-related alterations in parathyroid function. Studies of healthy men and women across the adult age range show an increase in circulating levels of parathyroid hormone with advancing age [15,16]. As parathyroid hormone is metabolized, fragments accumulate in the blood and are excreted via the kidney. Radioimmunoassays that detect intact hormone as well as these inactive fragments indicate an 80 percent increase in the circulation level of parathyroid hormone from age 30 to age 80. When assays sensitive only for intact hormone are employed, the increase is limited to 30 percent. This discrepancy probably relates to the decrease in renal function that accompanies normal aging and the associated reduced excretion of the non–biologically active fragments of parathyroid hormone. This increase in circulation levels of parathyroid hormone is not accompanied by a change in total serum calcium but rather by a slight reduction in ionized calcium, the major stimulus of parathyroid hormone release.

There are two possible major physiologic mechanisms underlying the increase in parathyroid hormone level with age. The decrease in renal function with aging might lead to decreased phosphate excretion and increases in serum phosphorus. This would result in a slight decrease in ionized calcium and subsequent stimulation of parathyroid hormone. This mechanism is unlikely, since serum phosphate levels do not rise with age but are actually slightly lower in the elderly. The more likely possibility is that aging is associated with a mild "secondary" hyperparathyroidism induced by the well-documented, age-related decrease in intestinal calcium absorption [17]. Decreases in circulation levels of 1,25-dihydroxy vitamin D_3 are probably responsible for the decreases in calcium absorption with age [18]. The resultant slight decline in ionized calcium might then normally lead to an increase in parathyroid hormone release and a mild form of secondary hyperparathyroidism, including the modest decrease in serum phosphate seen with age.

NORMOCALCEMIC HYPERPARATHYROIDISM

The age-related increase in parathyroid hormone levels led to speculation that osteoporosis is due to exaggeration of the normal aging process. Parathyroid hormone levels in postmenopausal osteoporosis have generally been found to be lower than in age-matched controls. However, a small proportion of individuals with osteoporosis are found to have very elevated serum parathyroid hormone levels despite normal serum calcium levels [16]. Such "normocalcemic" hyperparathyroidism is an uncommon but treatable cause of metabolic bone disease and should not be overlooked. This can be diagnosed by measurement of serum parathyroid hormone levels or by a "thiazide challenge test." Since thiazide diuretics decrease renal excretion of calcium, they tend to increase serum calcium levels. In the presence of excess circulating parathyroid hormone, individuals given thiazides for a short 10-day to 2-week course will often develop clear-cut hypercalcemia when serum calcium levels were previously borderline high. Such thiazide-induced hypercalcemia coupled with elevated parathyroid hormone levels and osteoporosis identifies patients who are appropriate candidates for parathyroid surgery.

HYPERPARATHYROIDISM

A clinical consequence of the increases in serum parathyroid hormone level with age, regardless of the type of assay used, is the need to consider age-related norms for parathyroid hormone levels in diagnosing hyperparathyroidism.

There are important differences between the presentation of hyperparathyroidism in young and old adults. Serum calcium is often lower in older than in younger individuals and the clinical presentation is frequently dominated by altered mental status [19]. Modest elevations in serum calcium, often to levels of between 11 and 12 mg/dl, may result in substantial alterations of mental status in the elderly, particularly in the presence of preexisting, mild central nervous system disease. Dramatic improvement in mental status may occur after removal of parathyroid adenomas in elderly individuals who had had only modest degrees of hypercalcemia. Hypercalcemia is thus an important treatable cause of mental failure in the elderly.

Parathyroid surgery is well tolerated by the elderly, and the clinical results are often gratifying [19]. The surgery may in fact be technically easier than in many young patients since elderly patients, despite their lack of very high serum calcium levels, are more often found to have larger adenomas than younger adults. The incidence of parathyroid carcinoma does not appear to be increased in the elderly.

If parathyroid surgery is contraindicated because of the coexistence of severe cardiac or respiratory disease, elderly patients can often be satisfactorily managed, with maintenance of serum calcium within or near the normal range, with conservative therapy. Conservative management includes removal of thiazide diuretics, because of their tendency to increase serum calcium, and administration of furosemide or ethacrynic acid, because of their calciuric effects. Often patients will have coexisting congestive heart failure or hypertension and thus have other indications for the use of these potent diuretics. If diuretics are not indicated for other reasons, they should nonetheless be administered along with a high-salt diet, which is often very effective in suppressing hypercalcemia. An additional useful medical measure is administration of phosphates by mouth. The dose should be titrated in order to keep serum calcium within the normal range and avoid diarrhea, which is a troublesome side effect of oral phosphates.

Posterior Pituitary Gland
ANTIDIURETIC HORMONE OVERSECRETION

Perhaps the most serious and least well-recognized electrolyte disorder in geriatric patients is their tendency for development of water intoxication. The clinical presentation of hyponatremia is nonspecific, with depression, confusion, lethargy, anorexia, and weakness the most common findings. When hyponatremia is severe (serum sodium concentration below 110 mEq/L), seizures and stupor may be seen. It is not unusual for geriatric patients to become hyponatremic in the setting of any stress, including surgery, fever, or acute viral illness.

Clinical evaluation of the elderly hyponatremic patient usually reveals a constellation of findings consistent with oversecretion of antidiuretic hormone (ADH) as a cause of the water retention. These include, in addition to the low serum sodium, evidence of good renal function (low BUN), mild extracellular fluid expansion (normal to slightly full neck veins, trace edema), and evidence of inappropriate renal water retention (urine osmolality greater than maximally dilute and in many cases more concentrated than serum). In addition, reduction in aldosterone secretion and elevation of glomerular filtration rate (GFR) is associated with the presence of modest to large amounts of salt in the urine.

Excess ADH secretion is commonly associated with pneumonia, tuberculosis, stroke, meningitis, subdural hematoma, and a variety of other pulmonary and central nervous system disorders [20]. Although all age groups may develop hyponatremia in these settings, the elderly seem particularly prone to this complication. This may also hold true for drug-induced ADH excess. In one study, elderly patients accounted for most cases of hyponatremia developing from use of chlorpropamide [21]. The stress of anesthesia and surgery have also been shown to result in water intoxication with excess ADH secretion, a complication seen most often in elderly patients [22]. Elderly patients may develop hyponatremia with laboratory concomitants of excess ADH secretion in a variety of viral illness. While hyponatremic, these patients are unable to excrete a water load, but after resolution of the acute illness water metabolism is normal. In many cases the same patient returns several weeks or months later with another acute illness and again develops hyponatremia. (Causes of hyponatremia other than excess ADH secretion, and management of hyponatremia, are discussed in Chapter 11.)

Autonomic Nervous System

Interest in a possible relation between aging and the sympathoadrenal system has recently been fostered by the availability of reliable techniques for the measurement of catecholamines in plasma and increasing knowledge of their physiologic effects.

BASAL SYMPATHETIC ACTIVITY

In an early report utilizing modern assay techniques, Cristensen [23] reported that basal plasma norepinephrine rose approximately twofold, from 200 pg/ml to 400 pg/ml between the ages of 20 and 70. This initial report has since been confirmed by several other laboratories. It seems certain at the present time that basal circulating norepinephrine is not decreased with normal aging, and it is likely that it is increased. The physiologic significance of such an increase might relate to several age-related physiologic changes, including decreased end-organ responsiveness or central nervous system changes, resulting in less tonic inhibitory input into the brain stem areas regulating sympathetic outflow.

SYMPATHETIC RESPONSIVENESS

The bulk of the available data indicates an age-related increase in sympathetic responsivity. Plasma norepinephrine response to several diverse stimuli, including upright posture, oral glucose, cold pressor test, and isometric exercise increases with age [24]. Of particular interest is the finding that norepinephrine persists at high levels for a longer time after the patient has been in an upright posture or has received oral glucose in old subjects than in young subjects. Since age has no effect on the disappearance of norepinephrine from plasma, the persistence of these high levels suggests that sympathetic response is not only greater but also more sustained in the elderly [25].

CARDIOVASCULAR RESPONSIVENESS
The well-established, age-related reduction in cardiovascular response to sympathetic stimulation, when coupled with the increase with age in post-stimulation norepinephrine levels, suggests that the reduced cardiovascular response reflects decreased target tissue sensitivity. The magnitude of the tissue resistance is such that the increased catecholamine response after stress generally results in either equivalent or reduced blood pressure and pulse changes in healthy old individuals compared to their younger counterparts.

ADRENAL MEDULLA
Adrenal medullary function, as estimated by circulating epinephrine values, does not appear to be influenced greatly by age, either under basal conditions or after a variety of physiologic stimuli.

PARASYMPATHETIC FUNCTION
While there is a need for more studies in this area, present evidence suggests that parasympathetic function declines slightly with age, a fact that is of questionable clinical significance.

SYMPATHETIC NERVOUS SYSTEM DYSFUNCTION
It has long been held that an age-related decline in sympathetic nervous system function underlies the increasing frequency of disorders such as accidental hypothermia and orthostatic hypotension in the elderly. As can be seen from the data already reviewed, current evidence indicates that sympathetic activity probably increases and certainly does not decrease as a consequence of normal aging. Thus, these disorders, while they may be based in part on autonomic nervous system dysfunction, should be viewed as pathologic in nature and do not represent extensions of the normal aging process. In addition, if sympathetic activity increases substantially with age, this might play an important role in the increased prevalence of disorders such as hypertension, carbohydrate intolerance, and fragmented sleep in otherwise healthy elderly individuals.

Accidental Hypothermia
Accidental hypothermia (AH) is the unintentional drop of body temperature below 95°F. The provocative cold stress is generally not exposure to

freezing air. Rather, the aged afflicted patients become hypothermic while at home in mildly cool environments (as warm as 65°F), although most episodes are initiated by temperatures below 60°F.

Incidence. The frequency of AH is difficult to assess. In Britain, 3.6 percent of elderly persons admitted to hospitals during the winter months are found to be hypothermic [26]. If American figures are comparable, nearly 50,000 old people may be entering our hospitals annually with occult hypothermia. A comprehensive survey [27] showed a lack of correlation between low body temperature and living alone, being housebound, lack of central heating, and lack of indoor plumbing, all suggesting that increasing urbanization does not reduce the risk of hypothermia in the elderly.

Signs and symptoms. The symptoms of AH are insidious and transient. While elderly people with temperatures between 95° and 97°F usually complain of being cold, patients with frank AH do not. The clinical findings are numerous but nonspecific, and without suspicion of AH they suggest stroke or metabolic disorder. The patient feels cool to the touch and has a history of progressive confusion. Neurologic signs of thick, slow speech; ataxic gait; depressed or pathologic reflexes, or both; and seizures may all occur. Body temperature, once falling below 95°F, continues to fall, slowly but inexorably; and death is inevitable unless treatment is instituted.

Although shivering may occur at temperatures greater than 95°F, most reports find shivering strikingly absent in elderly patients with AH [28]. Instead, marked rigidity with a generalized increase in muscle tone, occasionally accompanied by a fine tremor, may be found.

Although many people have cold extremities in winter, a hypothermic patient has a cold abdomen and back as well. The skin has a cadaveric pallor and chill, and pressure points show erythematous, purpuric, or bullous patches. Subcutaneous tissues are firm, probably from edema, which also produces a puffy appearance, especially of the face.

The cardiovascular system is initially stimulated by cold, resulting in peripheral vasoconstriction, tachycardia, and blood pressure elevation; frank hypothermia depresses the myocardium, producing progressively slow sinus bradycardia and hypotension [29]. Severe hypothermia can reduce blood pressure and heartbeat to barely detectable levels, sometimes leading to erroneous pronouncement of death. The bradycardia, uninfluenced by atropine or vagotomy, is thought to be a result of direct myocardial depression. In addition to sinus bradycardia, a variety of cardiac arrhythmias have been reported during AH, including atrial fibrillation or flutter, often with ventricular premature beats, and idioventricular rhythm as temperature drop continues. Death usually occurs from cardiac standstill or ventricular fibrillation.

The gastrointestinal tract responds to AH with decreased peristalsis, producing abdominal distention, decreased or absent bowel sounds, and, less often, acute gastric dilation with vomiting.

Pulmonary findings include depression of respiration and cough reflex. Atelectasis is universal and pneumonia common enough to be expected. Pulmonary edema during recovery may be related to vascular permeability as well as congestive heart failure.

Early in AH, cold suppresses secretion of antidiuretic hormone and diminishes tubular responsiveness to its action, provoking a diabetes insipidus–like diuresis. Later, as glomerular filtration and renal blood flow diminish as a result of volume depletion, oliguria and tubular necrosis may follow.

Risk factors. (1) *Decreased heat production.* Hypothyroidism has classically been associated with AH. Hypopituitarism, hypoglycemia, starvation, and malnutrition all reduce heat production. Shivering increases heat production several-fold, and is the major acute protective response against AH when ambient temperature falls. The shivering response is usually absent or severely impaired in the elderly, particularly during AH. Forced or voluntary inactivity as in parkinsonism, arthritis, paralysis, and dementia decreases heat production and increases risk of AH.

(2) *Increased heat loss.* Inflammatory skin disease, alcohol-induced vasodilation, exposure, and Paget's disease all increase heat loss.

(3) *Impaired thermoregulation.* Central hypothalamic temperature regulation can be disturbed by a variety of direct anatomic insults to the brain, including stroke, subarachnoid hemorrhage, brain tumor, and subdural hematoma. Several classes of drugs, including phenothiazines, tricyclic antidepressants, benzodiazepines, barbiturates, reserpine, and narcotics depress central thermoregulation and predispose to AH. Chlorpromazine is the best-known offender, also inhibiting shivering. Many other drugs, when taken in excessive doses or combined with alcohol, can produce the same effect.

Perhaps the most common problem predisposing to AH in the elderly is diminution of the normal vasoconstrictor response to cold, which, along with shivering, is the body's primary physiologic defense. It appears that defects in the autonomic nervous system are common in individuals who develop AH.

Diagnosis. Diagnosis of AH depends on the ability to measure body temperature below 95°F. Clinical custom with ill patients is to search for and exclude fever, and body temperature is recorded as high or normal. The standard clinical thermometer is calibrated from 94° to 108°F, but in common use it is rarely shaken down below 95°F—the highest temperature of the hypothermic patient. A rectal thermometer reading from 84° to 108°F is available through most hospital suppliers, although it is not in common use. In the absence of a low-reading thermometer, more expensive thermistors or thermocouples have been used.

Most clinical laboratory data are not specific for hypothermia. Hemoconcentration, dehydration, leukocytosis, lactic acidosis, bronchopneumonia, ileus, and thrombocytopenia are all common.

There are a few distinctive indicators of hypothermia. The electrocardiogram (ECG) can exhibit a major diagnostic clue. The junctional or "J" wave is a small deflection early in the ST segment, positive in the left and negative in the right ventricular leads. Although present in only one-third of AH patients, when found it always signifies hypothermia [30]. Another more common ECG finding is the fine regular oscillation of the baseline produced by the imperceptible tremor and increased muscle tone frequently found in the nonshivering hypothermic patient.

The blood glucose findings in AH have been a point of confusion. Hypothermia produces hyperglycemia by increasing gluconeogenesis via increased steroid and catecholamine secretion. Additionally, although insulin secretion is stimulated, cold interferes with its action, further raising glucose concentrations. When hypothermic patients are hypoglycemic, the causality is reversed, that is, hypoglycemia, usually drug-induced, produces hypothermia.

Management. Treatment of AH includes either slow spontaneous rewarming (SSR) or rapid active rewarming (RAR). SSR allows body temperature to rise slowly to normal by conserving the heat still being produced and has been the standard treatment for elderly patients with AH. RAR applies heat, either to the body surface or to the core, to raise the temperature quickly to normal. RAR is standard treatment for otherwise healthy young adults suffering from intense exposure-induced hypothermia, but the dogma has been that RAR can contribute to the death of aged hypothermic patients by inducing profound and irreversible hypotension.

The technique commonly used has been to insulate the patient in a warmed room to conserve what heat is being produced and to minimize further loss. Body temperature is monitored and allowed to rise 1°F per hour. Even using SSR, a more rapid rise of temperature may produce hypotension. In the patient who is hypothermic because of primary hypoglycemia, restoration of blood glucose will usually result in rapid return of normal temperature.

In one report [31], RAR under optimal intensive care unit (ICU) monitoring has been advocated as the preferred treatment for AH in the elderly, especially if initial SSR efforts produce inadequate temperature rise. Such ICU care would include familiarity with and readiness to use tracheal intubation with full ventilatory assistance, temporary cardiac pacing, pharmacologic circulatory support, and intracardiac pressure monitoring.

Insulin effectiveness declines progressively with temperature fall, and the hyperglycemia of AH is absolutely unresponsive to insulin in the patient whose body temperature is below 85°F. Therefore, insulin should be used cautiously in the hypothermic diabetic who is being rewarmed in order to avoid rebound hypoglycemia as temperature rises and insulin effectiveness increases. If the hyperglycemic AH patient is not known to have diabetes, insulin should not be given unless glucose is very high (greater than 350 mg/dl), since in the nondiabetic, hyperglycemia will often disappear spontaneously during rewarming as endogenous insulin becomes effective.

No studies have supported the routine use of corticosteroids, antibiotics, anticoagulants, or thyroid hormone in the absence of specific indications.

Conclusion. Prevention of AH is preferable to treatment. Since survival correlates with a milder degree of hypothermia, educating the elderly, particularly those with known risk factors, to seek medical attention earlier would reduce mortality and also prevent some cases. Old people with identifiable, predisposing problems should have thermostats set at 65°F or higher, and should keep a reliable thermometer separate from the thermostat and check it daily, especially during very cold weather. Additional indoor clothing, particularly covering for exposed areas such as hands, feet, and head, should be worn. Frequent periods of exercise can increase heat production, and adequate fluid and calorie intake are of prime importance.

References

1. Roth, G. S. Hormonal receptor and responsiveness changes during aging: genetic modulation. *Birth Defects* 14:365, 1978.
2. Andres, R. A., and Tobin, J. D. Aging and the disposition of glucose. *Adv. Exp. Med. Biol.* 61:239, 1975.
3. Gerich, J., Martini, M. M., and Recant, L. Clinical and metabolic characteristics of hyperosmolar–non-ketotic coma. *Diabetes* 20:228, 1971.
4. Arieff, A. I., and Kleeman, C. R. Studies on mechanisms of cerebral edema in diabetic comas. *J. Clin. Invest.* 52:571, 1973.
5. Shock, N. W., et al. Age differences in water content of the body as related to basal oxygen consumption in males. *J. Gerontol.* 18:1, 1963.
6. Ingbar, S. H. The Influence of Aging on the Human Thyroid Hormone Economy. In R. B. Greenblatt (Ed.), *Geriatric Endocrinology*. New York: Raven Press, 1978.
7. Davis, P. J., and Davis, F. G. Hyperthyroidism in patients over the age of 60 years. Clinical features in 85 patients. *Medicine* 53:161, 1974.
8. Dobbie, J. W. Adrenal cortical nodular hyperplasia: the aging adrenal. *J. Pathol.* 9:1, 1969.
9. Andres, R., and Tobin, J. D. Endocrine systems. In C. E. Finch and L. Hayflick (Eds.), *Handbook of the Biology of Aging*. New York: Van Nostrand Reinhold, 1977.
10. West, C. D., et al. Adrenal cortical function and cortisone metabolism in old age. *J. Clin. Endocrinol.* 10:1197, 1961.
11. Blichert-Toft, N., Blichert-Toft, B., and Jensen, H. K. Pituitary adrenal corticoid stimulation in the aged as reflected in levels of plasma cortisol and compound S. *Acta Med. Scand.* 136:665, 1970.
12. Blichert-Toft, N. The Adrenal Glands in Old Age. In R. B. Greenblatt (Ed.), *Geriatric Endocrinology*. New York: Raven Press, 1978.
13. Flood, C., et al. The metabolism and secretion of aldosterone in elderly subjects. *J. Clin. Invest.* 46:960, 1967.
14. Weidmann, P., et al. Effect of aging on plasma renin and aldosterone in normal man. *Kidney Int.* 8:325, 1975.
15. Wiske, T. S., et al. Increases in immunoreactive parathyroid hormone with age. *N. Engl. J. Med.* 300:1119, 1979.
16. Gallagher, J. C., et al. The effect of age on serum immuno reactive parathyroid hormone in normal and osteoporotic women. *J. Lab. Clin. Med.* 95:373, 1980.

17. Bolamore, J. R., et al.   Effect of age on calcium absorption. *Lancet* 2:535, 1970.
18. Gallagher, J. C., et al.   Intestinal calcium absorption and serum vitamin D metabolites in normal subjects and osteoporotic patients. *J. Clin. Invest.* 64: 729, 1979.
19. Mannix, H., et al.   Hyperparathyroidism in the elderly. *Am. J. Surg.* 139: 581, 1980.
20. Schwartz, W. B.   Disorders of Fluid Electrolyte and Acid Base Balance. In P. B. Beeson, W. McDermott, and J. Wyngaarden (Eds.), *Textbook of Medicine* (15th ed.). Philadelphia: Saunders, 1979.
21. Weissman, P. N., Shankman, L., and Gregerman, R. I.   Chlorpropamide hyponatremia. *N. Engl. J. Med.* 284:65, 1971.
22. Deutsch, S., Goldberg, M., and Dripps, R. D.   Post-operative hyponatremia with the inappropriate release of antidiuretic hormone. *Anesthesiology* 27:250, 1966.
23. Christensen, N. J.   Plasma noradrenaline and adrenaline in patients with thyrotoxicosis and myxoedema. *Clin. Sci. Mol. Med.* 45:163, 1973.
24. Rowe, J. W., and Troen, B. R.   Sympathetic nervous system and aging in man. *Endocr. Rev.* 1:167, 1980.
25. Young, J. R., et al.   Enhanced plasma norepinephrine response to upright posture and oral glucose administration in elderly human subjects. *Metabolism* 29:498, 1980.
26. Goldman, A., et al.   A pilot study of low body temperatures in old people admitted to hospital. *J. R. Coll. Physicians* 11:291, 1977.
27. Fox, R. H., et al.   Body temperatures in the elderly: A national study of physiological, social, and environmental conditions. *Br. Med. J.* 1:200, 1973.
28. MacLean, D., and Emslie-Smith, D.   *Accidental Hypothermia.* London: Blackwell, 1977.
29. Keatings, W. R.   *Survival in Cold Water: The Physiology and Treatment of Immersion Hypothermia and of Drowning.* London: Blackwell, 1969.
30. Emslie-Smith, D.   Accidental hypothermia: A common condition with a pathognomonic electrocardiogram. *Lancet* 2:492, 1958.
31. Nicolas, F., et al.   Vingt-quatre observations d'hypothermies accidentelles. *Anesth. Analg.* 31:485, 1974.

10. Reproductive System

Male Reproductive System
PHYSIOLOGY
The possible existence of a male climacteric analogous to the female menopause has long attracted substantial attention. Recent studies on healthy men
from across the adult age range have shown no effect of age on circulating
levels of total testosterone, free (unbound) testosterone, or the major metabolic product of testosterone, dihydrotestosterone (DHT) [1,2]. These normal blood levels may still reflect age-related decreases in secretion of androgens, since androgen clearance falls with advancing age [3]. The remarkable
increases in gonadotropic hormones (LH, FSH) that occur with menopause
are not seen in men, and LH and FSH are increased only slightly in elderly
men [1,2]. While sperm counts do fall late in life, fertility persists in many
men.

PROSTATE
Benign Prostatic Hypertrophy
Benign hyperplasia of the prostate gland, or benign prostatic hypertrophy
(BPH), is exceedingly common in elderly men. The well-documented absence of BPH in castrated men has long pointed to an endocrine basis for
the development of this disorder. It now appears certain that BPH is related
to the intraprostatic accumulation of DHT, a major metabolic product of
testosterone and a potent growth factor for prostatic tissue [4]. Men with
BPH show increased serum and prostatic levels of DHT and specific alterations in the metabolism of testosterone that result in prostatic DHT accumulation [5].

Estrogens seem to play an important role in the development of benign
prostatic hypertrophy. Estradiol production increases with age, and physiologic levels of this estrogen enhance the growth-promoting effects of DHT
in the prostate. Thus absence of estrogens will retard DHT-induced development of BPH. Recent advances in our understanding of the endocrine
pathogenesis of BPH open the door for trials of various therapeutic modalities to control this important geriatric disorder.

Prostatic hypertrophy and subsequent obstruction are important causes of
renal failure in elderly men and must be excluded carefully whenever
azotemia is encountered. While the symptoms of urinary obstruction due to
the prostatic hypertrophy—including urgency, frequency, and nocturia—are
well recognized, many cases progress to the silent development of obstructive
nephropathy, azotemia, and uremia. While most patients with obstructive
urinary symptoms from BPH are shown to have an enlarged prostate on rectal
examination, urethral obstruction may result from asymmetrical hypertrophy
that is not detectable on rectal examination.

Management. The most effective management of prostatic hypertrophy is surgical excision of the prostate, either by the transurethral route or by a more definitive procedure. The specific surgical approach employed is largely dictated by the patient's condition and the degree of symptoms. Different surgical procedures are associated with varying rates of postoperative incontinence. In patients in whom surgery is contraindicated because of severe, coexisting cardiac, respiratory, or central nervous system disease, a trial of pharmacologic doses of estrogens is indicated. Diethylstilbestrol in doses of 2 mg per day is often effective in shrinking hypertrophied prostate glands and in relieving or at least ameliorating symptoms of obstruction. Prolonged estrogen administration is associated with cardiovascular complications and should be avoided if possible.

Prostatic Carcinoma

Prostatic carcinoma is a geriatric disease of which over 95 percent of cases occur in elderly men. Although there is no clear-cut relationship between prostatic carcinoma and BPH, both disorders are clearly endocrine-dependent. The incidence of prostatic carcinoma is markedly lower in castrated men, and the disease is encouraged by excess testosterone and inhibited by estrogens. Most prostatic cancers are subcapsular, and rectal examination is an important diagnostic maneuver. One-half of all palpable prostatic nodules will prove to be cancerous. If a nodule is palpated, urologic consultation and biopsy are indicated. Urinary cytology is of no value in diagnosing prostatic carcinoma. Since the disease is clinically silent in its early stages, most cases (80 percent) have metastasized by the time of diagnosis. Metastasis is generally to the lumbar spine, pelvis, and local nodes. Radiologic manifestations of bone metastases include osteosclerosis, which can be confused with Paget's disease. Acid phosphatase is a useful screening test for the presence of prostatic carcinoma and, contrary to common belief, is not influenced by previous rectal examination.

Management. Management of prostatic carcinoma in patients who have no evidence of metastasis includes radical surgery, with removal of the prostate and seminal vesicles. In the presence of metastases, local symptoms of urethral obstruction can be managed with transurethral resection of the prostate. If surgery is contraindicated but cure appears possible, radical radiation therapy may be effective. Although this is associated with a reasonably high incidence of radiation proctitis, this disturbing complication is self-limited.

Endocrine manipulations are important in the management of prostatic carcinoma. At least two-thirds of prostatic carcinomas are endocrine-responsive. In patients with metastases to bone, bilateral orchiectomy will decrease pain and symptoms of urinary obstruction in two-thirds of cases, often over the course of several days [6]. Estrogen administration (diethylstilbestrol, 2 mg/day) has an effect similar to orchiectomy and, when used in conjunction with orchiectomy, provides further inhibition of tumor growth [6]. Long-term use of estrogens is associated with a high rate of cardiovascular complications, especially in the very elderly [7]. In cases of relapse after treatment with endocrine ablation and estrogens, therapy has little effect, although a number of cytotoxic agents have been tried with limited success.

The results of surgery in the treatment of prostate carcinoma are not influenced by the age of the patient. External beam or radiation therapy also is effective in managing carcinoma of the prostate regardless of age. General experience has been that patients with prostatic carcinoma in the younger age groups generally die of their disease, often with obstructive uropathy and debilitating bone disease, whereas older patients with prostatic carcinoma will generally die from causes other than prostatic carcinoma [8]. This is particularly important to keep in mind in view of the cardiovascular complications of estrogen therapy. The physician must carefully weigh the relative benefits and risks of estrogen therapy in elderly patients with prostatic carcinoma, particularly those with preexisting cardiovascular disease.

Female Reproductive System

Menopause is perhaps the most widely recognized and most studied age-related change in all of biology. The mean age of menopause, or the cessation of menstrual cycling, has increased steadily to the present age of approximately 50 years. Menopause occurs earlier in women who are heavy smokers. During the reproductive years age has marked influence on length and variability of the menstrual cycle. During the first six years after menarche and during the years preceding the end of menstruation, the usual cycle length varies substantially and is considerably longer than during the major reproductive years of ages 20 to 40, during which time it is remarkably stable [9].

The perimenopausal period is characterized by longer menstrual cycles, persistently high FSH and LH levels, lower estradiol levels, and low progesterone levels, which are probably the cause of infertility. The primary defect appears to be inadequate development of a corpus luteum, a characteristic seen not only in aging women but also in those afflicted with obesity and hirsutism.

Investigation of women with regular cycles reveals a regular progression of the physiologic changes with advancing age. At about age 40, levels of LH, FSH, and progesterone are not importantly different from those of younger women and estrogens are slightly lower. In 50-year-old women with regular cycles, one sees elevations of FSH along with decreases in estrogen levels and persistence of normal progesterone. At age 50, regular cycles characterized by normal progesterone are probably fertile cycles. As a woman enters menopause one sees the admixture of long cycles that are either anovulatory or associated with inadequate luteal phases and shorter, probably fertile cycles in which progesterone levels are normal. During this period of mixed long and shorter cycles gonadotropin levels are consistently elevated. This persistence of high gonadotropins despite some normal fertile ovulatory cycles focuses the defect in menopause as being a loss of the suppressive regulatory control of gonadotropin secretion or an uncoupling of the relationship between gonadotropins and the sex hormones [10].

TREATMENT OF ESTROGEN DEFICIENCY IN MENOPAUSE
Estrogen insufficiency has been clearly associated with three clinical sequelae, including atrophy of genital tissues, hot flashes, and osteoporosis. In addition, changes in skin and psychologic disturbances are thought to be related to menopause.

Genital Atrophy
The most clinically important reflection of the atrophy of the genital tissues during menopause is the development of atrophic vaginitis, with its secondary complications of infection, dyspareunia, and, perhaps, incontinence secondary to associated atrophy of the urethral epithelium. The development of atrophic vaginitis, as based on cytologic readings, is often quite delayed after menopause and is not a precipitous event. Many women retain normal vaginal cytology for several years after menopause; sufficient cytologic change to be termed atrophy is present in only 50 percent of individuals by 10 years after menopause [11]. The treatment of atrophic vaginitis includes careful diagnosis and local treatment of superinfection, including fungal as well as bacterial infection, and the administration of vaginal estrogen suppositories or nonhormone-containing, water-soluble lubricants. Many postmenopausal women with severe vaginal atrophy may experience urge incontinence as a reflection of the atrophy of the urethral epithelium. Urethral epithelium is responsive to estrogen treatment, and vaginal estrogens may be of some value in some elderly patients with urge incontinence.

Hot Flashes
Hot flashes occur in between two-thirds and three-quarters of postmenopausal women. In 80 percent of affected women, the symptoms will persist for greater than one year and in between 20 and 50 percent, hot flashes persist for more than five years. Hot flashes are highly integrated events triggered on a central basis, probably at the hypothalamic level. In a typical episode the subject identifies that a hot flash is beginning before any peripheral physiologic changes can be detected. About one minute thereafter reproducible increases in skin conductance (indicating increased perspiration) and in skin blood flow (indicating vasodilatation) and decreases in core temperature (indicating heat loss secondary to the peripheral events) can be detected in association with a 10 to 15 percent increase in pulse. Simultaneously there is a pulse release of LH from the pituitary [12]. Indi-

viduals who have suffered pituitary ablation from disease or radiation may still experience hot flashes, despite the total lack of LH, indicating that the LH release is not the cause of hot flashes but merely an associated event.

The clinical significance of hot flashes is often underestimated. Recent evidence suggests that hot flashes play an important role in sleep disturbances. Studies have shown that hot flashes frequently result in the woman awakening from sound sleep. The awakening occurs in association with LH surge but before the changes skin conductance or peripheral blood flow.

Osteoporosis
The pathophysiology and management of osteoporosis associated with menopause is discussed in Chapter 15.

ADMINISTRATION OF ORAL ESTROGENS
TO POSTMENOPAUSAL WOMEN
In some regions of the United States, over half of the postmenopausal women receive oral estrogen therapy [13]. These agents are prescribed in the belief that their benefit either in terms of the relief or prevention of symptoms of estrogen deficiency exceeds their risk. That estrogens relieve hot flashes and atrophic changes in genital tissues is beyond dispute. The protective effect of estrogens on retardation of bone loss, while less evident, seems to be well established [14].

On the other hand, there has been considerable uncertainty regarding the risks associated with estrogen administration. The occurrence of breakthrough bleeding in individuals on constant estrogen is well recognized. Presently available data fail to support an association between estrogen use and the occurrence of myocardial infarction, stroke, or thromboembolic phenomena in postmenopausal women. Similarly, the risk of breast or ovarian cancer does not seem to be increased [15]. It appears clear, however, that oral estrogens do increase the risk of gallbladder disease [16]. This complication is secondary to the effects of estrogen on the liver; these effects are enhanced by oral estrogen administration since this results in a high estrogen concentration in portal blood. The dose of estrogens required to induce changes in bile composition appears to be lower than that required to alleviate hot flashes or to increase intestinal calcium absorption. Thus one cannot identify a useful dose of estrogen for oral administration that is likely to be free of the increased risk of gallstone formation. Other available routes of estrogen administration, including vaginal and cutaneous, are currently under study. Vaginal administration has the dual advantage of providing local relief for atrophic vaginitis as well as prompt absorption into the systemic circulation for more distant effects.

The possible relationship between estrogen use and endometrial carcinoma has been the focus of intensive study. Current evidence supports the view that constant estrogen use is associated with a clear increase in the risk of endometrial carcinoma [15]. The risk is possibly related to dose and is clearly related to the length of estrogen administration. It appears that there is a latent period of three to six years after which risk increases rapidly. Cyclical use of estrogens in association with progesterone appears to protect against the estrogen-associated risk of endometrial carcinoma and is also effective in controlling breakthrough bleeding [17]. The addition of progesterone does not carry with it the necessity of increasing the estrogen dose in order to control hot flashes.

In view of these complications, one should limit estrogen therapy to patients with clear indications for it and use the lowest dose possible. In the patient with an intact uterus, estrogen should be cycled with progestational agents and the patient followed carefully for evidence of endometrial carcinoma. Some physicians prefer an annual endometrial biopsy as a means of surveillance of patients on long-term estrogen replacement. In patients who are on estrogens for control of hot flashes, it is important to recognize that the medication may be discontinued after two to five years without recurrence of the symptoms. This is particularly important in geriatric patients. Often patients are continued on the estrogen replacement for many years, sometimes decades, on the same dose when the agent might easily have been either stopped or reduced in amount.

The final point relates to the possible effect of estrogens on incontinence. Vaginal estrogen has beneficial effects on patients with atrophic vaginitis and may also be of use in some patients with urge incontinence. This is thought to be related to sensitivity of the urethral epithelium to estrogen and the possible atrophic changes that occur in the urethral epithelium postmenopausally.

References

1. Sparrow, D., Bosse, R., and Rowe, J. W. The influence of age, alcohol consumption and body build on gonadal function in man. *J. Clin. Endocrinol. Metab.* 51:508, 1980.
2. Harman, S. M., and Tsitouras, P. D. Reproductive hormones in aging men: I. Measurement of sex steroids, basal luteinizing hormone and Leydig cell response to human chorionic gonadotropin. *J. Clin. Endocrinol. Metab.* 51:35, 1980.
3. Vermuelen, A., Rubens, R., and Verdonck, L. Testosterone secretion and metabolism in male senescence. *J. Clin. Endocrinol. Metab.* 34:730, 1972.
4. Moore, R. J., et al. Concentration of dihydrotestosterone and androstenediol in naturally occurring and induced prostatic hyperplasia in the dog. *J. Clin. Invest.* 64:1003, 1979.
5. Morimoto, I., Edmiston, A., and Horton, R. Alteration in the metabolism of dihydrotestosterone in elderly men with prostate hyperplasia. *J. Clin. Invest.* 66:612, 1980.

6. Byar, D. P. Proceedings of the Veteran's Administration Cooperative Urological Research Group Studies of cancer of the prostate. *Cancer* 32:1126, 1973.
7. Blackard, C. E., et al. Incidence of cardiovascular disease and death in patients receiving diethylstilbestrol for carcinoma of the prostate. *Cancer* 26:249, 1970.
8. Correair, J. N., Curna, J. L., and Murphy, J. J. Prognosis in patients with carcinoma of the prostate. *Cancer* 25:911, 1970.
9. Treloar, S. E., et al. Variation of the human menstrual cycle throughout reproductive life. *Int. J. Fertil.* 12:77, 1967.
10. Jaffe, R. B. The menopause and perimenopausal period. In S. C. Yen and R. B. Jaffe (Eds.), *Reproductive Endocrinology*. Philadelphia: Saunders, 1978.
11. Meisels, A. The menopause: a cytohormonal study. *Acta Cytol.* 10:49, 1966.
12. Tataryn, I. V., et al. LH, FSH, and skin temperature during menopausal hot flash. *J. Clin. Endocrinol. Metab.* 49:152, 1979.
13. Weirs, N. S., Szekaly, D. R., and Austin, D. F. Increasing incidence of endometrial cancer in the United States. *N. Engl. J. Med.* 294:1259, 1976.
14. Lindsay, R., et al. Long-term prevention of postmenopausal osteoporosis by oestrogen: evidence of an increased bone mass after delayed onset of oestrogen treatment. *Lancet* 1:1038, 1976.
15. Weinstein, M. C. Estrogen use in postmenopausal women—costs, risks, and benefits. *N. Engl. J. Med.* 303:308, 1980.
16. Surgically confirmed gallbladder disease, venous thromboembolism and breast tumors in relation to postmenopausal estrogen therapy: a report from the Boston Collaborative Drug Surveillance Program, Boston University Medical Center. *N. Engl. J. Med.* 290:15, 1979.
17. Hammond, C. B., et al. Effects of long-term estrogen replacement therapy. *Am. J. Obstet. Gynecol.* 133:537, 1979.

II. Renal System

John W. Rowe

Renal Anatomy

Advancing age is associated with progressive loss of renal mass in humans, with renal weight decreasing from 250 to 270 g in young adulthood to 180 to 200 g by the eighth decade. In the absence of hypertension or marked vascular disease, the senescent kidney maintains its relatively smooth contour. The loss of renal mass is primarily cortical, with relative sparing of the renal medulla. The total number of identifiable glomeruli decreases with age, roughly in accord with the changes of renal weight. The number of hyalinized or sclerotic glomeruli identified on light microscopy increases from 1 to 2 percent during the third to fifth decade, to as high as 30 percent in some apparently healthy 80-year-olds; mean prevalence after age 70 is approximately 10 to 12 percent [1,2].

Aging is associated with a loss of lobulation of the glomerular tuft, thus decreasing the effective filtering surface. Although the total number of nuclei per glomerulus is unchanged with age, the filtering surface is further diminished by a progressive increase in the number of mesangial cells and a reciprocal decrease in the number and percent of epithelial cells. The glomerular basement membrane thickens with age, and studies of glomerular filtration characteristics, as estimated by dextran clearance, indicate no change in permeability with age [3].

Several changes have been documented in the renal tubule with age. Of particular interest is the observation by Darmady and coworkers [4] that diverticuli of the distal nephron, which are essentially absent in kidneys from young individuals, become increasingly prevalent with advancing age, reaching a frequency of three diverticuli per tubule at age 90 years. It has been suggested that these diverticuli represent the origin of the simple retention cysts commonly seen in the elderly.

It is generally agreed from histologic studies that normal aging, independent of hypertension or renal disease, is associated with variable sclerotic changes in the walls of the larger renal vessels. These sclerotic changes do not encroach on the lumen and are augmented in the presence of hypertension. Smaller vessels appear to be spared, with only 15 percent of senescent kidneys from nonhypertensive individuals displaying arteriolar changes [2,5,6].

Radiographic studies in normotensive individuals demonstrate an increasing prevalence after the seventh decade of abnormalities similar to those seen in hypertension, including abnormal tapering of interlobar arteries, abnormal arcuate arteries, increased tortuosity of intralobular arteries, and a predilection for age-related vascular abnormalities to occur in the polar region.

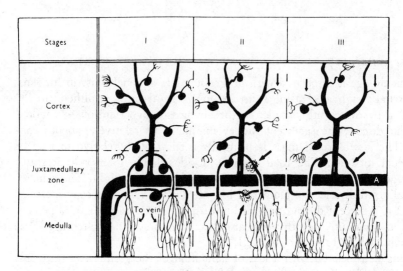

Figure 11-1. Diagram shows changes in the intrarenal arterial pattern with age. Stage I. Basic adult pattern shows glomerular arterioles. Stage II. Partial degeneration of some glomeruli. Two cortical afferent arterioles ramify into remnants of glomerular tufts (small arrows). Two juxtamedullary arterioles pass through partially degenerated glomeruli (large arrows). There is a slight spiraling of interlobular arteries and afferent arterioles. Stage III. Two cortical afferent arterioles now end blindly (small arrows), and two juxtamedullary arterioles are a glomeruli (large arrows). The corresponding glomerular tufts have degenerated completely. The spiraling of interlobular arteries and afferent arterioles is now more pronounced. (A, arcuate artery; I, interlobular artery.) (From A. Ljungqvist and C. Lagergren. Normal intrarenal arterial pattern in adult and aging human kidney. *J. Anat.* 96:285, 1962. By permission of Cambridge University Press.)

Combined microangiographic and histologic studies have identified two very distinctive patterns of change in arteriolar-glomerular units with senescence [7,8] (Figs. 1, 2). In one type (Fig. 11-1), hyalinization and collapse of the glomerular tuft is associated with obliteration of the lumen of the preglomerular arteriole and a resultant loss in blood flow. This type of change is seen primarily in the cortical area. The second pattern (Fig. 11-2), seen primarily in the juxtamedullary area, is characterized by the development of anatomic continuity between the afferent and efferent arterioles during glomerular sclerosis. The end point is thus loss of the glomerulus and shunting of blood flow from afferent to efferent arterioles. Blood flow is maintained to the arteriolar rectae verae, the primary vascular supply of the medulla, which are not decreased in number with age.

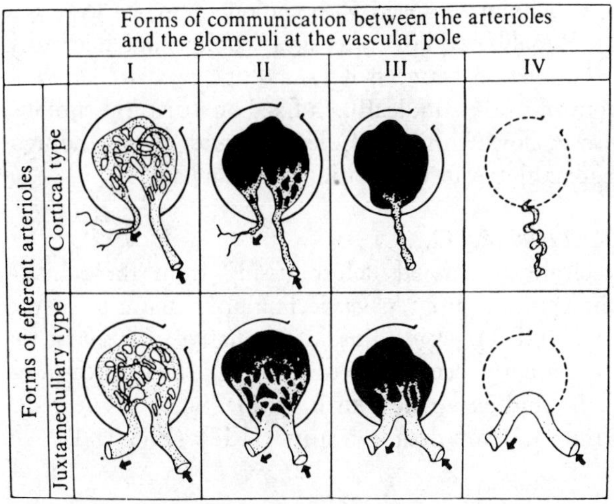

Figure 11-2. Diagram of the degenerative process in the cortical and juxta-medullary nephrons. (Reprinted from *Kidney International*. From E. Takazakura, et al. Intrarenal vascular changes with age and disease. *Kidney Int.* 2:224, 1972.)

Renal Physiology
RENAL BLOOD FLOW

A progressive reduction in renal plasma flow from 600 ml per minute in young adulthood to 300 ml per minute by 80 years of age is well established. Factors contributing to this decrease include an age-related decline in cardiac output and the reduction in the renovascular bed already outlined. Xenon washout studies in healthy potential renal donors ranging in age from 17 to 76 years indicate that the age-related decrease in flow is not purely a reflection of decreased renal mass, but that flow per gram of tissue falls progressively after the fourth decade [9]. There is a highly significant decrease with advancing age in the cortical component of blood flow, with preservation of medullary flow—a finding consistent with the histologic studies showing selective loss of cortical vasculature. These cortical vascular changes probably account for the patchy cortical defects commonly seen on renal scans in healthy elderly adults [10]. This histologic and functional demonstration of selective decrease in cortical flow may explain the observation that filtration fraction (the fraction of renal plasma flow that is filtered at the glomerulus) actually increases with advancing age since outer cortical nephrons have a lower filtration fraction than juxtamedullary nephrons.

In order to clarify the relative contributions of functional "spasm" to the observed change in blood flow, Hollenberg and associates [9] studied young and old subjects before and during intraarterial administration of acetylcholine and angiotensin. If age-related functional spasm was present, maximal renal blood flow after acetylcholine-induced vasodilation might be expected to be independent of age. Renal blood flow after acetylcholine was markedly influenced by age, and the relation between flow and age was similar after acetylcholine as in the control studies, indicating a fixed or structural etiology for the observed decrease in flow with age. Consistent with these findings, vasoconstrictor response to angiotensin was not influenced by age.

GLOMERULAR FILTRATION RATE

The major clinically relevant functional defect arising from these histologic and physiologic changes is a progressive decline after maturity in the glomerular filtration rate (GFR). Age-adjusted normative standards for creatinine clearance have recently been established (Fig. 11-3). Creatinine clearance is stable until the middle of the fourth decade, when a linear decrease of about 8.0 ml/min/1.73 m²/decade begins [11,12] (Fig. 11-4).

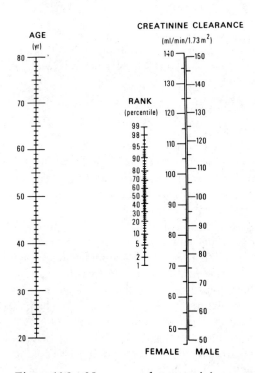

Figure 11-3. Nomogram for ascertaining age-adjusted percentile rank in creatinine clearance. Nomogram is constructed for use with creatinine clearance and with creatinine determinations done by automated "total chromogen" method. A line through the subject's age and creatinine clearance intersects the percentile rank line at a point indicating the subject's age-adjusted percentile rank. (From J. W. Rowe, et al. Age-adjusted normal standards for creatinine clearance in man. *Ann. Intern. Med.* 84:567, 1976.)

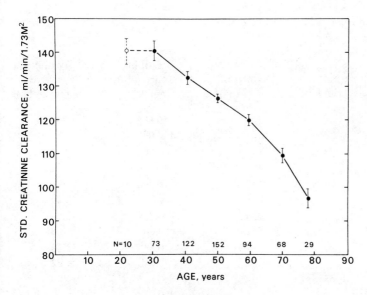

Figure 11-4. Cross-sectional differences in standard creatinine clearance with age. The number of subjects in each age group is indicated above the abcissa. Values plotted indicate mean ± SEM. (From J. W. Rowe, et al. The effect of age on creatinine clearance in man: a cross-sectional and longitudinal study. *J. Gerontol.* 31:155, 1976.)

The argument that entire nephrons drop out with advancing age is supported by the rather striking parallel declines with age in GFR and several proximal tubular functions, including maximum excretion of paraaminohippurate and diodrast and maximal absorption of glucose. Additional observations regarding glucose absorption indicate that the renal threshold for glycosuria, which relates inversely to the degree of "splay" in reabsorptive capacity of individual nephrons, increases with age. A healthy older individual is less likely than his younger counterpart to show a false-positive urinary glucose test in postprandial screening for diabetes. Likewise, glucose will appear in the urine of a young diabetic patient at a lower blood glucose than in an elderly diabetic.

SERUM CREATININE
Since muscle mass, from which creatinine is derived, falls with age at roughly the same rate as GFR, the rather drastic age-related loss of GFR is not reflected in an elevation of serum creatinine (Table 11-1). Thus, serum creatinine overestimates GFR in the elderly. A healthy 80-year-old man with a creatinine clearance 32 ml per minute less than his 30-year-old counterpart will have the same serum creatinine. Depressions of GFR so severe as to

Table 11-1. Cross-Sectional Age Differences in Creatinine Clearance, Serum Creatinine, and 24-Hour Creatinine Excretion

Age (years)	No. of Subjects	Creatinine Clearance (ml/min/ 1.73 m²)*	Serum Creatinine Concentration (mg/dl)	Creatinine Excretion (mg/24 hr)
17–24	10	140.2 ± 3.7	0.808 ± 0.026	1,790 ± 52
25–34	73	140.1 ± 2.5	0.808 ± 0.010	1,862 ± 31
35–44	122	132.6 ± 1.8	0.813 ± 0.009	1,746 ± 24
45–54	152	126.8 1.4	0.829 ± 0.008	1,689 ± 18
55–64	94	119.9 ± 1.7	0.837 ± 0.012	1,580 ± 22
65–74	68	109.5 ± 2.0	0.825 ± 0.012	1,409 ± 25
75–84	29	96.9 ± 2.9	0.843 ± 0.019	1,259 ± 45

* Values indicate mean ± 1 SEM

result in elevation of serum creatinine above 1.5 mg/dl are rarely due to normal aging and so indicate the presence of a disease state. In clinical practice, the doses of many drugs excreted primarily by the kidneys are routinely adjusted to compensate for alteration in renal function (Table 11-2). This is particularly true of digoxin preparations and aminoglycoside antibiotics. Unfortunately, these adjustments are usually based on serum creatinine values, with the resultant predictable overdose in elderly patients. Dose adjustments should ideally be based on creatinine clearances, and when only serum creatinine is available the influence of age must be considered. Also of clinical relevance is the fact that the decreased GFR in the elderly serves to augment potential injury secondary to hypotension or induced by angiographic or pyelographic contrast agents.

Fluid and Electrolyte Balance

Under normal circumstances age has no effect on plasma sodium or potassium concentrations, plasma, pH, or the ability to maintain normal extracellular fluid volume. However, adaptive mechanisms responsible for maintaining constancy of the volume and composition of the extracellular fluid

Table 11-2. Common Renally Excreted Drugs for Which Dose Adjustment in Normal Elderly Persons May Be Required

Aminoglycoside antibiotics
Gentamicin
Kanamycin
Tobramycin
Amikacin
Vancomycin
Nitrofurantoin
Tetracycline
Digoxin
Hypoglycemic agents
Acetohexamide
Chlorpropamide
Procainamide
Cephaloridine

are impaired in the elderly. Because of these physiologic changes, acute illness in geriatric patients is often complicated by development of derangements in fluid and electrolyte balance that delay recovery and prolong hospitalization. These changes in homeostasis are best understood in terms of renal sodium and water excretion after acute alterations in salt and fluid intake.

SODIUM BALANCE
Sodium Deficiency
The aged kidney's response to sodium deficiency is blunted. Studies on the renal response to acute reduction in salt intake (100-mEq to 10-mEq sodium diet) have shown that although aged patients are capable of sodium conservation and reaching salt balance on this markedly restricted intake, their response is sluggish when compared to younger adults. In the studies of Epstein and Hollenberg [13], the half-time for reduction of urinary sodium after salt restriction was 17.6 hours in the young and 30.9 hours in old subjects (Fig. 11-5). The cumulative sodium deficit before daily renal losses equal intake is thus greater in the elderly. Since old patients are more likely to experience confusion, loss of sense of thirst, and disorientation when acutely ill, this "salt-losing" tendency is aggravated by failure of adequate salt intake, leading to further depletion of the extracellular fluid volume and impaired cardiac, renal, and mental function. This vicious cycle is too often continued in the hospital when physicians, dreading pulmonary edema, are reluctant to administer substantial amounts of sodium-containing fluids intravenously to the acutely ill, volume-depleted geriatric patients.

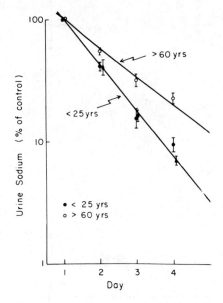

Figure 11-5. Response of urinary sodium excretion to restriction of sodium intake in normal humans. The mean half-time for eight subjects over 60 years of age was 30.9 ± 2.8 hours, exceeding the mean half-time of 17.6 ± 0.7 hours for subjects under 25 years of age (P = 0.01). (Reprinted from Epstein, M. *Federation Proceedings* 38:168, 1979.)

This salt-losing tendency of the senescent kidney is due to both nephron loss, with increased osmotic load per nephron and resultant mild osmotic diuresis, and also to the important age-related alterations that occur in the renin-aldosterone system. Basal renin, whether estimated by plasma renin concentration or renin activity, is diminished by 30 to 50 percent in the elderly in the face of normal levels of renin substrate. This basal difference between young and old is magnified by maneuvers designed to augment renin secretion, such as salt restriction, diuretic administration, or upright posture [14,15].

The lowered renin levels are associated with 30 to 50 percent reductions in plasma concentrations of aldosterone, as well as significant reductions in the secretion and clearance rates of aldosterone [16]. That aldosterone deficiency of old age is a function of the coexisting renin deficiency and not secondary to intrinsic adrenal changes is suggested by studies showing that plasma aldosterone and cortisol responses after adrenocorticotropic hormone (ACTH) stimulation are not impaired with advancing age [15].

The impact of normal aging on plasma renin must be considered when assigning hypertensive patients to specific pathophysiologic groups based on renin levels. A geriatric hypertensive patient, or occasionally a normotensive patient with the normal elevation of systolic blood pressure seen with advancing age, may be labelled as having "low renin hypertension" when actually the renin level is not low but normal for the patient's age.

The management of sodium depletion and its resultant deleterious effects on cardiac, central nervous system, renal, and intestinal function includes the prompt administration of sodium chloride. If extracellular depletion is mild, oral administration of fluids and foods with high sodium content over several days is often sufficient. If volume depletion is more marked, as reflected by decreased blood pressure, tissue turgor, or orthostatic hypotension, intravenous administration of isotonic saline is indicated. The administration of hypotonic fluids, such as 5% glucose in water, will lead to hyponatremia while failing to correct the salt depletion and may aggravate the patient's overall condition.

Sodium Excess

Just as volume depletion is more likely to develop in old patients who are salt- and water-deprived, volume expansion is a commonly encountered problem. Primarily because of its lower glomerular filtration rate, the senescent kidney is less able to excrete an acute salt load than the younger kidney. Geriatric patients, with or without preexisting myocardial disease, are thus at risk for expansion of the extracellular fluid volume when faced with an acute salt load (from inappropriate intravenous fluids, dietary indiscretions, or, as commonly happens, after the administration of sodium-rich radiographic contrast agents such as those used in intravenous pyelography).

The mainstay of management of acute volume expansion with pulmonary congestion remains the intravenous administration of potent diuretics such as furosemide or ethacrynic acid. However, in the absence of preexisting cardiomegaly, administration of excess fluid generally does not result in the precipitation of acute congestive heart failure, but rather in modest weight gain and the appearance of mild peripheral edema. Over the course of several days, this excess salt is generally excreted. The administration of oral diuretics can be helpful if the volume expansion aggravates preexisting heart failure or hypertension.

POTASSIUM BALANCE
Hyperkalemia

The age-related decreases in renin and aldosterone mentioned earlier contribute to the elderly patient's increased risk of developing hyperkalemia in a variety of clinical settings. Through its action on the distal renal tubule, aldosterone increases sodium reabsorption and facilitates the renal excretion of potassium. Aldosterone represents one of the major protective mechanisms that prevent hyperkalemia during periods of potassium challenge. Since glomerular filtration rate (another major determinant of potassium excretion) is also impaired in old patients, serious elevations of plasma potassium are likely to develop, especially in the presence of gastrointestinal bleeding (a major source of potassium) or when potassium salts are given intravenously. This tendency toward hyperkalemia is further aggravated in any clinical setting associated with acidosis, since the senescent kidney is sluggish in its response to acid loading, resulting in prolonged depression of pH and concomitant potassium elevation. Similarly, diuretics such as spironolactone or triamterene, which impair renal potassium excretion, should be administered with caution to the elderly, and the concomitant administration of these agents and potassium should be avoided.

The initial management of hyperkalemia includes discontinuation of any sources of potassium in the diet, discontinuation of potassium-sparing diuretics, and the prompt maximization of renal function in patients with volume depletion or heart failure. Severe hyperkalemia, which is reflected in electrocardiographic abnormalities, including symmetrically peaked T waves and widened QRS complexes, requires prompt treatment with intravenous calcium salts (calcium chloride or calcium gluconate), which directly antagonize the effect of hyperkalemia on the myocardium and often normalize the ECG. Also indiated are sodium bicarbonate, glucose, and insulin. Because such emergency treatment is of only temporary benefit in controlling serum potassium and has no effect on total body potassium, simultaneous with these emergency efforts should be the initiation of efforts toward total-body potassium depletion. These include the oral or rectal administration of sodium-potassium exchange resin (Kayexalate) and potent intravenous diuretics such as furosemide or ethacrynic acid.

WATER BALANCE
Dehydration
The clinical impact of the aged kidney's inability to regulate salt balance properly under stress is compounded by similar abnormalities in water metabolism. The capacity of elderly individuals to conserve water and elaborate a concentrated urine under conditions of either water deprivation or infusion of antidiuretic hormones is impaired [17,18]. The cause of the decreased concentrating capacity of the aged kidney is unclear but probably relates to the concomitant decline in GFR and an age-related decrease in renal response to antidiuretic hormone (ADH).

Although the decline in water-conserving capacity is not so severe as to have clinical significance under conditions of free access to water, it may become important when fluid intake is limited in the presence of exaggerated insensible losses such as with fever. Under such conditions elevations of the serum sodium concentration to levels that impair mental function (greater than 160 mEq/L) is commonly seen in the geriatric age group. Both the salt-and-water-losing tendencies of the senescent kidneys contribute to the common clinical presentation of acutely or subacutely ill elderly patients with hypertonic volume depletion.

In the initial management of the patient with severe hypertonic volume depletion, it is important to focus on volume repletion as potentially life-saving and to treat such patients with rapid intravenous infusion of isotonic saline until cardiovascular stability is attained. In the presence of marked hypernatremia, these isotonic fluids are actually "hypotonic" relative to the patient's plasma, and serum sodium will begin to fall as volume is expanded. Once blood pressure and intravascular volume are corrected, hypotonic fluids should be administered until the serum sodium is below 150 mEq/L. Severe hypertonic dehydration in the elderly is uniformly associated with marked alterations in consciousness. Although the volume and the composition of the extracellular fluid may be normalized within 72 hours of admission, mental state alterations commonly persist for some time and slow recovery over two weeks is not infrequent. This persisting confusion despite normal electrolytes should not necessarily precipitate invasive clinical evaluation. Patience is often rewarded in such cases, and the complications of lumbar punctures and sophisticated radiologic procedures avoided.

Water Intoxication
Perhaps the most serious and least well-recognized electrolyte disorder in geriatric patients is their tendency to develop water intoxication. The clinical presentation of hyponatremia is nonspecific, with depression, confusion, lethargy, anorexia, and weakness the most common findings. When hyponatremia is severe (serum sodium concentrations below 110 mEq/L), seizures and stupor may be seen, and central nervous system damage may be irreversible. It is not unusual for geriatric patients to become hyponatremic in the setting of any stress, including surgery, fever, or acute viral illness.

Clinical evaluation of the elderly hyponatremic patient usually reveals one of two general causes. One is decreased renal capacity to excrete water as a consequence of acute or chronic reductions in renal blood flow. This is seen in patients with extracellular volume depletion, congestive heart failure, hypoalbuminemia associated with cirrhosis or nephrosis, or drug-induced hypotension. In addition to the evidence on history and physical examination of the possible presence of any of these disorders, a laboratory examination is often helpful. In this category of patients, laboratory examination reveals prerenal azotemia with blood urea nitrogen (BUN) elevations out of proportion to the elevations in serum creatinine.

A second group of patients with hyponatremia reveals a constellation of findings consistent with oversecretion of antidiuretic hormone as a cause of the water retention. These include low serum sodium, evidence of good renal function (low BUN), mild extracellular fluid expansion (normal to slightly full neck veins, trace edema), and evidence of inappropriate renal water retention (urine osmolality greater than maximally dilute and in many cases more concentrated than serum). In addition, excess ADH secretion, because of the slight extracellular fluid (ECF) expansion and subsequent reduction in aldosterone secretion and elevation of glomerular filtration rate, is associated with the presence of modest to large amounts of sodium in the urine (greater than 20 mEq/L).

Excess ADH secretion is commonly associated with pneumonia, tuberculosis, stroke, meningitis, subdural hematoma, and a variety of other pulmonary and central nervous system disorders. As discussed in Chapter 9, the elderly seem particularly prone to this complication. This may also hold true for drug-induced ADH excess. In one study, elderly patients accounted for most cases of hyponatremia developing from use of chlorpropamide [19]. Elderly patients may develop hyponatremia in a variety of clinical settings including fever, psychological stress, general anesthesia, and acute viral illness [20]. While hyponatremic, these patients are unable to excrete a water load, but, after resolution of the acute illness, water metabolism is normal. In many cases the same patient returns several weeks or months later with another acute illness, and again develops hyponatremia.

One must maintain a high degree of suspicion for hyponatremia in geriatric patients, particularly in view of the slow, insidious nature of the development of water intoxication and its nonspecific clinical presentation. Physicians caring for the elderly should be cautious when prescribing medications known to increase ADH secretion, such as chlorpropamide and barbiturates (Table 11-3), as well as in the administration of hypotonic fluids in the setting of recent surgery or any acute illness.

Management of water intoxication is dictated by the level and rate of fall of the serum sodium, the clinical manifestations, and the cause. In all cases, strict water restriction is appropriate. Medications possibly associated with water intoxication such as diuretics or agents that increase ADH (Table 11-3) should be withheld promptly. In patients in whom hyponatremia is associated with reduced renal blood flow, therapy should be aimed at maximizing renal function by either correction of congestive heart failure, vol-

Table 11-3.   Drugs Known to Impair Water Excretion and Induce Hyponatremia

Vasopressin	Amitriptyline
Oxytocin	Thiothixene
Chlorpropamide	Aspirin
Vincristine	Acetaminophen
Cyclophosphamide	Narcotics
Fluphenazine	Barbiturates
Clofibrate	Haloperidol
Carbamazepine	

ume repletion of patients with extracellular fluid depletion, or restoration of blood pressure to normal in hypotensive patients.

In cases of excess ADH secretion, fluid restriction alone generally results in a slow return of plasma osmolality toward normal levels. In resistent cases or where fluid restriction is impractical, the water-retaining effects of ADH can be inhibited by oral administration of dimethyl chlorotetracycline in doses of 300 mg two or three times a day. This nephrotoxic agent induces a state of partial nephrogenic diabetes insipidus and predictably results in correction of hyponatremia over the course of several days. Since it is a nephrotoxic agent, the serum creatinine and BUN levels should be followed closely.

Severe hyponatremia (serum sodium concentrations less than 115 mEq/L) that is associated with seizures or major central nervous system abnormalities requires prompt correction. The most effective approach is the administration of hypertonic saline; 500 ml of 3% sodium chloride can safely be administered intravenously to most patients over 12 hours and will generally increase the serum sodium 8 to 10 mEq/L and place the patient out of immediate danger while other therapeutic modalities are initiated.

Acute Renal Failure

Age influences renal disease by either altering the prevalence of specific diseases or by affecting the presentation, course, and response to treatment of conditions seen in both early and late adult life. Acute renal failure is seen more frequently in old patients simply because the common inciting events, including hypotension associated with marked volume depletion, major surgery, sepsis, major angiographic procedures, or the injudicious use of antibiotics, are more common in multiply impaired elderly, who are often at increased risk because of preexisting moderate renal insufficiency.

The management of acute renal failure in the elderly is a complex and demanding task worthy of the effort. The aged kidney retains the capacity to recover from acute ischemic or toxic insults over the course of several weeks. While the usual acute tubular necrosis (ATN) with 2 to 10 days of oliguria followed by a diuretic phase preceding recovery of function is seen in the elderly, "nonoliguric" acute renal failure is being recognized with increasing frequency. In these cases, renal function, as reflected in serum BUN and creatinine levels, is impaired for several days after a brief hypotensive episode associated with surgery, sepsis, overmedication, or volume depletion, or after the administration of nephrotoxic radiographic contrast agents. After this brief period of azotemia, renal function gradually returns to its previous level. Despite this transient and reversible loss of renal function, oliguria is not a prominent component of the clinical picture. Since the clinical hallmark of renal failure is generally thought to be a dramatic reduction in urine output, cases of nonoliguric acute renal failure may go unrecognized.

This may result in an inadvertent overdose being given to patients during the period of impaired renal function of medications excreted predominantly via renal mechanisms, including digitalis preparations and aminoglycoside antibiotics such as gentamicin.

The management of elderly patients with full-blown acute renal failure complicated by oliguria is guided by the same general principles employed in younger patients. The most important principle is the careful exclusion of urinary obstruction as a cause of the renal failure. This is particularly true in men with prostatic hypertrophy or prostatic carcinoma or in women with gynecologic malignancy.

The major causes of death during acute renal failure are volume overload precipitating acute pulmonary edema, hypertensive crisis, hyperkalemia, and infection. Dialysis, whether it be hemodialysis or peritoneal dialysis, is effective in the elderly, and the complication rate seems to be dictated more by coincident cardiovascular disease than by the patient's age. Dialysis often substantially simplifies management; thus, one should not wait until an emergency situation is present before initiating dialysis in a patient with acute renal failure. It is more prudent to initiate dialysis early in patients in whom it is very likely that renal function will not return before the dialysis will be needed. The immediate indications for emergency dialysis include pulmonary edema unresponsive to diuretics, hyperkalemia, uremic pericarditis, and seizures or uncontrolled bleeding on a uremic basis. The use of intravenous catheters placed in the femoral vein for dialysis has been a recent major advance in the management of elderly patients with acute renal failure. These catheters are easily placed, may be left in for several days to a week with a very low incidence of infection or thrombosis, and circumvent the need for implantation of arteriovenous shunts for access for dialysis in acute renal failure.

Aside from the initiation of dialysis, careful attention to the balance of several factors is necessary. Water and salt balance must be monitored carefully. Due to catabolism, the usual patient with acute renal failure will lose about one pound of body mass per day. Attempts to keep body weight constant will result in the gradual expansion of the extracellular fluid and the consequent increase in blood pressure and risk of precipitation of cardiac failure. Similarly, overzealous fluid restriction will impair the patient's general condition and central nervous system function and may delay the recovery of renal function. In general, the administration of approximately 600 cc of fluid a day, in addition to insensible losses, provides adequate fluid balance.

Potassium balance is crucial and hyperkalemia must be avoided if possible and treated promptly if present. Acidosis progresses with the length and degree of renal failure and sodium bicarbonate should be administered in an effort to maintain circulating bicarbonate levels in the range of 15 to 19 mEq/L. Administration of sodium bicarbonate may expand extracellular fluid volume, and thus patients should be watched carefully for the presence of congestive failure.

Infection is a common and lethal complication of acute renal failure. Urinary infection secondary to unnecessary urinary catheterization is particularly common. Little is gained from placing a urinary catheter in an oliguric patient in whom volume status and serum levels of BUN, creatinine, and potassium are better guides to progress and treatment than his urinary output. Infection of intravenous lines is also common, and these should be scrupulously monitored and discontinued when possible.

Additional routine measures include the administration of oral phosphate-binding agents in an effort to minimize the elevation of serum phosphorus associated with acute renal failure and the administration of diet limited in protein content in order to blunt the rise in BUN. Of major importance is careful attention to the alteration in dose-interval of medications excreted via the kidney and recognition of the enhanced sensitivity of elderly uremic patients to psychotropic medications such as hypnotics and major tranquilizers.

Chronic Renal Failure

Many forms of chronic renal failure are seen more commonly late in life because the renal disease is secondary to other age-dependent diseases. Examples include prostatic hypertrophy or cancer leading to hydronephrosis, renovascular hypertension or renal failure secondary to atherosclerosis, multiple myeloma, drug-related causes of renal insufficiency, and, perhaps most common, prerenal azotemia from congestive heart failure or volume depletion.

RECOGNITION

While the general principles of the management of renal failure are similar in young and old adults, the geriatric patient with chronic renal insufficiency presents several special considerations. With regard to diagnosis, serum creatinine generally fails to rise to as high levels in the elderly as in the young despite equivalent levels of residual renal function. This is because muscle mass, the ultimate source of creatinine, falls with age, particularly in the presence of nutritional deficits such as those seen in uremia. Since serum creatinine underestimates the degree of renal failure, many debilitated, uremic elderly patients will not be recognized as uremic since their creatinine levels may be less than 10 mg/dl, whereas substantially higher levels are common in younger uremic patients.

Another factor that often delays recognition of chronic renal failure in the elderly is the presentation of renal failure as decompensation of a previously impaired organ system before the emergence of specific symptoms of uremia. Examples include worsening of preexisting heart failure or hypertension due to inability to excrete salt and water, gastrointestinal bleeding in the presence of previous gastrointestinal malignancy or ulcer, or mental confusion in a borderline demented patient who becomes increasingly azotemic.

DIAGNOSIS

Once the presence of chronic renal failure is established, the definitive cause should be identified. Most renal failure in the elderly is due to chronic glomerulonephritis, hypertensive and atherosclerotic vascular disease, diabetes, or, in some cases, late-presenting polycystic kidney disease. The most important diagnostic consideration is strict exclusion of potentially reversible causes, such as urinary tract obstruction, particularly in men with symptoms of prostatism; renal arterial occlusion that may be reparable; hypercalcemia; or the administration of nephrotoxic agents.

MANAGEMENT

If no reversible component is identified, the patient should be followed closely so that the rate of loss of renal function can be judged accurately. Appropriate adjustments to account for the renal failure should be made in the doses and dose schedules of all medications, especially digoxin. Hypertension should be controlled carefully. As serum phosphate rises, phosphate-binding antacids should be given, with meals, in order to suppress parathyroid hormone and its resultant adverse effects on bone. As serum phosphate falls in response to treatment, serum calcium will generally rise toward the normal range. If hypocalcemia persists after normalization of phosphate, this should be treated with preparations of vitamin D or its congeners (vitamin D_1, 50,000-unit tablets, two or three times a day; dihydrotachysterol, 0.2–0.4 mg twice a day; 1,25-dihydroxy vitamin D_3, 0.25–0.5 mg twice a day) in order to increase intestinal calcium absorption.

Anemia associated with chronic renal failure often requires more aggressive management in elderly patients because of coexisting cardiac disease. Red cell indices are not a reliable estimate of iron deficiency in uremia. Iron deficiency should be excluded by evaluation of serum iron and ferritin and oral or parenteral iron supplements administered if indicated. In the absence of iron deficiency, the anemia of chronic renal failure will respond to monthly injections of androgens (nandrolone decanlate, 200 mg intramuscularly). If symptomatic anemia persists, which it often does, regular transfusions of red cells are indicated.

Dietary management of elderly patients with chronic renal failure is often overdone, compounding the nutritional impact of the disease. Protein and salt restriction is often needed in young individuals to suppress the volume expansion and BUN elevations. Many elderly patients ingest only 60 to 70 g of protein daily and 4 to 5 g of salt under normal conditions, and strict limitations of these dietetic constituents is often unnecessary. Similarly, hyperkalemia should be avoided and dietary potassium controlled, but the reductions required in the elderly are often moderate. Acidosis should be controlled with the addition of oral sodium bicarbonate tablets with the aim to keep serum bicarbonate levels near 18 to 20 mEq/L. The best approach to these modifications is careful alteration of the diet to the proved needs of the individual patient.

Pruritus is a major problem in elderly uremic patients, especially in the presence of coexisting xerosis. In addition to skin moisteners, ultraviolet treatments have been found effective and safe for elderly uremic patients. Administration of so-called antipruritic agents such as antihistamines in ataractics are rarely helpful since they act primarily by causing sedation and may produce adverse nervous system effects in the elderly.

DIALYSIS IN THE ELDERLY

Chronic maintenance dialysis—generally hemodialysis but occasionally chronic ambulatory peritoneal dialysis—remains the mainstay of treatment of elderly uremic patients. Elderly patients often do very well on dialysis, with the frequency of complications seemingly more related to the coexisting extrarenal disease than to age itself. Psychologically, elderly patients often are more able to adapt to chronic dialysis than are their younger counterparts. Once it is clear that a patient will need dialysis at some time in the near future, early creation of an arteriovenous fistula for access to hemodialysis is important. This is particularly so in the elderly patient since such fistulas often mature rather slowly. At present renal transplantation is generally not considered in individuals over the age of 60.

Nephrotic Syndrome

Nephrologists have traditionally taught that age plays an important role in the etiology of nephrotic syndrome, with the likelihood of lipoid nephrosis decreasing and amyloidosis increasing with advancing age. In 1971, Fawcett and coworkers [21] reviewed 100 consecutive "biopsied" adults with nephrotic syndrome, 25 of whom were over 60 years of age. They found no impact of age on the frequency of any specific histologic type of glomerular change. In particular, minimal-change disease and amyloidosis were seen with equal frequency in young and old patients, and, additionally, there was no impact of age on the generally excellent response of patients with minimal-change disease to corticosteroids. Thus, age has no specific impact on the diagnosis or management of nephrotic syndrome.

Acute Glomerulonephritis

Acute glomerulonephritis is receiving increasing attention as a disease in which presentation and prognosis are clearly age-related. In children and young adults, acute glomerulonephritis is frequently associated with recent streptococcal infection and, less commonly, with one of a wide variety of conditions, including Schönlein-Henoch purpura, crescentic nephritis with or without pulmonary hemorrhage, hemolytic-uremic syndrome, or generalized vasculitis. The presentation, regardless of etiology, is fairly uniform with hematuria, heavy proteinuria, edema, hypertension, and the development, in many cases, of pulmonary congestion. The prognosis is generally good in poststreptococcal disease in young patients, with a variable outcome in non-poststreptococcal cases.

In old patients, acute glomerulonephritis is manifestly different [22,23]. The presentation is nonspecific, with nausea, malaise, arthralgias, and a rather striking predilection for pulmonary infiltrates initially. Commonly, the clinical picture is believed to represent worsening of a preexisting illness, especially congestive heart failure. Proteinuria is generally moderate. Hypertension or edema, although unusual, usually indicates a poststreptococcal etiology and favorable prognosis; otherwise, the prognosis is poor, with crescentic glomerulonephritis with focal, segmental necrotizing and fibrosing glomerulitis the most frequent histologic finding [24]. Although management is presently controversial, some patients respond to a combination of corticosteroids and immunosuppressive agents, including azathioprine or cyclophosphamide.

References

1. McLachlan, M. S. F., et al. Vascular and glomerular changes in the aging kidney. *J. Pathol.* 121:65, 1977.
2. Tauchi, H., Tsuboi, K., and Okutomi, J. Age changes in the human kidney of the different races. *Gerontologie* 17:87, 1971.
3. Artursen, G., Groth, T., and Grotte, G. Human glomerular membrane porosity and filtration pressure: dextran clearance data analyzed by theoretical models. *Clin. Sci.* 40:137, 1971.
4. Darmady, E. M., Offer, J., and Woodhouse, M. S. The parameters of the aging kidney. *J. Pathol.* 109:195, 1973.
5. McLachlan, M. S. F. The aging kidney. *Lancet* 2:143, 1978.
6. Griffiths, G. J., Cartwright, G. O., and McLachlan, M. S. F. Loss of renal tissue in the elderly. *Clin. Radiol.* 26:249, 1975.
7. Takazakura, E., et al. Intrarenal vascular changes with age and disease. *Kidney Int.* 2:224, 1972.
8. Ljungqvist, A., and Lagergren, C. Normal intrarenal arterial pattern in adult and aging human kidney. *J. Anat.* 96:285, 1962.
9. Hollenberg, N. K., et al. Senescence and the renal vasculature in normal man. *Circ. Res.* 34:309, 1974.
10. Friedman, S. A., et al. Functional defects in the aging kidney. *Ann. Intern. Med.* 76:41, 1972.
11. Rowe, J. W., et al. Age-adjusted normal standards for creatinine clearance in man. *Ann. Intern. Med.* 84:567, 1976.
12. Rowe, J. W., et al. The effect of age on creatinine clearance in man: a cross sectional and longitudinal study. *J. Gerontol.* 31:155, 1976.

13. Epstein, M., and Hollenberg, N. K. Age as a determinant of renal sodium conservation in normal men. *J. Lab. Clin. Med.* 87:411, 1976.
14. Crane, M. G., and Harris, J. J. Effect of aging on renin activity and aldosterone excretion. *J. Lab. Clin. Med.* 87:947, 1976.
15. Weidmann, P., et al. Effect of aging on plasma serum and aldosterone in normal man. *Kidney Int.* 8:325, 1975.
16. Flood, C., et al. The metabolism and secretion of aldosterone in elderly subjects. *J. Clin. Invest.* 46:960, 1967.
17. Rowe, J. W., Shock, N. W., and DeFronzo, R. The influence of age on urine concentrating ability in man. *Nephron* 17:279, 1976.
18. Lindeman, R. D., et al. Influence of age, renal disease, hypertension, diuretics and calcium on the anti-diuretic response to suboptimal infusion of vasopressin. *J. Lab. Clin. Med.* 68:206, 1966.
19. Weissman, P. N., Shenkman, L., and Gregerman, R. I. Chlorpropamide hyponatremia. *N. Engl. J. Med.* 284:65, 1971.
20. Deutsch, S., Goldberg, M., and Dripps, R. D. Postoperative hyponatremia with the inappropriate release of antidiuretic hormone. *Anesthesiology* 27:250, 1966.
21. Fawcett, I. W., et al. Nephrotic syndrome in the elderly. *Br. Med. J.* 2:387, 1971.
22. Arieff, A., et al. Acute glomerulonephritis in the elderly. *Mod. Geriatr.* 3:77, 1973.
23. Boswell, D. C., and Eknoyan, G. Acute glomerulonephritis in the aged. *Geriatrics* 23:73, 1968.
24. Potvliege, P. R., DeRoy, G., and Dupuis, F. Necropsy study on glomerulonephritis in the elderly. *J. Clin. Pathol.* 28:891, 1975.

12. Cardiovascular System

Edward G. Lakatta
Gary Gerstenblith

Cardiovascular Gerontology

In the year 1982 more than 11 percent of the population in the United States is aged 65 years or older. In this age group heart disease is the leading cause of death worldwide and is also the most frequent reason for hospitalization. In addition to specific pathologic changes, the cardiovascular system also undergoes several physiologic alterations with advancing age. Since the diagnosis of cardiac disease in an individual is dependent on the determination that an individual's cardiac status differs from normal, age-adjusted criteria for clinically important parameters of cardiac function must be defined. While these "normal" age-related changes usually cause no symptoms, they do provide an altered substrate on which specific cardiovascular pathologic conditions are superimposed; thus, the signs, symptoms, and clinical course of cardiac disease may be modified to a significant extent by physiologic aging of the cardiovascular system.

Experimentation in normal men and animals has elucidated some of the mechanisms responsible for the age-related differences in cardiovascular performance [1]. In this discussion, the term *normal* will refer to aged humans and animals in whom, by best available criteria, specific cardiovascular pathologic disease states are absent. The extent to which the results of such investigations reflect the normal aging process is determined by the level of certainty regarding the absence of specific disease, that is, occult coronary disease. Additional selective criteria, such as the limit of blood pressure regarded as normal at a given age, level of physical fitness, nutrition, and life-style should also be considered in the interpretation of the results of investigations of normal aging of the cardiovascular system.

ANATOMY AND FUNCTION AT REST

Autopsy and echocardiographic studies (Fig. 12-1) indicate that the mammalian heart hypertrophies with advancing age [2]. Although the amount of fibrous tissue increases with age, this constitutes only a small portion of the increase in heart mass, and marked fibrosis is not the rule. Amyloid infiltrates, although common in advanced age, are not extensive and when present are usually in the atrium [3]. Studies in animal hearts demonstrate that the hypertrophy results from an increase in the size of muscle cells. Although the stimulus for the mild but definite cardiac hypertrophy that occurs with advanced age has not been clearly defined, other forms of hypertrophy result from increased loading conditions. Peripheral vascular resistance in humans is increased in advanced age. Possible mechanisms include: (1) diminished peripheral demand for flow due to a decrease in basal metabolic rate, (2) a diminution in the area of the total capillary bed, (3)

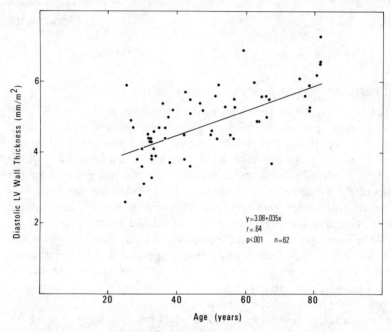

Figure 12-1. Linear regression plot depicting the relationship between age and diastolic left ventricular (LV) wall thickness (mm/m²). Increased age is associated with increased diastolic wall thickness. (From G. Gerstenblith, et al. Echocardiographic assessment of a normal adult aging population. *Circulation* 56:273, 1977. By permission of the American Heart Association, Inc.)

altered arteriolar reactivity to neurohumoral stimuli, (4) anatomic changes in elastin and collagen, and (5) the presence of medial calcification.

These changes in peripheral vasculature are reflected in elevations in systolic and, to a lesser extent, diastolic blood pressure [4], and impose a greater load on the heart. Aortic dilatation seen with advanced age may also present a greater load to the heart in that a larger volume of blood in the aorta must be accelerated before left ventricular ejection can occur. These gradual persistent changes in the peripheral vasculature may be the stimulus for cardiac hypertrophy with advancing age.

The early diastolic left ventricular filling rate is reduced markedly with increasing age in resting normal humans [5] (Fig. 12-2). This is also observed in hypertrophied hearts at any age and is often attributed to diminished ventricular compliance. That diminished compliance is the cause of the diminished filling rate in the aged heart is supported by animal studies in both intact hearts [6] and isolated cardiac muscle [7,8] that demonstrate increased muscle stiffness in senescence. Alternatively, age-related changes

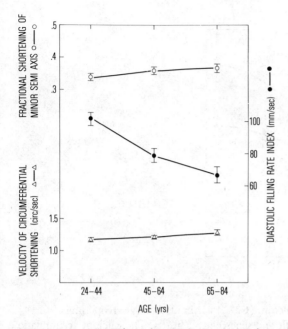

Figure 12-2. The effect of increasing age on echocardiographic indices of
ventricular performance determined in individuals free of cardiovascular disease.
Diastolic filling rate index, the E-F slope of the anterior mitral valve leaflet, is
significantly decreased with increasing age, $P < 0.01$, regression analysis of
variance. Fractional shortening of the minor semi axis, an index of ejection
fraction or pump performance, and velocity of circumferential fiber shortening,
an index of muscle performance, are unaltered by age. (Redrawn from
G. Gerstenblith et al. Echocardiographic assessment of a normal adult aging
population. *Circulation* 56:273, 1977.)

in the mitral valve itself may impede ventricular filling. In addition the
prolonged time course of isovolumic relaxation in both humans and several
animal models may affect filling of the senescent heart [9]. Relaxation on
the cellular level is effected by the removal of Ca^{++} from the contractile
proteins resulting from Ca^{++} sequestration by the sarcoplasmic reticulum.
Sarcoplasmic reticulum isolated from senescent animal hearts accumulates
Ca^{++} at a slower rate than that from adult hearts [10] (Fig. 12-3), and
this change may therefore be responsible for diminished early ventricular
filling in the senescent heart. Although the number of capillaries relative
to muscle fibers is decreased in normal humans [11], there are no data
regarding the relationship between coronary blood flow and age. In animals,
total coronary flow is unchanged in senescence, but flow adjusted for heart
weight is mildly reduced [12]; this correlates with a reduction in the capil-
lary-to-fiber ratio in the rat model [13].

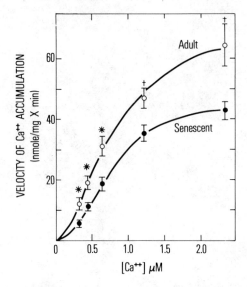

Figure 12-3. Velocity of calcium (Ca^{++}) accumulation by sarcoplasmic reticulum isolated from adult and senescent rat hearts. The calcium accumulation velocity is significantly diminished in sarcoplasmic reticulum from senescent hearts as compared to the adult heart ($+$, $P < 0.01$; $*$, $P < 0.02$). (Redrawn from J. P. Froehlich et al. Studies of sarcoplasmic reticulum function and contraction duration in young adult and aged rat myocardium. *J. Mol. Cell. Cardiol.* 10:427, 1978.)

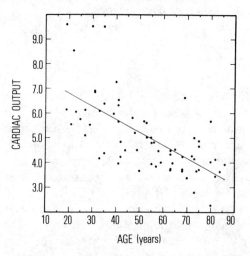

Figure 12-4. The effect of age on cardiac output at rest as determined by the dye dilution technique in ambulatory male patients aged 19 to 86 years. (From M. Brandfonbrener et al. Changes in cardiac output with age. *Circulation* 12:557, 1955. By permission of the American Heart Association, Inc.)

Cardiac output is determined by heart rate, loading conditions, autonomic tone, and intrinsic cardiac muscle performance, and when the cardiovascular system is functioning normally, output is matched to the demands of the organism. Resting heart rate is not influenced by age. The decrease in cardiac output (Fig. 12-4), reflecting a decreased stroke volume with age, appears to be due to extrinsic factors such as age differences in preload, afterload, or autonomic tone [14–16]. The age difference in output at rest measured with the person in the supine position is eliminated when measurements are obtained with him in the upright position [16]. Intrinsic cardiac muscle performance and pump function at rest, measured as velocity of circumferential shortening and ejection fraction index, respectively, are not age-related [5,17] (see Fig. 12-2). Furthermore, in response to stress the senescent heart can increase its output several-fold.

PERFORMANCE DURING STRESS

An informative means of testing overall cardiovascular function is to subject human, animal, or the cardiac muscle isolated from animals to studies that increase the demand placed on the performance of cardiac muscle or of the cardiovascular system. We shall now proceed to discuss age-related similarities and differences over a spectrum of cardiovascular performance ranging from basal to maximal levels.

The extent to which age-related changes in cardiovascular performance can be attributed to the tendency to become sedentary with advanced age deserves consideration. Maximum oxygen consumption (Vo_2max), the product of maximal cardiac output and the maximal arteriovenous oxygen difference, adjusted for body weight, is used as a measure of cardiovascular performance [18]. A summary of 17 studies clearly indicates that maximum oxygen consumption progressively declines with age [19] (Fig. 12-5).

Longitudinal studies reveal that this decline with age can be retarded by physical conditioning, but even when compared at optimum levels of physical conditioning, an age decline still persists [20]. The decline in overall cardiovascular performance with age, then, cannot be entirely attributed to the deconditioning of a more sedentary life-style; it must reflect in part age-related changes in other factors that regulate cardiovascular performance. In utilizing Vo_2max to assess cardiovascular performance in advanced age, the contribution of age changes in O_2 exchange in the lungs and in tissue utilization of O_2 should be assessed. Although lean body, and therefore muscle mass, declines with advanced age, this does not account for the decline in Vo_2max since this decline, although lessened, persists when Vo_2max is corrected for lean muscle mass [21]. Age changes in the distribution of blood flow to organs that extract differential quantities of O_2 could in part alter the maximum arteriovenous oxygen, and thus limit Vo_2max. In the context of the present discussion, this might be considered not as a differ-

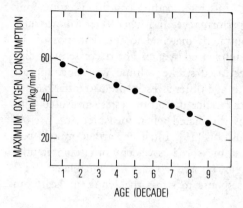

Figure 12-5. The effect of age on maximum oxygen consumption. The points represent data recalculated from 700 observations from 17 different studies in the literature made by Dehn and Bruce [19]. The line represents the regression of these points as a function of age. (Redrawn from M. M. Dehn and R. A. Bruce. Longitudinal variations in maximal oxygen uptake with age and activity. *J. Appl. Physiol.* 33:805, 1972.)

ence in tissue utilization per se, but as a difference in the vascular regulation of utilization.

The increase in cardiovascular performance in response to stress is achieved by an increase in heart rate and stroke volume and a decrease in total peripheral vascular resistance. The heart rate increase in response to static and to maximum dynamic [22] exercise in the form of handgrip, even when matched for strength and duration of the exercise [23], is diminished in the elderly. Overall, this response is mediated by an increase in sympathetic tone and a withdrawal of vagal stimulation of the heart. Little is known regarding the latter in aged humans. Elaboration of catecholamines during this response, however, does not decrease with age and therefore cannot explain the age-related decrement in heart rate [24]. However, intravenous infusion of isoproterenol elicits less of a heart rate increase in aged men, as compared with adult men [25], and the maximum response to infused isoproterenol is diminished in the senescent as compared to the adult awake beagle [26]. Other forms of stress that are in part catecholamine-mediated, including hypoxia and hypercarbia, also elicit a diminished heart rate response in senescent as compared with adult men [27].

In addition to heart rate, maximum cardiac performance in the elderly is also limited by stroke volume. Factors that affect stroke volume are preload, afterload, and intrinsic muscle performance. Little is known about the effect of age on venous return during maximum dynamic exercise. However, the relative afterload during exercise may be age-related because peripheral vascular resistance does not drop to the same extent in the aged as in adult men during maximal work loads [28]. Although some studies indicate that age changes during the developmental period alter the vasodilatory responsiveness to catecholamines, no comparable studies have compared senescent with adult individuals [29]. Thus, it is unknown at present whether age-dependent differences in the response to catecholamines modify the peripheral vascular response to exercise. In addition, other aspects of the characteristic vascular input impedence of a stiffer arterial system, such as that found in advanced age, may limit performance.

Pulmonary wedge pressure, which reflects left ventricular end diastolic pressure, is increased in aged as compared to young men during cycling exercise [16]. This may reflect either an increase in end diastolic volume, which results from diminished ejection, or an unchanged end diastolic volume with altered compliance, due to myocardial and/or pericardial factors. Diminished ejection could result from either an increase in afterload as discussed above, or diminished intrinsic muscle performance during stress, or both. Regardless of the mechanism of this effect, catecholamines have an important role since age difference in stroke volume during maximum exercise are decreased in the presence of beta-blockade [30].

Information pertinent to cardiac muscle performance in the senescent myocardium during stress is available in the aging rat model [31]. Under control or basal conditions, force production and rate of force production, when measured over a range of resting muscle lengths, are not age-related. Force production depends on Ca^{++} activation of the contractile proteins, and when the concentration of calcium in the bathing milieu is increased [32] (Fig. 12-6A) performance is enhanced to a similar extent in both adult and senescent muscle. In this model, then, maximum muscle performance is not limited in senescence. Beta-adrenergic stimulation, however, fails to elicit as great a response in senescent as in adult myocardium [32] (Fig. 12-6B). Since the increase in force production after stimulation results from an increased amount of Ca^{++} available for contraction, and since the response to an increase in Ca^{++} is not altered in senescence, the diminished response to catecholamines in the senescent heart appears to be related to those mechanisms that mediate the catecholamine-induced enhancement of Ca^{++} transport.

Recent studies demonstrate that age changes are not present at the level of the receptor, as both the affinity and number of receptors are unaltered in the senescent heart [33]. Furthermore, the age difference in force production persists when the agonist is dibutyryl cAMP, which mediates the contractile response without stimulating the beta-receptor. In addition, cAMP stimulation and protein kinase activation in these hearts is not age-related [33]. The diminished contractile response to catecholamines in senescence seems to be related then to diminished phosphorylation of endogenous intracellular proteins, such as sarcoplasmic reticulum and sarcolemma, which

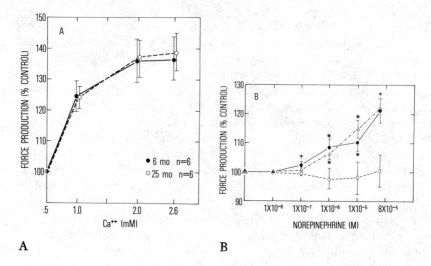

A   B

Figure 12-6. (A) The effect of age on the response of force production to increasing calcium (Ca^{++}) concentrations in the perfusate in left ventricular muscle from adult (6 months old) and senescent (25 months old) rats. (B) The effect of age on the response of force production to increasing norepinephrine concentrations in the perfusate in left ventricular muscle from adult (6 months and 12 months old) and senescent (25 months old) rats (* = P < 0.05; ‡ = P < 0.01 vs. 25-month-old rats). (Redrawn from E. G. Lakatta et al. Diminished inotropic response of aged myocardium to catecholamines. *Circ. Res.* 36:262, 1975.)

result in relatively less of an increase in Ca^{++} transport after beta-adrenergic stimulation.

In summary, a feature common to several facets of the age-related decrease in overall cardiovascular performance in response to stress is a diminished response to catecholamines. This appears to be the common mechanism linking the age differences in each of these components.

AGE CHANGES IN THE CONDUCTION SYSTEM AND ELECTROPHYSIOLOGY

Beginning at age 60 years, there is a pronounced decrease in the number of pacemaker cells in the sinoatrial node, and by age 75 less than 10 percent of the cells found in the young adult remain [34]. The functional significance of this pronounced anatomic age-related change is not clear. A sinus rate of less than 50 beats per minute, which is often present in the elderly, does not necessarily imply that sinus node disease is limiting heart rate, since exercise and pharmacologic agents have been shown to increase sinus rate significantly in elderly individuals [35]. However, it is interesting to note that the intrinsic sinus rate, i.e., in the presence of both sympathetic and parasympathetic blockade, is significantly diminished with age. At age 20 the average intrinsic heart rate is 104 beats per minute as compared with 92 beats per minute in persons in the 45 to 55 age group [36]. Variation in sinus rate with respiration is diminished with advancing age [37], but the possible effect of cardiac disease on this phenomenon has not been elucidated.

Information on the transmembrane action potential is provided by studies in animal models. In rat ventricular nonworking cardiac muscle, the duration of the action potential and the electrical refractory period are not changed significantly from adulthood to senescence [9]. In Purkinje's fibers from dogs, the amplitude of phase zero of the action potential decreases from adulthood (63.7 months) to senescence (up to 130 months) [38].

Cardiovascular Diseases in the Aged
CORONARY ARTERY DISEASE
The major cause of death in the 65-plus age group worldwide is heart disease, and in a typical Western nation ischemic heart disease accounts for 80 to 90 percent of all cardiac deaths. Fifty percent of deaths from all causes in western countries can be attributed to either a coronary or cerebrovascular event. These estimates lead us to the obvious question of whether vascular changes represent disease or are part of the natural aging process. Vascular intimal changes (atherosclerosis) increase progressively with age [39] (Fig. 12-7), as do changes in the vessel media [40] (Fig. 12-8).

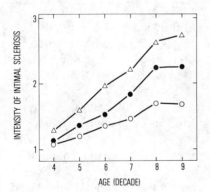

Figure 12-7. The effect of age on the severity of atherosclerosis in the anterior descending (top line, triangles), circumflex (middle line, solid circles), and left coronary (bottom line, open circles) arteries. In each decade 100 hearts were obtained from routine consecutive autopsies on men; they represented persons dying from many and varied causes. The severity was expressed by a grade ranging from 1 (minimal sclerosis) to 4 (complete occlusion of the lumen). (Redrawn from N. K. White et al. The relationship of the degree of coronary atherosclerosis with age, in men. *Circulation* 1:645, 1950.)

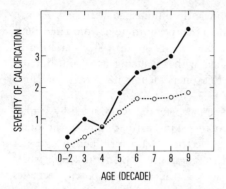

Figure 12-8. The effect of age on the severity of medial calcification in coronary arteries (solid lines) and aorta (dotted lines). (Redrawn from H. T. Blumenthal et al. The interrelation of elastic tissue and calcium in the genesis of arteriosclerosis. *Am. J. Pathol.* 26:989, 1950.)

Similar age changes include changes in the amount of fibrosis, the mean thickness of the intima, degeneration of the internal elastic membrane, luminal dilatation, and increased collagen content [40]. The relationship of age-related changes in the vessel media to those in the coronary intima, which result in luminal occlusion, is unknown. Although the relationship between altered lipid metabolism and coronary atherosclerosis has been recently stressed [41], the relation between age changes in the media and intimal disease has not been emphasized. The fact remains, however, that intimal changes, whether symptomatic or not, rise sharply with age and parallel the process that occurs in the vessel media, as noted in Figure 12-8. Presently we cannot resolve the question of whether the marked prevalence of coronary artery disease in the elderly is related to an effect of age per se or to another effect such as that of risk factors acting over time with no true age-specific component.

Most of the evidence supporting the emphasis of risk factors for acquiring coronary artery disease has been gathered in middle-aged populations. Recently the Pooling Project research group [41] published its final report on the combined incidence of coronary artery disease in five longitudinal studies in middle-aged white men. A typical example of risk factor analysis is given in Table 12-1. The most prominent feature of the systolic blood pressure risk factor analysis in a middle-aged population (ages 40–64) is the marked effect of age. This can be appreciated by reading across the age groups in a given percentile of risk. In fact, the risk in the 60 to 64 age group in the lowest percentile is as great or greater than that of the highest percentile in the younger age group (ages 40–44). This pattern is also seen when the other risk factors of diastolic blood pressure, cholesterol, smoking, obesity, and abnormal electrocardiogram parameters are examined.

Table 12-1. Systolic Blood Pressure as a Risk Factor for Developing Symptomatic Coronary Artery Disease

Systolic Blood Pressure (mm Hg)	Age at Risk*	
	40–44	60–64
< 120	2.0	54.2
120–130	10.4	80.0
130–138	12.2	74.1
138–150	18.7	93.0
> 150	47.0	146.0

Source: Modified from Pooling Project Research Group. Relationship of blood pressure, serum cholesterol, smoking habit, relative weight and ECG abnormalities to incidence of major coronary events: final report of the Pooling Project. *J. Chronic Dis.* 31:201, 1978.
* Risk of an event between the two ages per 1,000 men.

From the result of studies to date, it is clear that we cannot resolve the marked increase in coronary artery disease with age into an effect of age alone or an effect of the length of time during which a person had a risk factor before being monitored in such a study. If it were possible, though, the most effective manner by which a 40-year-old man could avoid symptomatic coronary artery disease in the next five years would be to remain the same age. To date, however, an understanding of the aging process and its important effect on the development of coronary artery disease have been virtually neglected.

Some epidemiologic studies have indicated that in the elderly hypertension, hyperglycemia, hypercholesterolemia, and obesity are not associated with the prevalence of coronary disease [42–44]. However, many of those younger persons who may have had risk factors may have developed coronary artery disease and died at a young age. The complex interaction of risk factors and age must be elucidated before we can test the real significance of risk factors at any age.

Two extreme estimates of the prevalence of significant coronary atherosclerosis come from postmortem and epidemiologic studies. Postmortem studies in people dying from random causes have found significant coronary narrowing in a major coronary vessel in up to 60 percent of hearts [39,45] (Fig. 12-9). It is interesting to note that this percentage levels off at ages 50 to 59 in men and a decade later in women. One interpretation of this figure is that people who are alive in their seventh, eighth, and ninth decades do not have a greater probability of having severe stenosis than their counterparts at age 50 to 60 years.

Epidemiologic studies (in people aged 32–90) based on history and resting electrocardiogram have found the prevalence of coronary artery disease

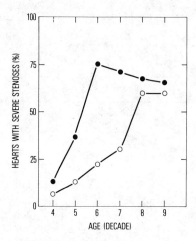

Figure 12-9. The effect of age on the prevalence of severe coronary stenosis (at least 60 percent narrowing) in autopsied hearts (100 hearts in each decade) from men (top line, solid circles) and women (bottom line, open circles). (Redrawn from N. K. White et al. The relationship of the degree of coronary atherosclerosis with age, in men. *Circulation* 1:645, 1950; and R. F. Ackerman et al. Relationship of various factors to the degree of coronary atherosclerosis in women. *Circulation* 1:1345, 1950.)

to range from 2 to 30 percent depending on the bracketing of the data for analysis [43,46]. These are relatively insensitive criteria for diagnosing coronary disease in a given patient and probably in a study population as well. The highest figures for the prevalence of coronary disease in the elderly (75-plus age bracket) for a population living in the community is about 30 percent [43]. This is still somewhat less than the 50 to 60 percent level expected from necropsy studies. The results of epidemiologic studies must be interpreted only as indicative of the prevalence of symptomatic coronary artery disease. The prevalence of asymptomatic disease as detected by stress testing is at least 18 percent [47].

In summary, it seems reasonable on the basis of information provided by autopsy and epidemiologic studies that the prevalence of coronary artery disease in Western societies in persons aged 45 to 60 years ranges from 40 to 60 percent and does not rise above this level with increasing age (Fig. 12-9). The incidence or the rate of new cases of coronary artery disease over a 16-year period as manifested by the combined incidence of uncomplicated angina, myocardial infarction, coronary insufficiency, and sudden death is about 35 percent in men who were 60 to 62 years old at the beginning of the study [48].

Treatment
The primary medications used in the treatment of angina in the elderly as in the young are nitrates and propranolol. Special consideration should be given to possible increased susceptibility to the hypotensive effects of nitrates due to altered cardiovascular reflexes and to increased plasma propranolol levels due to altered pharmacokinetics of this drug in elderly patients [63]. Elderly patients undergoing cardiac surgery no longer experience an increased mortality. At several centers the hospital mortality of those undergoing bypass surgery is less than five percent [64,65]. Thus, survival is similar to that of a younger population, and age should not be considered a deterrent for cardiac surgery when it is otherwise indicated.

MYOCARDIAL INFARCTION
It is difficult to determine whether the presenting symptoms of myocardial infarction differ in the adult and the elderly. Reports on the prevalence of chest pain associated with infarction in the elderly vary from 20 percent in a chronically institutionalized population [49] to 89 percent in those admitted to the coronary care unit from outside of the hospital [50]. The reason why some people do not have chest pain with infarction is unknown. A diminished sensitivity to ischemic pain is possible but difficult to document. Dyspnea is often a more prominent symptom than pain in the elderly. The effect of the ischemic-induced decrease in ventricular compliance is additive to that of diminished compliance in the normal aged heart, as described earlier.

Mortality associated with myocardial infarction in persons older than age 70 is twice that in those younger than age 70 [51]. These estimates are based on studies in which the patients were not matched with respect to clinical status. Several prognostic indices of in-hospital mortality of patients who had myocardial infarctions have also suggested that increasing age is associated with an unfavorable prognosis [52–54]. It should be pointed out, however, that in devising these prognostic parameters, the interaction between age and other variables such as the severity and duration of disease have not been taken into account, and although these indices may be of practical usefulness, the independent effect of age per se cannot be determined.

It has been demonstrated that the mortality for those presenting with myocardial infarction of a severe clinical class is definitely greater than for those presenting with a mild clinical class [55,56]. When elderly and young adults are matched for clinical status and other variables, including previous infarction, age differences in mortality are either lessened [57] or obliterated [58]. Since the elderly usually present with a more severe clinical status [50,58], they are more likely to develop the complications of infarction during hospitalization than their younger adult counterpart.

Congestive heart failure, pulmonary edema, and cardiogenic shock occur more frequently in the aged [50,59]. It cannot be determined, however, whether the elderly have larger infarctions, acute infarctions of similar size but additional myocardial loss from previous infarcts, poor ventricular reserve in noninfarcted muscle, or a combination of all of these factors. The diminished response to catecholamines associated with aging, as discussed earlier, may have a role in the diminished cardiovascular response to the stress of a myocardial infarction. While some studies found that second degree or third degree heart block was twice as common in people over age 70 (35 percent versus 17 percent) [50], others found no age trend in the tendency to develop block [51]. Premature atrial contractions are prevalent in those over age 70 who have acute myocardial infarction. The incidence of ventricular premature beats and ventricular fibrillation is not influenced by age [6].

Cardiac rupture complicating acute myocardial infarction is much more common in older than younger patients [60,61]. There is some uncertainty regarding the role of hypertension in increasing the tendency to rupture. Other factors could include an age difference in the extent of infarction and an alteration of the inflammatory response with age. In spite of the more serious clinical status of the elderly with infarction, several studies indicate that the acute mortality of the elderly admitted from the community is about 30 to 40 percent [50,52]. Mortality rates on the order of 80 percent [59] appear to reflect what might be expected in a clinically institutionalized population and is not necessarily a sequela of aging per se, but of the multiple diseases and poor conditions of such institutionalized populations.

The pure effect of age itself on mortality and complications after myocardial infarction cannot be measured with precision. It is not clear whether specific changes in the present routine therapy for acute myocardial infarction would reduce the increased mortality from this disease in aged individuals. Certainly no person on the basis of age alone should be excluded from medical care in a coronary care unit. The long-term survival (after discharge from the hospital) relative to that in age-matched controls is not changed or is even greater than in younger adults [43,56,62].

HYPERTENSION

Blood pressure, primarily systolic, increases with advancing age. In fact, a large proportion of the population aged 62 years and greater would be declared hypertensive if the criterion of greater than 150/90 were used (see Fig. 12-2). However, there is no number that serves as a dividing line between what is a normal and an abnormal blood pressure. In considering whether a person's blood pressure is elevated, however, his or her age, sex, and activity at the time of measurement should be considered. Controlled trials have shown that in men and women patients whose diastolic pressures are above 110, and in men with diastolic pressures between 90 and 114, treatment reduces morbidity and mortality [66,67]. The mean ages in the latter study were 52.0 and 50.5 years in the controlled and treatment groups, respectively. Comparable studies of the effect of treatment in an elderly population with hypertension have not been performed. However, the risk associated with hypertension was examined in the Framingham Study [68]. Men and women were followed for 18 years for the development of cardiovascular mortality in relation to their blood pressure. The incidence in hypertensive men who reached 65 to 74 years of age during the study was 2.4 times greater than in normotensive men and in women the risk was almost eight times as great in those with hypertension.

Despite these results, it is uncertain who should be treated and how vigorous treatment should be. The moderate incidence of postural blood pressure changes in the elderly as well as diminished cardiac reserve and overall sympathetic responsiveness described earlier would render the elderly particularly susceptible to side effects of antihypertensive medication. Given the tremendous importance of cardiovascular events in this population and the strong correlation with blood pressure, a trial assessing the benefit of therapy is urgently needed. Furthermore, the mechanisms for the age-associated anatomic changes in vasculature and in vascular reactivity that may be responsible for the increase in blood pressure in the elderly need to be elucidated so that treatment can be directed in a more physiologic and rational manner.

CONGESTIVE HEART FAILURE

The prevalence of heart failure increases nearly exponentially with increasing age, and about 75 percent of all ambulatory patients with congestive heart failure are over the age of 60 years [69,70]. The diagnosis and etiology of the heart failure in elderly individuals are often obscure. Failure symptoms of dyspnea or ankle edema may be due to noncardiac disease. Alternatively, a person who is sedentary because of physical limitations imposed by other disease, such as degenerative arthritis, may not be able to exercise sufficiently to be aware of symptoms when congestive heart failure is present.

The clinical signs of failure may also be difficult to interpret. Abnormalities of the thoracic cage may make palpation of the apex difficult and displace its position. If palpable, the characteristics of the impulse have the same implications in the elderly as in the younger population. A fourth heart sound is often heard in elderly individuals regardless of whether they have overt cardiac disease [71]. This is probably because decreased left ventricular compliance results in a shorter S4-S1 interval, allowing summation of the low frequency vibrations to behave as one sound of longer duration that would be easier to hear [72]. Rales often result from chronic lung disease. A low diaphragm may be responsible for a palpable liver edge. The venous pulse is one of the most reliable indicators of right heart failure since it is easy to observe; however, the right side of the neck should be used, since left-sided venous drainage may be compressed between an elongated, unfolded aortic arch and the back of the sternum.

Pathologic studies of hearts from elderly patients with clinically evident failure show a 50 percent occurrence of ischemic heart disease followed by calcific valvular degenerative changes and hypertensive disease [3]. However, since many of these changes also occur in individuals in whom failure is not present, it is uncertain whether these changes are sufficient in and of themselves to result in failure, and it has been argued that it is the presence of several coexisting pathologic processes that is most responsible for heart failure in advanced age [73].

Alternatively, some studies have found no specifically identifiable pathology in patients diagnosed as having heart failure. Rose and Wilson [74] examined hearts from 50 patients over 70 years of age who died of heart failure in whom no adequate clinical cause of failure was apparent. In 36 percent, no pathologic finding was identified, suggesting an "obscure weakening" of the myocardium with age, or a "senile cardiomyopathy" unassociated with any visible pathologic change. However, the concept of a pathologic disorder related solely to aging that results in clinical failure is hard to justify. In normal hearts, age changes occur that diminish the response to stress, and the presence of a given amount of stress associated with a fever, tachycardia, and hyperthyroidism may induce failure in an old but not in a young individual [75]. Although it is difficult to ascertain whether the stresses imposed on the cardiovascular system by everyday living are sufficient to induce failure in old individuals, it is likely that age-associated changes alter the clinical presentation of failure in the setting of specific pathologic disease.

Treatment

The pharmacology of digoxin, one of the primary drugs used to treat failure, is altered with increasing age. Digoxin is moderately well absorbed, bound only slightly to albumin, and excreted by the kidney in nearly its original form. Its steady state plasma concentration would tend to be influenced by the reduced volume of distribution and decline in creatinine clearance. Following acute intravenous and oral administration of digoxin, the half-life is longer and serum levels higher in the elderly [76,77]. In humans, some data suggest greater toxicity in the elderly but this can be accounted for largely by higher serum levels. In awake, intact beagles, the serum level of acetylstrophanthidin at the onset of ventricular tachycardia was not different in senescent as compared with the adult animal [78]. The inotropic effect in both intact dogs and isolated rat myocardium is diminished in senescence [78,79]. This effect cannot be attributed to an age difference in Na-K adenosine triphosphatase (ATPase) inhibition.

The effect of age on the inotropic response to cardiac glycosides in humans is not known. However, several recent studies have demonstrated that in patients in sinus rhythm with chronic congestive heart failure, most of whom are elderly, digitalis can be withdrawn without any change in clinical status [80,81]. In fact, the inotropic efficacy of glycosides given on a long-term basis in patients of any age remains to be proved. Considering the considerable toxicity associated with glycoside administration in the elderly, it may be wise to treat failure symptoms with diuretics or possibly vasodilators. It is important to realize, however, that elderly patients may be more prone to develop hyponatremia (due to an inability to excrete free water and conserve sodium), hyperglycemia, and hyperuricemia from diuretic therapy [63,82], and impaired cardiovascular reflex mechanisms may make them more susceptible to the hypotensive effects of vasodilators. In addition, no information on the efficacy of these agents in the elderly is currently available. Much more information is needed before we can rationally use these agents to treat disease in the elderly.

VALVULAR HEART DISEASE

Rheumatic mitral valve disease is the most common cause of mitral pathology in the elderly population. Patients with rheumatic disease survive to old age not because of a later onset of disease but because they have suffered fewer recurrences of rheumatic activity. The complications of rheumatic disease are atrial fibrillation and emboli. Of elderly patients with rheumatic disease and atrial fibrillation, 60 percent have evidence of heart failure, whereas 25 percent of those in sinus rhythm will be in failure [83]. This may be related to an age-associated decrease in left ventricular compliance, resulting in a greater reliance on atrial contribution to ventricular filling in the elderly. Although emboli may be present, thrombosis is a much more common cause of occlusion of systemic arteries in these patients and the differential between the two may be difficult. The prognosis of mitral disease in the elderly depends on the cardiac rhythm and the presence or absence of failure. Those in sinus rhythm with no evidence of failure do not have reduced life expectancy [83]. If atrial fibrillation or heart failure is present, however, survival is reduced.

Calcification of the mitral annulus and mucoid degeneration of the mitral valve are conditions peculiar to elderly individuals [73]. Calcification occurs in the area of the ring and is the only cardiovascular abnormality in old age that is more common in women than in men. It can be diagnosed by the inverted C shape of calcium seen on chest x-ray and by the heavy calcification seen in the region on the echocardiogram. The usual murmur is that secondary to mitral insufficiency. Although it is usually of no clinical significance, in extensive cases it may prevent proper closure or opening of the valve and result in incompetence or stenosis. Calcification may also extend into the His bundle and peripheral bundle branches and result in conduction disturbances. It can also ulcerate the atrial surface of the cusps and the endocardium and result in a site for the development of endocarditis.

The suspicion of aortic valve disease is frequently encountered because systolic ejection murmurs are present at the base and/or apex in 60 percent or more of patients 70 years of age or older [84]. They are thought to originate primarily in the aortic area and to be secondary to calcification of the aortic valve ring or sclerosis of the aortic cusps. One distinction between those murmurs that are and are not clinically important can be made by listening in late systole. Nonpathologic ejection murmurs will exhibit markedly diminished intensity or become absent during this time.

Aortic stenosis is not uncommon in elderly individuals and the etiology varies with the age of the patient. In those under 60 years of age, rheumatic disease is most common. In those aged 60 to 75 years, the most common etiology is calcification on a congenitally bicuspid valve. In those greater than 75 years, degenerative calcification of an aortic valve is most frequent [73]. It is often impossible to distinguish between various etiologies in the clinical situation.

The examination in the presence of significant aortic stenosis is basically the same as that in a younger individual, with the exception that the slow anacrotic pulse and reduced pulse pressure may not be present because of the increased stiffness of the central arteries associated with advanced age. This condition should be differentiated from aortic valvular sclerosis and idiopathic hypertrophic subaortic stenosis (IHSS). Significant disease is distinguished from aortic valvular sclerosis by the characteristics of the murmur (as discussed previously), those of the second heart sound, and evidence of left ventricular hypertrophy. It is important to obtain age-adjusted values for left ventricular wall thickness since mild hypertrophy is present in normal old individuals [5]. As in younger adults IHSS can be diagnosed by the echocardiogram. The medical treatment of valvular heart disease in the elderly does not differ from that in the younger individual. The mortality of those aged 65 or greater undergoing aortic and mitral valve replacement at Johns Hopkins Hospital between 1974 and 1978 was only 4.9 percent and 4.3 percent, respectively [64].

ARRHYTHMIAS AND ABNORMALITIES OF THE CONDUCTION SYSTEM

In nonselected populations, both resting electrocardiogram and Holter monitoring demonstrate an increase in ectopic activity with age [46,85] that is highly correlated with the increased prevalence of coronary artery disease. Long-term recording of the electrocardiogram in a population free of cardiovascular disease showed that the incidence of ectopic activity increases between age 20 and 70 years [86].

The prevalence of atrial fibrillation increases with age and ranges from 3 percent of people living at home to 10 to 15 percent of elderly patients hospitalized for a long period of time; in some instances, atrial fibrillation occurs in the absence of other classifiable cardiac disease [87].

The prolongation in PR interval seen with age [88] may be related to the muscle cell loss, increase in fibrous and adipose tissue, and amyloid infiltrates

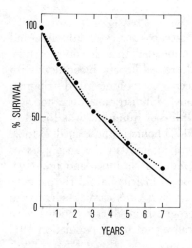

Figure 12-10. The survival in patients over 80 years of age with a permanent pacemaker inserted for complete heart block (dotted line) and that in the general age-matched population (solid line). (Redrawn from H. Siddons. Death in long-term paced patients. *Br. Heart J.* 36:1201, 1947.)

that occur in this region with advancing age [34]. In most hearts after the age of 60 there is a loss of as many as 50 percent of the fascicles that connect the main bundle of His to the left bundle [34]. This is also often accompanied by a slight decrease in the distal connecting fibers. While these changes occur frequently in senescent hearts, left bundle block occurs in two percent or less of unselected populations over the age of 62 [87]. The leftward shift in the QRS axis [88] may be related to fibrosis in the anterior division, myocardial fibrosis, mild hypertrophy of the left ventricle, and/or a change in the spatial orientation of the heart in the chest.

The prevalence of complete heart block in the elderly is strikingly low, less than one percent in both unselected populations [87] and those in clinical facilities [89]. Carotid sinus massage is often employed in the evaluation of individuals with supraventricular tachycardias. In this regard, it should be remembered that older patients have an increased frequency and degree of response to this maneuver than younger patients do [90].

In contrast to the normal age-related changes that occur in the conduction system, severe bundle branch fibrosis and degenerative calcification extending from the aortic and mitral valve rings occur in a relatively small number of hearts. These changes, which are not the norm for age and which should be considered pathologic, appear to be responsible for one-third of the cases of complete heart block in the elderly. Other common causes of complete heart block are coronary artery disease, cardiomyopathy, and calcific valvular disease.

Treatment

The effect of age of the patient on the pharmacokinetics of lidocaine and quinidine has been investigated. It is recommended that the dose of lidocaine be reduced in the elderly because of decreased hepatic blood flow with increasing age [91,92]. In healthy volunteers, the volume of distribution and serum levels measured after intravenous administration were not age-related [92]. However, the elimination half-life of quinidine was found to be 9.7 hours in those aged 60 to 69 years and 7.3 hours in those aged 23 to 29 years. Total quinidine clearance was 2.64 ml/kg/min in the aged persons and 4.04 ml/kg/min in the younger. The reduced clearance and prolongation of elimination half-life could predispose to toxicity in elderly patients.

Recent experience with permanent pacemakers and cardiac surgery in aged individuals is good. The long-term prognosis in elderly patients with pacemakers is identical to that of a general, age-matched population [93] (Fig. 12-10).

References

1. Gerstenblith, G., Lakatta, E. G., and Weisfeldt, M. L.   Age changes in myocardial function and exercise response. *Progr. Cardiovasc. Dis.* 19:1, 1976.
2. Lakatta, E. G.   Alterations in the cardiovascular system that occur in advanced age. *Fed. Proc.* 38:163, 1979.
3. Pomerance, A.   Pathology of the heart with and without cardiac failure in the aged. *Br. Heart J.* 27:697, 1965.
4. Hamilton, M., et al.   The aetiology of essential hypertention: I. The arterial pressure in the general population. *Clin. Sci.* 13:11, 1954.
5. Gerstenblith, G., et al.   Echocardiographic assessment of a normal adult aging population. *Circulation* 56:273, 1977.
6. Templeton, G. H., et al.   Influence of aging on left ventricular hemodynamics and stiffness in beagles. *Circ. Res.* 44:189, 1979.
7. Spurgeon, H. A., et al.   Increased dynamic stiffness of trabeculae carneae from senescent rats. *Am. J. Physiol.* 232:H373, 1977.
8. Weisfeldt, M. L., Loeven, W. A., and Shock, N. W.   Resting and active mechanical properties of trabeculae carneae from aged male rats. *Am. J. Physiol.* 220:1921, 1971.
9. Lakatta, E. G., et al.   Prolonged contraction duration in aged myocardium. *J. Clin. Invest.* 55:61, 1975.
10. Froehlich, J. P., et al.   Studies of sarcoplasmic reticulum function and contraction duration in young adult and aged rat myocardium. *J. Mol. Cell. Cardiol.* 10:427, 1978.
11. Hort, W.   Quantitative Untersuchungen uber die Capillarisierung des Herzmuskels in Erwachsenen und Greisenalter. *Virchows Arch. Pathol. Anat.* 327:560, 1955.
12. Weisfeldt, M. L., et al.   Coronary flow and oxygen extraction in the perfused heart of senescent male rats. *J. Appl. Physiol.* 30:44, 1971.
13. Rakusan, K., and Pupa, O.   Capillaries and muscle fibers in the heart of the old rats. *Gerontologia* 9:107, 1964.

14. Brandfonbrener, M., Landowne, M., and Shock, N. W.   Changes in cardiac output with age. *Circulation* 12:557, 1955.
15. Lewis, W. J., Jr.   Changes with age in the cardiac output in adult men. *Am. J. Physiol.* 121:517, 1938.
16. Strandell, T.   Circulatory studies on healthy old men. With special reference to the limitation of the maximal physical working capacity. *Acta Med. Scand.* 175:(Suppl.)414, 1964.
17. Yin, F. C. P., et al.   Age-associated decrease in ventricular response to hemodynamic stress during beta-adrenergic blockade. *Br. Heart J.* 40:1349, 1978.
18. Rowell, L. B.   Human cardiovascular adjustments to exercise and thermal stress. *Physiol. Rev.* 54:75, 1974.
19. Dehn, M. M., and Bruce, R. A.   Longitudinal variations in maximal oxygen intake with age and activity. *J. Appl. Physiol.* 33:805, 1972.
20. Hartley, L. H., et al.   Physical training in sedentary middle-aged and older men: III. Cardiac output and gas exchange at submaximal and maximal exercise. *Scand. J. Clin. Lab. Invest.* 24:335, 1969.
21. Tzankoff, S. P.   Age-related determinants of muscular work perfusion and capacity. (In preparation.)
22. Robinson, S.   Experimental studies of physical fitness in relation to age. *Arbeitsphysiologie* 10:251, 1938.
23. Petrofsky, J. S., and Lind, A. R.   Isometric strength, endurance, and the blood pressure and heart rate responses during isometric exercise in healthy men and women, with special reference to age and body fat content. *Pfluegers Arch.* 360:49, 1975.
24. Ziegler, M. G., Lake, C. R., and Kopin, I. J.   Plasma noradrenaline increases with age. *Nature* 261:333, 1976.
25. Yin, F. C. P., et al.   Age-associated decrease in chronotropic response to isoproterenol. *Circulation* 54:II–167, 1976.
26. Yin, F. C. P., et al.   Age-associated decrease in heart rate response to isoproterenol in dogs. *Mech. Ageing Dev.* 10:17, 1979.
27. Kronenberg, R. S., and Drage, C. W.   Attenuation of the ventilatory and heart rate response to hypoxia and hypercapnia with aging in normal man. *J. Clin. Invest.* 52:1812, 1973.
28. Julius, S., et al.   Influence of age on the hemodynamic response to exercise. *Circulation* 36:222, 1967.
29. Fleisch, J. H., and Hooker, C. S.   The relationship between age and relaxation of vascular smooth muscle in rabbit and rat. *Circ. Res.* 38:243, 1976.
30. Conway, J., Jr.   Changes with age in the cardiac output in adult men. *Am. J. Physiol.* 121:517, 1938.
31. Lakatta, E. G.   Excitation-Contraction. In M. L. Weisfeldt (Ed.), *The Heart in Old Age: Its Function and Response to Stress. Aging,* Vol. 12. New York: Raven Press, 1980.
32. Lakatta, E. G., et al.   Diminished inotropic response of aged myocardium to catecholamines. *Circ. Res.* 36:262, 1975.
33. Guarnieri, T., et al.   Contractile and biochemical correlates of β-adrenergic stimulation of the aged heart. *Am. J. Physiol.* 239(Heart Circ. Physiol.). 8:H501, 1980.

34. Davies, M. J.   Pathology of the Conduction System. In F. I. Caird, J. L. C. Dall, and R. D. Kennedy (Eds.), *Cardiology in Old Age.* New York: Plenum Press, 1976.
35. Agruss, N. S., et al.   Significance of chronic sinus bradycardia in elderly people. *Circulation* 46:924, 1972.
36. Jose, A. D.   Effect of combined sympathetic and parasympathetic blockade on heart rate and cardiac function in man. *Am. J. Cardiol.* 18:476, 1966.
37. Davies, H. E. F.   Respiratory change in heart rate, sinus arrhythmia in the elderly. *Gerontol. Clin.* 17:96, 1975.
38. Rosen, M. R., et al.   Age-related changes in Purkinje fiber action potentials of adult dogs. *Circ. Res.* 43:931, 1978.
39. White, N. K., Edwards, J. E., and Dry, T. J.   The relationship of the degree of coronary atherosclerosis with age, in men. *Circulation* 1:645, 1950.
40. Blumenthal, H. T., Lansing, A. I., and Gray, S. H.   The interrelation of elastic tissue and calcium in the genesis of arteriosclerosis. *Am. J. Pathol.* 26:989, 1950.
41. Pooling Project Research Group. Relationship of blood pressure, serum cholesterol, smoking habit, relative weight and ECG abnormalities to incidence of major coronary events: final report of the Pooling Project. *J. Chronic Dis.* 31:201, 1978.
42. Goldstein, J. L., et al.   Hyperlipidemia in coronary heart disease: I. Lipid levels in 500 survivors of myocardial infarction. *J. Clin. Invest.* 52:1533, 1973.
43. Kennedy, R. O., Andrews, G. R., and Caird, F. I.   Ischemic heart disease in the elderly. *Br. Heart J.* 39:1121, 1977.
44. Kitchin, A. H., and Milne, J. S.   Longitudinal survey of ischemic heart disease in randomly selected sample of older population. *Br. Heart J.* 39:889, 1977.
45. Ackerman, R. F., Dry, T. J., and Edwards, J. E.   Relationship of various factors to the degree of coronary atherosclerosis in women. *Circulation* 1:1345, 1950.
46. Kannel, W. B., Gordon, T., and Offutt, D.   Left ventricular hypertrophy by electrocardiogram. Prevalence, incidence, and mortality in the Framingham Study. *Ann. Intern. Med.* 71:89, 1969.
47. Gerstenblith, G., et al.   Stress testing redefines the prevalence of coronary artery disease in epidemiologic studies. *Circulation* 62:III–308, 1980.
48. Kannel, W. B., and Feinleib, M.   Natural history of angina pectoris in the Framingham Study. Prognosis and survival. *Am. J. Cardiol.* 29:154, 1972.
49. Pathy, M. S.   Clinical presentation of myocardial infarction in the elderly. *Br. Heart J.* 29:190, 1967.
50. Williams, B. O., et al.   The elderly in a coronary unit. *Br. Med. J.* 2:451, 1976.
51. Kincaid, D. T., and Botti, R. E.   Acute myocardial infarction in the elderly. *Chest* 64:170, 1973.
52. Librach, G., et al.   Immediate and long-term prognosis of acute myocardial infarction in the aged. *J. Chronic Dis.* 29:483, 1976.
53. Marx, H. J., and Yu, P. N.   Prognostic Factors in Acute Myocardial Infarction. In E. Corday and H. J. C. Swan (Eds.), *Myocardial Infarction.* Baltimore: Williams & Wilkins, 1973.
54. Norris, R. M., et al.   A new coronary prognostic index. *Lancet* 1:274, 1969.

55. Killip, T., and Kimball, J. T. Treatment of myocardial infarction in a coronary care unit. *Am. J. Cardiol.* 20:457, 1967.
56. Kitchin, A. H., and Pocock, S. J. Prognosis of patients with acute myocardial infarction admitted to a coronary care unit: I. Survival in hospital. *Br. Heart J.* 39:1163, 1977.
57. Honey, G. E., and Truelove, S. C. Prognostic factors in myocardial infarction. *Lancet* 1:1155, 1957.
58. Schnur, S. Mortality rates in acute myocardial infarction: III. The relation of patient's age to prognosis. *Ann. Intern. Med.* 44:294, 1954.
59. Harris, R., and Piracha, A. R. Acute myocardial infarction in the aged: prognosis and management. *J. Am. Geriatr. Soc.* 18:893, 1970.
60. Biorck, G., Sievers, J., and Blomqvist, G. Studies on myocardial infarction in Malmo 1935–1954: III. Follow-up studies from a hospital material. *Acta Med. Scand.* 162:81, 1958.
61. Zeman, F. D., and Rodstein, M. Cardiac rupture complicating myocardial infarction in the aged. *Arch. Intern. Med.* 105:431, 1960.
62. Sievers, J., Blomqvist, G., and Biorck, G. Studies on myocardial infarction in Malmo 1935–1954: VI. Some clinical data with particular reference to diabetes, menopause and heart rupture. *Acta Med. Scand.* 169:95, 1961.
63. O'Malley, K., and O'Brien, E. Management of hypertension in the elderly. *N. Engl. J. Med.* 302:1397, 1980.
64. Gardner, T. J. Personal communication, 1980.
65. Meyer, J., et al. Coronary artery bypass in patients over 70 years of age: indications and results. *Am. J. Cardiol.* 36:342, 1975.
66. Veterans Administration Cooperative Study Group on Antihypertensive Agents. Effects of treatment on morbidity in hypertension: results in patients with diastolic blood pressures averaging 115 through 129 mm Hg. *J.A.M.A.* 202:1028, 1967.
67. Veterans Administration Cooperative Study Group on Antihypertensive Agents. Effects of treatment on morbidity in hypertension: II. Results in patients with diastolic blood pressure averaging 90 through 114 mm Hg. *J.A.M.A.* 213:1143, 1979.
68. Kannel, W. B. Blood Pressure and the Development of Cardiovascular Disease in the Aged. In F. I. Caird, J. L. C. Dall, and R. D. Kennedy (Eds.), *Cardiology in Old Age.* New York: Plenum Press, 1976.
69. Klainer, L. M., Gibson, T. C., and White, K. L. The epidemiology of cardiac failure. *J. Chronic Dis.* 18:797, 1965.
70. McKee, P. A., et al. The natural history of congestive heart failure: the Framingham Study. *N. Engl. J. Med.* 285:1441, 1971.
71. Spodick, D. H., and Quarry, V. M. Prevalence of the fourth heart sound by phonocardiography in the absence of heart disease. *Am. Heart J.* 87:11, 1974.
72. Kino, M., Shahmatpour, A., and Spodick, D. Auscultatory perception of the fourth heart sound. *Am. J. Cardiol.* 37:848, 1976.
73. Pomerance, A. Pathology of the Myocardium and Valves. In F. I. Caird, J. L. C. Dall, and R. D. Kennedy (Eds.), *Cardiology in Old Age.* New York: Plenum Press, 1976.
74. Rose, G. A., and Wilson, R. R. Unexplained heart failure in the aged. *Br. Heart J.* 21:511, 1959.

75. Dock, W.   Cardiomyopathies of the senescent and senile. *Cardiovasc. Clin.* 4:362, 1972.
76. Ewy, G. A., et al.   Digoxin metabolism in the elderly. *Circulation* 39:449, 1969.
77. Triggs, E. J., and Nation, R. L.   Pharmacokinetics in the aged: a review. *J. Pharmacokinet. Biopharm.* 3:387, 1975.
78. Guarnieri, T., et al.   Diminished inotropic response but unaltered toxicity to acetylstrophanthidin in the senescent beagle. *Circulation* 60:1548, 1979.
79. Gerstenblith, G., et al.   Diminished inotropic responsiveness to ouabain in aged rat myocardium. *Circ. Res.* 44:517, 1979.
80. Dobbs, S. M., Kenyon, W. I., and Dobbs, R. J.   Maintenance digoxin after an episode of heart failure: placebo-controlled trial in outpatients. *Br. Med. J.* 1:749, 1977.
81. Fleg, J. L., Gottlieb, S. H., and Lakatta, E. G.   Is digitalis really useful in the therapy of chronic congestive heart failure? *Circulation* 60:(Suppl. 2)II–178, 1979.
82. Rowe, J. W.   Fluid and Electrolyte Disturbances in the Elderly. In R. Harris (Ed.), *Geriatric Medicine,* Unit 1, Lesson 4. New York: Physician Program Inc., 1979.
83. Bedford, P. D., and Caird, F. I.   *Valvular Disease of the Heart in Old Age.* London: Churchill Livingstone, 1960.
84. Burch, G. E., and Depasquale, N. P.   Geriatric cardiology. *Am. Heart J.* 78:700, 1969.
85. Chiang, B. N., et al.   Relationship of premature systoles to coronary heart disease and sudden death in the Tecumseh epidemiologic study. *Ann. Intern. Med.* 70:1159, 1969.
86. Raftery, E. B., and Cashman, P. M.   Long-term recording of the electrocardiogram in a normal population. *Postgrad. Med. J.* 52(Suppl. 7):32, 1976.
87. Caird, F. I., and Kennedy, R. D.   Epidemiology of Heart Disease in Old Age. In F. I. Caird, J. L. C. Dall, and R. D. Kennedy (Eds.), *Cardiology in Old Age.* New York: Plenum Press, 1976.
88. Simonson, E.   *Differentiation Between Normal and Abnormal in Electrocardiography.* St. Louis: Mosby, 1961.
89. Bhat, P. K., et al.   Conduction defects in the aging heart. *J. Am. Geriatr. Soc.* 22:517, 1974.
90. Sigler, L. H.   Hyperactive cardioinhibitory carotid sinus reflex. A possible aid in the diagnosis of coronary disease. *Arch. Intern. Med.* 67:177, 1941.
91. Harrison, D. C.   Should lidocaine be administered routinely to all patients after acute myocardial infarction? *Circulation* 58:581, 1978.
92. Ochs, H. R., et al.   Reduced quinidine clearance in elderly persons. *Am. J. Cardiol.* 42:481, 1978.
93. Siddons, H.   Death in long-term paced patients. *Br. Heart J.* 36:1201, 1947.

Suggested Reading

Abu-Erreish, G. M., et al.   Fatty acid oxidation by isolated perfused working hearts of aged rats. *Am. J. Physiol.* 232:E258, 1977.

Fleg, J. L., and Kennedy, H. L.   Cardiac arrhythmias in a healthy elderly population. Detection by 24-hour ambulatory electrocardiography. *Chest* (in press).

Lakatta, E. G.   Age-related alterations in the cardiovascular response to adrenergic mediated stress. *Fed. Proc.* 39:3173, 1980.

Lakatta, E. G.   Determinants of cardiovascular performance: modification due to aging. *J. Chronic Dis.* (in press).

Weisfeldt, M. L.   *The Aging Heart: Its Function and Response to Stress. Aging,* Vol. 12. New York: Raven Press, 1980.

Yin, F. C. P., Weisfeldt, M. L., and Milnor, W. R.   Role of aortic input impedance in the decreased cardiovascular response to exercise with aging in dogs. *J. Clin. Invest.* 68:28, 1981.

13. Altered Blood Pressure

High Blood Pressure

The prevalence of high blood pressure coupled with widespread recognition of its importance as a precedent for cardiovascular disease and the availability of effective, safe therapy has made management of hypertension a centerpiece of the practice of modern medicine. It is surprising therefore that, despite these advances, generalized uncertainty persists regarding the proper management of high blood pressure in the elderly.

INFLUENCE OF AGE ON BLOOD PRESSURE

Numerous cross-sectional and longitudinal studies in Western countries have demonstrated similar trends for changes in blood pressure after adulthood (Fig. 13-1). The increase in systolic blood pressure is generally linear from age 30 to old age, whereas the increase in diastolic blood pressure is less prominent and peaks in the midfifties in men and early sixties in women, declining slightly thereafter [1]. As a result of this pattern, pulse pressure increases in late life in both men and women. While trends for blood pressure with age are similar in many Western societies, the well-documented lack of a rise of blood pressure with age in less-developed countries [2] clearly indicates that the increases in blood pressure do not represent an inevitable consequence of normal human aging but rather are caused by some genetic or environmental factor common to developed countries. While early studies suggested that differences in salt intake between primitive and developed countries might account for the changes in blood pressure with age, current evidence does not support this hypothesis [3]. Within Western societies longitudinal studies have shown that increases in blood pressure over time are more related to the initial blood pressure level and to subsequent weight gain than to age itself [4].

PATHOPHYSIOLOGIC MECHANISMS UNDERLYING AGE-RELATED INCREASES IN BLOOD PRESSURE

The fact that systolic blood pressure rises despite coincident decreases in cardiac output and stroke volume clearly points to changes in the peripheral vascular system as underlying the changes in blood pressure with age. While peripheral vascular resistance clearly increases with age, this change alone would be expected to result in rises in both systolic and diastolic blood pressure. Increases in pulse pressure with age, as well as a specified change in the arterial pressure waves such as flattening of the dicrotic notch, indicate the importance of losses of vascular distensibility and elastic recoil [5].

DEFINITION AND PREVALENCE OF HYPERTENSION IN THE ELDERLY

Blood pressure is a continuous variable, with increasing levels associated with increasing cardiovascular risk and with no apparent threshold for the

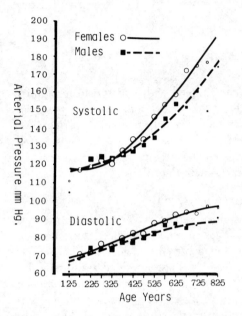

Figure 13-1. Systolic and diastolic pressures for females and males for each five-year age group of the population sample, together with the fitted curves. The area of each circle or square is proportional to the number of subjects in that age group.

onset of the risk. The definition of any particular level as abnormal-pathologic must thus be empiric and varies from clinic to clinic and study to study. The definition of hypertension in the elderly can be approached in two general ways. One approach is to apply the same criteria for hypertension to all age groups. In this way one applies increasingly stringent criteria for high blood pressure in older age groups. Thus, if the definition of hypertension is systolic pressure over 160 or diastolic pressure over 95, as in the Framingham Study [6], one finds that 22 percent of men and 34 percent of women aged 65 to 74 can be considered hypertensive. Using the slightly lower cutoffs of 150 systolic and 95 diastolic, one finds the prevalence of hypertension to increase from 25 percent at age 50 to over 70 percent between ages 85 to 95 [7]. A second approach views the increasing blood pressure with age as normative and employs age-adjusted criteria for the definition of hypertension. With such an approach the percent of any given age cohort considered to be hypertensive will not change (for instance one-half of one standard deviation) but the level needed to reach this cutoff will increase with age. While this takes into account the "normal" distribution of blood pressures in the elderly, it overlooks the fact that while increases in blood pressure are normal in a statistical sense this does not indicate that they are harmless. Since strong epidemiologic data support the view that increases in blood pressure are associated with an increased risk of cardiovascular disease, it would appear that the more appropriate definition of hypertension is the establishment of some empiric but reasonable cutoff, such as 160 systolic and 95 diastolic, and application of these criteria regardless of age.

RISKS OF HIGH BLOOD PRESSURE

There is clear evidence from several large-scale epidemiologic studies that increasing levels of blood pressure are associated with increased risk of morbidity and mortality from stroke, congestive heart failure, coronary heart disease, and peripheral vascular disease. The bulk of the present evidence indicates that the "riskiness" of high blood pressure persists into old age, that systolic blood pressure is a better predictor of risk than diastolic pressure, and that the risk associated with increasing levels of blood pressure is roughly equivalent for elderly men and women and may increase abruptly at systolic levels over 180 [8–10]. While the risk of a stroke or other adverse cardiovascular event is greater in a hypertensive individual with already established end organ damage such as left ventricular hypertrophy, the risks in individuals without end organ damage is also considerable and they deserve careful attention and appropriate treatment [11] (Fig. 13-2). Among the various cardiovascular events that have been studied, hypertension carries the greatest increase in risk as compared to normal blood pressure for the development of stroke and seems to have the least impact on occlusive peripheral vascular disease. However, since the prevalence of coronary heart disease is so much greater than stroke, the absolute occurrence of coronary heart disease death or related morbid events is much greater than that for stroke, even in hypertensive individuals.

ISOLATED SYSTOLIC HYPERTENSION IN THE ELDERLY

Since the increases in systolic blood pressure after age 60 are not accompanied by further increases in diastolic pressure, pulse pressure increases and the prevalence of isolated systolic hypertension (systolic pressure greater than 160 and diastolic pressure less than 95) increases dramatically in the elderly. In the Framingham Study the prevalence of isolated systolic hypertension rose from 5 percent at age 60 in both men and women to 30 percent in women and 10 percent in men by age 70 [12]. The cause for the higher prevalence in women than men is uncertain. The proper management of systolic hypertension thus becomes of major importance to the geriatrician.

One of the many myths enveloping geriatric medicine is the commonly held view that elevations of systolic pressure, unaccompanied by elevations of diastolic pressure, are not harmful in the elderly. Nothing could be further from the truth. All major studies have shown that systolic rather than

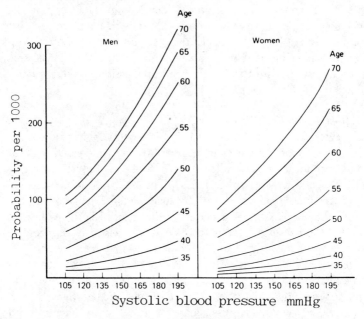

Figure 13-2. Probability of cardiovascular disease in an eight-year period according to systolic blood pressure at specified ages in each sex. Low-risk subjects: those with serum cholesterol less than 185 mg/dl, nonsmokers, no glucose intolerance, no ECG evidence of left ventricular hypertrophy (Framingham Heart Study—18-year follow-up).

diastolic or mean arterial blood pressure is the most potent risk factor for morbidity or mortality from cardiovascular disease. In addition, there is no a priori reason why one would expect that the diastolic blood pressure should be more damaging to vessels than the systolic pressure, which is indeed the pressure at which stress factors are placed on the vessel wall. In elderly individuals with systolic blood pressures over 160 and diastolic pressures less than 95, there is a two-fold to five-fold increase in the risk of death from cardiovascular events and a four-fold increase in cardiovascular morbidity [12]. In the Chicago Stroke Study elderly individuals with isolated systolic hypertension (which was defined in the study as systolic pressure over 160 and diastolic pressure less than 80) were over three times more likely to suffer stroke within three years than were age-matched normotensive individuals (those with systolic pressure less than 140) and twice as likely as those with systolic pressures between 140 and 160 [13]. Recently the Framingham Study has shown that systolic pressure is a much more potent predictor of stroke than age or changes in the dicrotic notch, which are reflective of arterial rigidity [12]. Thus, the commonly expressed view that the intraluminal pressure is not as important as the changes in vessel walls would appear to be myth.

MANAGEMENT OF HYPERTENSION

The increased variability of blood pressure in the elderly requires that at least three determinations be made in order to establish a reliable baseline before the initiation of treatment. As with hypertension in younger adults, the standard therapy of hypertension in the elderly involves lifelong administration of oral antihypertensive medications. Other treatments, such as weight loss, while exerting some beneficial effect are rarely corrective and generally only decrease the amount of medication needed. In addition, weight loss and other nonmedication-related therapies are very difficult to accomplish in the elderly. One nonmedical treatment of hypertension in the elderly that merits special attention, however, is surgical correction of renal vascular disease. In elderly individuals with severe occlusive vascular disease that has led to major losses in renal function and hypertension, operative vascular reconstruction in carefully selected individuals has met with surprising success, resulting in correction of blood pressure and return of renal function toward normal. The best candidates for this surgery are individuals with prominent collateral circulation on arteriography, which thus allows the non-functioning renal mass to maintain viability. Another major favorable prognostic finding is a proximal renal artery occlusion with a clear main renal artery distal to the occlusion. Some patients have undergone operative reconstruction months to years after loss of renal function and have recovered dramatically, often over long periods of time, to eventually become normotensive and gain considerable renal function [14,15].

A large body of data is accruing indicating the value of proper management of hypertension. The importance of strict control of blood pressure for the prevention of cerebral hemorrhage from intracerebral aneurysms, at any age, is unquestioned [16]. While most studies of essential hypertension do not focus particularly on the elderly, the data available on geriatric patients suggest, but do not establish, that the benefits of treatment extend into old age. In the Veterans Administration Cooperative Trial of blood pressure in men with diastolic pressure between 90 and 114, approximately 20 percent of the men were over 60 years old. In this older group, treatment was over 50 percent effective and decreased the likelihood of morbid cardiovascular events [17].

The Hypertension Detection and Follow-up Program has recently reported that long-term reduction of elevated diastolic blood pressure to levels below 90 mm Hg is associated with significant reductions in the incidence of fatal and nonfatal stroke in men and women aged 65 to 74 at initiation of treatment [18]. However, the benefit of treatment is less clear in very old institutionalized patients. A randomized controlled trial of methyldopa treatment of nursing home residents (mean age 80 years) in England failed to demonstrate any difference in mortality between treated hypertensive patients, nontreated controls, and normotensive individuals [18a].

As with pharmacotherapy of many disorders in old age, a sensible approach to the management of hypertension in the elderly employs a limited number of agents in as simple a regimen as possible in as low a dose as effective. The elderly are at particular risk for the development of confusion and stroke from hypotension secondary to overenthusiastic antihypertensive therapy [19,20]. Another major risk is the development of orthostatic hypotension and its adverse orthopedic sequelae from diuretic-induced volume depletion. The special vulnerability of the elderly is due in part to an age-related decrease in baroreceptor sensitivity, so that cardio-acceleration in response to posture-induced decreases in pressure is blunted [21]. An additional important factor in the genesis of hypotension-induced central nervous system changes are the dual effects in elderly hypertensives of decreased cerebrovascular autoregulatory capacity coupled with an increased threshold level for the initiation of autoregulatory changes [22,23]. The proper use of specific antihypertensive agents in the elderly is discussed in Chapter 4.

Orthostatic Hypotension

Complaints of dizziness and lightheadedness upon arising from bed or chair are very common among the elderly, particularly those who are chronically ill or the recipients of numerous medications. Unsteadiness on arising is a major cause of morbidity in the elderly, since it leads to confusion, dangerous falls, and avoidance of activity due to insecurity in one's gait. While normal young individuals respond to the assumption of upright posture with a prompt increase in pulse and a slight increase in blood pressure, normal healthy elderly individuals have a blunted pulse increase after standing and a very modest if any increase in blood pressure. While the presence of significant orthostatic reductions in blood pressure among healthy young individuals is very low, a study among elderly persons in Scotland showed that 24 percent of community-dwelling elders experienced reduction of at least 20 mm Hg systolic and 10 mm Hg diastolic upon assuming upright posture [24]. The dramatic impact of age is even more evident when one considers that, in the same study, the prevalence of orthostatic hypotension rose from 16 percent between ages 65 to 74 to 30 percent in individuals over age 75.

Orthostatic hypotension in the elderly may appropriately be viewed as having two major components, the normal or physiologic component and the abnormal or pathologic component. Homeostatic mechanisms responsible for maintaining constancy of blood pressure upon standing are diminished in the elderly, but these changes are not adequate by themselves to result in symptomatic orthostatic hypotension. The elderly are clearly more vulnerable than young adults to the development of orthostatic hypotension when the homeostatic reflexes are further impaired by specific disease states or medications.

PHYSIOLOGIC CHANGES IN BARORECEPTOR MECHANISMS WITH AGE

Baroreceptor mechanisms play a major role in maintaining the adequacy of arterial pressure. Specialized baroreceptors in the carotid artery, aorta, atria, and pulmonary veins represent the afferent limb of the reflex that influences central nervous system regulation of tone of the sympathoadrenal system. The efferent limb includes the sympathetic nerve terminals in heart and blood vessels as well as the adrenal medulla, the source of circulating epinephrine. Advancing age is associated with a marked blunting of the baroreceptor reflex, with impairments in both cardioacceleration during hypotension [25,26] and in cardiac slowing in response to acute increases in blood pressure [21]. Recent studies attempting to evaluate various aspects of the baroreceptor reflex indicate that the responsivity of the sympathetic nervous system to standing, as reflected by circulating levels of plasma norepinephrine, is intact in the elderly [27]. Failure of adequate cardioacceleration thus appears to be related to age-related decreases in myocardial response to adrenergic stimuli. That this effect is stimulus-specific and not a general characteristic of the aging heart is suggested by the intact response of the senescent heart to electrical pacing at rates much greater than those achieved by maximal exercise [28].

PATHOPHYSIOLOGY OF ORTHOSTATIC HYPOTENSION IN THE ELDERLY

Clinically significant orthostatic hypotension can occur in elderly individuals whenever their already weakened cardioacceleratory reflex is joined by any factor that diminishes function of the autonomic nervous system. These abnormalities may occur at any level in the baroreceptor reflex—the afferent, central, or efferent. In addition, orthostatic hypotension may develop in the absence of a defect in autonomic nervous system function but in the presence of a cardiovascular abnormality so severe as to overwhelm the normal regulatory responses of the healthy elderly person. An additional compounding factor, of great importance among many chronically ill patients, is the physiologic deaccommodation that occurs in the autonomic nervous system during prolonged bed rest. Thus, an elderly individual with an intact—for his or her age—autonomic nervous system and a modest cardiovascular abnormality may develop significant orthostatic hypotension once confined to bed for a subacute or chronic illness.

Orthostatic hypotension can be conveniently divided, according to etiologies, into four separate categories (Table 13-1). First, and best understood, are a variety of central nervous system disorders with prominent involvement of the regulatory centers of the autonomic nervous system. Perhaps the best known but by no means the most common is the rather rare Shy-Drager syndrome, which presents with orthostatic hypotension and other sequelae of autonomic insufficiency, including abnormal sweating and decreases in

Table 13-1.   Classification of Orthostatic Hypotension in the Elderly

Autonomic insufficiency based on central nervous system lesions
  Shy-Drager syndrome
  Parkinson's disease
  Cerebrovascular disease
  Wernicke's disease
  Chronic alcoholism
  Medications: phenothiazine, tricyclic antidepressants, methyldopa, clonidine, and other centrally acting psychotropics and antihypertensives
Autonomic insufficiency based on peripheral lesions
  Diabetes mellitus
  Amyloidosis, vitamin deficiencies, paraneoplastic syndromes
  Medications: ganglionic blocking agents, sympatholytic agents
Cardiovascular abnormalities
  Heart block
  Severe varicose veins
  Intravascular volume depletion secondary to salt and water loss, diuretics
  Blood loss
  Medications: hydralazine, prasozin
Idiopathic orthostatic hypotension

sphincter tone. Other neurologic deficits follow after a period of from one to many years, including alterations in gait, muscular rigidity, and features suggestive of Parkinson's disease. Parkinson's disease itself is an important cause of orthostatic hypotension, but unlike the Shy-Drager syndrome the autonomic insufficiency of Parkinson's disease generally occurs late in the course.

Other important central nervous system disorders leading to orthostatic hypotension include multiple small or combined small and large cerebral infarctions, Wernicke's disease, as well as the effects of chronic alcoholism. Perhaps the most commonly encountered central nervous system origin for orthostatic hypotension is represented by the adverse side effects of psychotropic medication, including phenothiazines, tricyclic antidepressants, antianxiety agents, antihypertensive medications with predominantly central effects such as methyldopa and clonidine, and many other agents. The orthostatic hypotension associated with these medications may occur within the therapeutic range and poses a difficult clinical dilemma in patients in whom the target abnormality, whether it be abnormal behavior, depression, or hypertension, is under good control but the unwanted effect of orthostatic hypotension is bothersome.

The second major category of causes of orthostatic hypotension includes disorders of the peripheral autonomic nervous system. This includes diabetes mellitus, generally the rather severe insulin-dependent variety in which severe peripheral neuropathy and other end organ damage is evident, as well as less common entities such as amyloidosis, vitamin deficiencies, and the neuropathies associated with malignancies, particularly cancers of the lung and pancreas. As is the case with disorders of the central nervous system, drugs are an important contributing factor to orthostatic hypotension caused by lack of responsiveness of the peripheral autonomic nervous system, especially ganglionic blocking agents such as guanethidine, which is very dangerous in the elderly, and agents designed to block the peripheral actions of the sympathoadrenal system such as propranolol.

A third category includes those cases of orthostatic hypotension in which the autonomic nervous system appears intact but other cardiovascular factors override the capacity of the homeostatic mechanism. Included in this category are individuals with heart block who are unable to increase their pulse in response to adrenergic stimulation, individuals with severe varicose veins in whom pooling of blood upon standing limits cardiac output, and individuals receiving medications such as hydralazine or prasozin, which cause direct vasodilatation of peripheral vessels. Another important group in this category are individuals whose extracellular fluid and intravascular volume are inadequate secondary to poor salt and water intake, acute intestinal illness, injudicious use of diuretics, or blood loss.

The fourth category of orthostatic hypotension is the idiopathic group. In patients with this type, orthostatic hypotension may be accompanied by other evidence of autonomic dysfunction such as impaired sweating, but other neurologic findings are often absent. While both individuals with idiopathic hypotension without diffuse neurologic findings and individuals with Shy-Drager syndrome fail to increase circulating norepinephrine levels on standing, the basal values are generally low in the idiopathic group, whereas patients with Shy-Drager syndrome have been found to have basal norepinephrine levels within the normal range [29].

CLINICAL PRESENTATION
In many cases impressive reduction in systolic and diastolic blood pressure upon standing can be documented in individuals who steadfastly deny the presence of any symptoms. When symptoms are present they are generally independent of the etiologic basis of the orthostatic hypotension and will generally include dizziness and lightheadedness. While falling is an important consequence of serious reduction in blood pressure on standing, orthostatic hypotension has been found, in two large series, to account for only four percent of falls in the elderly [30,31]. Other symptoms that are occasionally seen are blurred vision, generalized weakness, slurred speech, and ataxia.

MANAGEMENT
The proper management of orthostatic hypotension begins with a clear definition of the presence of significant reductions in blood pressure upon standing. The clinician should not assume that an elderly individual com-

plaining of postural dizziness and lightheadedness is actually suffering from reductions in blood pressure but should measure blood pressure after the patient is recumbent for one hour and then after two minutes of quiet upright standing while carefully monitoring pulse rate. It is often helpful to obtain these measurements on several occasions to confirm the consistent reduction of blood pressure before the introduction of any therapy. The goal of therapy should be reduction or elimination of symptoms. This can often be achieved short of complete correction of orthostatic reductions in blood pressure.

Initial therapeutic considerations are nonpharmacologic and include careful review of any prescribed and over-the-counter medications the patient is taking in order to identify a possible offending agent. In addition, it is important to train individuals to arise slowly from bed as well as from a chair after a long period of recumbency or sitting. Isometric exercises, including handgrip, prior to standing are often very helpful in accelerating pulse and increasing blood pressure. Initiation of a high salt intake program may result in modest weight gain and significant blunting of symptoms of orthostatic hypotension in many individuals. The use of elastic stockings is generally ineffective unless they cover the thigh as well as the calf, and in some cases abdominal binders may be useful.

A wide variety of pharmacologic maneuvers have been attempted in elderly individuals with orthostatic hypotension. While most of these have either been found not to be effective or to require further study, one agent, fludrocortisone acetate, appears to be helpful [32]. This mineralocorticoid, given in daily doses of 0.1 to 1.0 mg, results in an increase in extracellular fluid volume and plasma volume and is accompanied by a modest increase in basal blood pressure. These physiologic changes appear to be adequate to circumvent the homeostatic defect on arising in many individuals with orthostatic hypotension, and a satisfactory response to this medication is seen in most individuals with mild or moderately severe symptoms. With the exception of occasional elevations of blood pressure beyond the acceptable range, complications in treatment are rare. The development of hypokalemia, a theoretical problem with large doses of mineralocorticoids, is rarely a practical problem. Other medications that are receiving increasing attention, but which are of unproved value in the management of orthostatic hypotension in the elderly, include inhibitors of prostaglandin synthesis such as indomethacin and other nonsteroidal, antiinflammatory agents. A variety of sympathomimetic agents have yielded inconsistent results. In very severe cases that are resistant to traditional therapeutic approaches, atrial pacing may be of value.

References

1. Gordon, T., and Shurtleff, D. Means at Each Examination and Interexamination Variation of Specified Characteristics: the Framingham Study.

In W. B. Kannel and T. Gordon (Eds.). Section 29, DHEW publication no. NIH 74478, 1974.

2. Page, L. P., and Sidd, J. J. Medical management of arterial hypertension. *N. Engl. J. Med.* 287:960, 1972.

3. Tudge, C. The biggest risk factor of them all? *World Med.* 13:21, 1978.

4. Harlan, W. R., et al. A thirty-year study of blood pressure in a white male cohort. In G. Onesti, K. E. Kim, and J. H. Moyer (Eds.), *Hypertension: Mechanisms in Management.* New York: Grune & Stratton, 1973.

5. O'Rourke, M. F. Arterial hemodynamics in hypertension. *Circ. Res.* 6(Suppl. 2):123, 1970.

6. Shurtleff, D. Some Characteristics Related to the Incidence of Cardiovascular Disease and Death. In W. B. Kannel and T. Gordon (Eds.), Framingham Study, 18-Year Followup. Section 30, DHEW publication no. NIH 74-599, 1974.

7. Russek, H. I., and Zohman, B. L. Normal blood pressure in senescence. *Geriatrics* 1:113, 1946.

8. Moore-Smith, B. The Management of Hypertension in the Elderly. In M. J. Denham (Ed.), *The Treatment of Medical Problems in the Elderly.* Baltimore: University Park Press, 1980.

9. Miall, W. E., and Chinn, C. Screen for hypertension; some epidemiologic observations. *Br. Med. J.* 35:95, 1974.

10. Dyer, A. R., et al. Hypertension in the elderly. *Med. Clin. North Am.* 61:513, 1977.

11. Kannel, W. B., et al. Epidemiologic assessment of the role of blood pressure in stroke—the Framingham Study. *J.A.M.A.* 214:301, 1970.

12. Kannel, W. B., et al. Systolic blood pressure, arterial rigidity, and risk of stroke. *J.A.M.A.* 245:1229, 1981.

13. Shekelle, R., Ostfeld, A., and Kao, A. Hypertension and risk of stroke in an elderly population. *Stroke* 5:71, 1974.

14. Besarab, B., et al. Reversible renal failure following bilateral renal artery occlusive disease. *J.A.M.A.* 235:2838, 1976.

15. Libertino, J. A., et al. Renal artery revascularization. *J.A.M.A.* 244:1340, 1980.

16. Pickering, G. Hypertension—definitions, natural history, and consequences. *Am. J. Med.* 52:570, 1972.

17. Veterans Administration Cooperative Study Group on Anti-hypertensive Agents. Effects of treatment on morbidity and hypertension: III. Influence of age, diastolic pressure, and prior cardiovascular disease—further analysis of side effects. *Circulation* 45:995, 1972.

18. Hypertension Detection and Follow-up Program Cooperative Group. Five-year findings of the Hypertension Detection and Follow-up Program. *J.A.M.A.* 247:633, 1982.

18a. Sprackling, M. E., et al. Blood pressure reduction in the elderly: a randomized controlled trial of methyldopa. *Br. Med. J.* 283:1151, 1981.

19. Graham, D. I. Ischemic brain damage of cerebral profusion. Failure after treatment of severe hypertension. *Br. Med. J.* 4:739, 1975.

20. Jackson, J., et al. Inappropriate anti-hypertensive therapy in the elderly. *Lancet* 2:1317, 1976.

21. Gribbin, B., et al.   Effect of age and high blood pressure on baroreflex sensitivity in man. *Circ. Res.* 29:424, 1971.
22. Skinhoj, E.   Hemodynamic studies within the brain during migraine. *Arch. Neurol.* 29:95, 1973.
23. Stranguaard, S., et al.   Autoregulation of brain circulation in severe arterial hypertension. *Br. Med. J.* 1:507, 1973.
24. Caird, R. L., Andrews, G. R., and Kennedy, R. D.   Effect of posture on blood pressure in the elderly. *Br. Heart J.* 35:527, 1973.
25. Collins, K. J., et al.   Functional changes in autonomic nervous responses with ageing. *Age Ageing* 9:17, 1980.
26. Minaker, K. L., Rowe, J. W., and Sparrow, D.   Impaired cardiovascular adaptation to vasodilation in the elderly. *Gerontologist* 25:162, 1980.
27. Young, J. B., et al.   Enhanced plasma norepinephrine response to upright posture and oral glucose administration in elderly human subjects. *Metabolism* 29:532, 1980.
28. Lakatta, E. G.   Alterations in the cardiovascular system that occur in advanced age. *Fed. Proc.* 38:163, 1979.
29. Ziegler, M. T., Lake, C. R., and Kopin, I. J.   The sympathetic nervous system defect in primary orthostatic hypotension. *N. Engl. J. Med.* 296:293, 1977.
30. Sheldon, J. H.   On the natural history of falls in old age. *Br. Med. J.* 2:1685, 1960.
31. Clark, A. N. G.   Factors in fracture of the female femur; clinical study of the environmental, physical, medical, and preventive aspects of this injury. *Gerontol. Clin.* 10:257, 1968.
32. Schatz, T. J.   Current management concepts in orthostatic hypotension. *Arch. Intern. Med.* 140:1152, 1980.

14. Peripheral Vascular Disease

Burt Alan Adelman

As the number of elderly persons in our society continues to grow, those conditions that result from advanced atherosclerosis will have an increasing impact on the national health. Although stroke, myocardial infarction, and peripheral vascular disease all too often leave a surviving individual unable to continue an independent life-style, recent medical and surgical advances permit many affected patients to continue to lead productive lives. Advances in the prevention and management of peripheral vascular disease will depend on an increased understanding of the process of atherosclerosis and its consequences. As complex treatment modalities are developed that aim at both prevention of the disease and amelioration of the secondary effects of diseased arteries, the practicing physician will be required to have a broad understanding of the pathobiology of atherosclerosis and its related complications.

This chapter will focus on the pathobiology of atherosclerosis, especially peripheral vascular disease, and its management in the elderly; cerebrovascular disease and coronary artery disease are discussed elsewhere in this book.

Normal Vascular Anatomy

Atherosclerosis is primarily a disease of the elastic arteries—the aorta and its major branches (subclavian, innominate, and proximal common carotid) and the muscular (distributing) arteries (renal, internal carotid, femoral, mesenteric). The wall of both elastic and muscular arteries consists of three concentric tunics: (1) the tunica intima, (2) tunica media, and (3) tunica adventitia.

The boundaries of the intima are formed by a single layer of endothelial cells on the luminal side and the internal elastic lamina on the vessel wall side (Fig. 14-1). In all arteries the endothelial cells lie on a thin, extracellular matrix called the subendothelium. In arteries free of vascular disease, the intima is a thin layer, and the media contains the bulk of the vessel wall. In muscular arteries, the media is composed of a thick band of smooth muscle cells and an extracellular matrix that contains collagen and elastin. In elastic arteries, the media is composed of circumferential bands of elastin between which are dispersed smooth muscle cells. In all arteries, the media provides the necessary strength to allow the vessel to withstand systolic pressure. The adventitia in both vessel types is composed primarily of fibroblasts and contains no smooth muscle cells. In both elastic and large muscular arteries, this coat of fibroblasts provides support for the nerve fibers that penetrate the vessels and the vaso vasorum (vessels of the vessel) that provide nourishment to the outer portion of the media. The adventitia cannot provide adequate physical support to the vessel if the media is weakened.

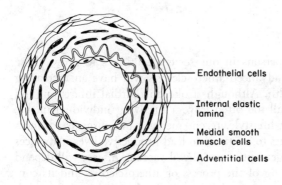

- Endothelial cells
- Internal elastic lamina
- Medial smooth muscle cells
- Adventitial cells

Figure 14-1.   Anatomy of the blood vessel wall.

CELL BIOLOGY OF VESSEL WALL
The Endothelial Cell

Both endothelial and smooth muscle cells are critical to the normal function of the vascular system. The endothelial cell, an important regulator of vascular function and integrity, provides a nonthrombogenic surface to passing blood, synthesizes von Willebrand's factor (an important constituent of the coagulation protein factor VIII), and secretes collagen into the underlying subendothelial basement membrane (contributing to the hemostatic and thrombogenic potential of the vessel wall) [1]. Endothelial cells produce prostaglandin I_2 (see section on prostaglandins and atherosclerosis, p. 229) and thereby contribute to the nonthrombogenic quality of the vessel surface [2]. In addition, endothelial cells maintain a tight barrier that prevents plasma constituents, notably lipid, from passing randomly into the vessel wall. After a fibrin clot forms within a vessel lumen, the endothelial cells are thought to initiate activation of plasminogen to plasmin and thereby facilitate fibrinolysis and clot removal. Clearly, disruption of this important cell will result in major alterations in vessel homeostasis.

Smooth Muscle Cells

Smooth muscle cells have a significant function in the vessel beyond that of establishing vascular tone. They produce many components of the extracellular matrix, including collagen, elastin, and a number of proteoglycans. Smooth muscle cells respond to vascular injury by migrating from the media into the intima, where they proliferate and at the same time produce extracellular matrix. Smooth muscle cell proliferation can also be initiated by low-density lipoproteins and by a platelet-derived mitogenic factor (platelet-derived growth factor). For these reasons smooth muscle cell activity plays an important role in the development of the atherosclerotic lesion [3–5].

Arteriosclerosis

Atherosclerosis is only one form of arteriosclerosis; arteriosclerosis includes all processes that result in loss of elasticity and "hardening" of the arteries. Other entities that are considered arteriosclerotic processes include thrombo-angiitis obliterans (Buerger's disease), Mönckeberg's medial calcinosis, and those changes strictly associated with aging. The word *atherosclerosis* is derived from the Greek word *athera* meaning "gruel" and is an apt description for the grumous, gruellike, material that is commonly found in the central portion of an atherosclerotic plaque.

AGE-RELATED CHANGES IN THE ARTERIAL WALL

Although atherosclerosis is commonly considered a disease of aging, it is not merely an age-related process. Only those biologic changes that affect all individuals in a progressive, irreversible fashion can be considered secondary to the aging process. Age-related vascular changes may predispose the individual to the development of atherosclerosis but are not specifically atherogenic.

Study of animal and human vascular tissue has identified specific histologic changes that occur with aging in the aorta and arteries. As aging progresses, most major vessels develop changes in mineral and protein content. The intima, a thin layer at birth, becomes thickened due to cellular proliferation and fibrosis. Elastin fibers, the extracellular material that gives arteries elasticity, become calcified, thinned, and fragmented. Collagen content increases in both the intima and media, and with time, this collagen becomes progressively rigid and insoluble due to nonenzymatic cross-linking. In addition, as the structural composition of the vessel wall changes, lipid accumulation increases. While the mechanism underlying these changes is not understood, one prominent hypothesis holds that they are a response to constant stress [6].

From a functional standpoint these age-related changes result in a progressive stiffening of vessels, which raises peripheral resistance and limits the capacity of the vascular system to increase organ blood flow. Further, baro-receptor function is impaired since stiff vessel walls dampen the transmission of the systolic pressure wave.

Epidemiology of Atherosclerotic Vascular Disease

Extensive epidemiologic study has identified several risk factors for the development of atherosclerosis. Atherosclerotic vascular disease is most prevalent in Western industrialized areas and is closely associated with dietary habits that contribute to elevated levels of serum cholesterol. Other important risk factors include cigarette smoking, hypertension, type A personality trait, diabetes, male sex, and hereditary influences [7]. Table 14-1, from the

Table 14-1. Incidence of Cardiovascular Events According to Age and Sex

| | Average Annual Incidence per 1,000 | | | | | | | |
| | Coronary Heart Disease | | Cerebrovascular Accident | | Peripheral Arterial Disease | | Congestive Heart Failure | |
Age	Men	Women	Men	Women	Men	Women	Men	Women
45 to 54	9.9	3.1	2.0	0.9	1.8	0.6	1.8	0.8
55 to 64	20.8	9.5	3.2	2.9	5.1	1.9	4.3	2.7
65 to 74	20.4	14.5	8.4	8.6	6.3	3.8	8.2	6.8

Source: Modified from W. B. Kannel and T. Gordon. Cardiovascular Risk Factors in the Aged: The Framingham Study. In S. G. Haynes and M. Feinleb (Eds.), *Epidemiology of Aging*. NIH Publication No. 80-969, 1980.

Framingham Study 20-year follow-up, shows the incidence of specific cardiovascular events according to age and sex.

While the incidence of cardiovascular disease continues to increase with age, the impact of some specific risk factors, including serum cholesterol levels, cigarette smoking, and diabetes, declines after age 65. Hypertension, however, remains a significant factor even in the elderly (see Chap. 13). Since no level of elevated blood pressure is without a discernible effect on risk, careful attention must be given to treatment of high blood pressure in

Table 14-2. Attributable Risk for Hypertension According to Age*

Age	Overall Mortality	Cardiovascular Mortality	Cardiovascular Morbidity
Men			
45 to 54	17.9	29.3	16.4
55 to 64	16.1	21.4	17.9
65 to 74	8.4	12.9	18.8
Women			
45 to 54	12.0	28.6	17.4
55 to 64	8.5	17.5	26.5
65 to 74	14.9	34.5	26.9

Source: Modified from W. B. Kannel and T. Gordon. Cardiovascular Risk Factors in the Aged: The Framingham Study. In S. G. Haynes and M. Feinleb (Eds.), *Epidemiology of Aging*. NIH Publication No. 80-969, 1980.
* Attributable risk = total population rate − non-hypertensive population rate/total population rate × 100.

Table 14-3. Average Annual Incidence of Intermittent Claudication According to Age and Sex, per 10,000

Age Group (yrs)	No. of Men	No. of Women
45 to 54	18	5
55 to 64	51	19
65 to 74	59	40

Source: From N. C. Peabody, W. B. Kannel, and P. M. McNamara. Intermittent claudication: surgical significance. *Arch. Surg.* 109:693, 1974.

Table 14-4. Subsequent Occurrence of Major Cardiovascular Events in Persons Aged 50 to 76 Years With Claudication

Years After Onset of Intermittent Claudication	Cumulative % with Cardiovascular Disease	
	Men	Women
2	7	20
4	25	34
6	43	39
8	47	45
10	56	66

Source: From N. C. Peabody, W. B. Kannel, and P. M. McNamara. Intermittent claudication: surgical significance. *Arch. Surg.* 109:693, 1974.

the elderly (Table 14-2). Interestingly, high-density lipoprotein (HDL) in both men and women up to the age of 80 continues to play an important role in inhibiting atherosclerosis.

PERIPHERAL VASCULAR DISEASE
Because the main clinical focus of this chapter is on peripheral vascular disease, some specific comments on its epidemiology are indicated. The incidence of intermittent claudication continues to rise with age in both sexes (Table 14-3). In addition there is a high correlation between the presence of peripheral vascular disease, as indicated by claudication, and the subsequent occurrence of a major cardiovascular event (Table 14-4).

All major studies of the epidemiology of peripheral vascular disease have identified cigarette smoking and diabetes as the most significant risk factors. In the Framingham Study a strong association was found between peripheral vascular disease and cigarette smoking in men of all ages and in women over 60. Between the ages of 60 and 69 the incidence of intermittent claudication in cigarette smokers is twice that of nonsmokers [8]. Diabetes imparts an even greater risk. The cumulative incidence of peripheral vascular disease following the diagnosis of diabetes is estimated to be 15 percent at 10 years and 45 percent at 20 years. In addition, among persistent smokers and diabetics, progression from stable claudication to advanced ischemia requiring amputation is quite high [9,10].

The Atherosclerotic Plaque
HISTOLOGY
The characteristic atherosclerotic lesion is a thickening of the intima that extends into the lumen. In extensive lesions the media is also involved. Within the plaque a number of distinct regions are seen. The roof of the plaque is composed of fibrous connective tissue containing collagen, smooth muscle cells, and amorphous extracellular material. Underlying the fibrous cap is the lipid-containing region, in which cholesterol crystals may be seen along with calcium deposits and fat-filled cells. Some plaques are predominantly fibrotic and others contain large amounts of grumous lipid material. The advanced plaque can further progress to a "complicated plaque" following any of a number of possible events: rupture of the fibrous cap, necrosis of the underlying media, or hemorrhage into the lesion. Such a lesion is highly thrombogenic and liable to promote embolization of its lipid contents or of adherent thrombus.

From this description of the atherosclerotic lesion, it becomes clear how this slowly progressing process can suddenly cause dramatic clinical events. Progressive encroachment on the vascular lumen by plaque formation causes the syndromes of angina pectoris and intermittent claudication. Transient ischemic attacks may be due to embolization of plaque contents, thrombus material, or intermittent vascular obstruction promoted by advanced lesions. In patients with amaurosis fugax, it is possible to visualize cholesterol emboli passing through the retinal vessels by direct ophthalmoscopy. These emboli are characteristically refractile in appearance. Stroke, myocardial infarction, gangrene of the extremities, and ischemic bowel syndromes may be due to any single or combined process. In the aorta the associated surface is highly thrombogenic and can promote the development of secondary thrombotic events, including obstruction of the distal aorta and embolization to the extremities. Aortic aneurysms result from extensive complicated plaque formation that compromises the mechanical strength of the vessel by extending into the media.

MECHANISM OF PLAQUE FORMATION
The leading hypothesis regarding the development of atherosclerosis is called the "response to injury" theory; it holds that the initiating event in the early development of the atherosclerotic lesion is endothelial cell injury, either desquamation of endothelial cells or alterations in their functional integrity

[11–13]. Desquamation would allow for platelet adhesion and secretion of the growth factor into the media where it would stimulate smooth muscle cell proliferation and migration into the intima. Entry of low-density lipoprotein into the media would also be facilitated by endothelial cell damage and would also cause smooth muscle cell proliferation.

The continuous repetition of these initiating events in the appropriate setting of hypertension, cigarette smoking, diabetes, and hypercholesterolemia would allow for the development of full-fledged atherosclerotic lesions. Experimental evidence from animal studies suggests that regrowth of endothelial cells over these early lesions in the presence of elevated serum cholesterol levels, can actually contribute to the trapping and concentrating of lipid within the arterial wall [14]. In humans the factors that cause the initial endothelial cell injury have not been identified specifically, but evidence from animal experiments supports the possible role of cigarettes, hypertension, antibody-antigen complexes, and cholesterol [15,16]. Finally, there are numerous hereditary factors, all of which are poorly understood, that determine an individual's overall response to any and all of these factors.

Prostaglandins and Atherosclerosis

It is clear from the preceding discussion that activation of the coagulation system is critical to the development of the atherosclerotic lesion and to the production of clinical disease [17]. Recently the possible role of various prostaglandins in vascular homeostasis has gained wide interest. These ubiquitous fatty acid compounds are produced in many tissues and can circulate throughout the body. Endothelial cells make a prostaglandin called prostaglandin I_2 (PGI_2, or prostacyclin), which acts as a vasodilator and potent inhibitor of platelet adhesion and aggregation. The continual production of PGI_2 by vascular endothelial cells is postulated to be important in modulating the reactivity of the vessel surface with circulating platelets [18,19]. Vascular smooth muscle cells also make PGI_2.

Platelets make a number of prostaglandins and related compounds, the most important of which is thromboxane A_2, a vasoconstrictor and platelet-aggregating agent. Thromboxane A_2 production is stimulated when platelets adhere to exposed collagen surfaces such as would occur after vascular injury. Thus, an important interplay may exist between endothelial cell production of PGI_2 and platelet production of thromboxane A_2, the net effect of which may modulate platelet activation [20].

The existence of a hypercoagulable state in patients with advanced atherosclerosis has often been suggested but never documented clearly. Current data suggest that vessels involved with atherosclerotic plaques produce less PGI_2, and that the platelets of hyperlipidemic individuals and diabetics may be more sensitive to aggregating agents, perhaps because they produce more thromboxane A_2 [21,22]. Although this evidence is still preliminary, it can serve to help identify drugs that should be tested in clinical trials.

Clinical Manifestations of Peripheral Vascular Disease

The primary cause of obstructive arterial disease affecting the lower extremities is atherosclerosis. When obstructed vessels cannot supply muscle, skin, and nerves adequately, ischemic complications develop. Although affected individuals commonly have diffuse vascular disease in both limbs at the time of presentation, clinical symptoms are usually a result of a critical narrowing in one particular part of the arterial tree [23,24].

CLINICAL PRESENTATION

The most characteristic clinical sign of atherosclerotic disease in the legs is pain on exertion that is relieved by rest, known as intermittent claudication. Although cramping pain is the most common complaint, individuals also report fatigue and weakness in affected legs. An important characteristic of intermittent claudication is the consistency of the precipitating event; the amount of exertion that produces symptoms in any one individual is constant, for example, cramping pain always occurs after walking the same number of city blocks.

Location of the critical stenosis often determines the specific symptoms. High aortic obstruction is associated with buttock and low back pain. Aorto-iliac disease may cause thigh and calf pain. Iliofemoral disease usually causes foot and calf pain, while popliteal and calf artery obstruction affects the foot. In general, calf pain is the most common symptom of individuals having disease above the popliteal artery.

The spectrum of clinical symptoms associated with occlusive vascular disease is determined by the relative adequacy of collateral flow around areas of critical stenosis, degree of exertion required by the patient to function satisfactorily, and by a host of systemic factors such as cardiac output, presence of anemia, blood viscosity, and recurrent embolization.

Rest Pain, Ulcers, Gangrene

Pain at rest results from advanced obstructive disease complicated by poor collateral flow. Affected individuals complain of pain that first begins in the toes and may progress to involve the entire lower leg. Painful ulcerations of the foot and ankle may also develop in these individuals. Ischemic neuropathy may accompany rest pain, causing patients to suffer various disturbing sensations, including numbness, burning, and electric shocks. In advanced diabetes, however, neuropathic changes may actually result in loss of pain sensation in the foot or lower leg. Gangrene is the most severe complication of ischemic vascular disease; its presence signifies total loss of blood flow to the affected area.

PHYSICAL EXAMINATION

A careful history and physical examination will help to identify arterial insufficiency as the cause of leg pain. Loss of normal or previously present pulses is helpful in localizing the distal side of a stenotic lesion. Bruits are also indicative of stenosis. Careful examination of the abdomen and popliteal vessels is performed to detect possible aneurysm formation.

Skin color may suggest vascular insufficiency. In severe disease the feet are often red or violacious, with areas of mottled discoloration; pallor on elevation and rubor on dependency are characteristic of arterial insufficiency in the legs. In normal individuals the plantar surfaces of the feet remain pink during elevation; in patients with vascular insufficiency and poor collateralization, the plantar surface develops pallor during this maneuver. If following elevation the patient is asked to place his feet in a dependent position, venous filling time can be estimated. In normal individuals venous filling occurs within 20 seconds; in the presence of severe arterial insufficiency, filling time may exceed 30 seconds.

Characteristic trophic changes include thinning of the skin, loss of hair, and thickening of the nails. The thinned skin is susceptible to fissure formation that often results in infection and ulceration. Muscle mass may decrease in ischemic areas and further contribute to patient complaints of weakness.

Additional diagnostic procedures may be undertaken to better define the extent and severity of disease or to assist in making a diagnosis in an unusual situation. Systolic pressure can be measured in the leg before and after exercise, and ultrasonography can be used to visualize the aorta. Segmental plethysmography allows measurement of blood volume and flow characteristics.

Angiography is rarely indicated as a diagnostic tool; its main usefulness is in evaluating patients before arterial reconstruction and in detecting emboli. Caution must be exercised in its use because elderly patients are particularly susceptible to the toxic effects of contrast media on the kidney.

DIFFERENTIAL DIAGNOSIS
In general, differentiation of occlusive atherosclerotic vascular disease from other entities causing leg pain or affecting blood flow in the extremities is not difficult. Vascular syndromes affecting the legs include thromboangiitis obliterans (Buerger's disease), arterial embolism, and venous disease.

Thromboangiitis Obliterans
Thromboangiitis obliterans is a poorly understood disorder characteristically affecting young men between the ages of 20 and 40. Affected individuals develop upper and lower extremity ischemia, and a high percentage of them have migratory thrombophlebitis. Vascular lesions show a characteristic pattern on biopsy. Unlike atherosclerotic disease, this disorder is not associated with diabetes mellitus, hypercholesterolemia, or hypertension but occurs almost solely in cigarette smokers. In patients who have thromboangiitis obliterans, symptoms of progressive vascular obstruction are often relieved by cessation of cigarette smoking [25].

Arterial Embolus

Symptoms associated with arterial embolus may vary from pain at rest to intermittent claudication; however, the onset of symptoms is almost always sudden. The sudden loss of a pulse in a patient with no other evidence of severe vascular disease should make the examiner suspicious of an embolic event, but a specific source for emboli must be identified before the diagnosis can be confirmed. The most common source of peripheral emboli is the heart, particularly in the setting of atrial fibrillation, recent myocardial infarction, or infective endocarditis. Less commonly, emboli will dislodge from a complicated atherosclerotic plaque in the aorta. In patients with advanced atherosclerosis, differentiating local thrombosis of an atherosclerotic plaque from embolic occlusion may be impossible. If thrombectomy is planned, definitive diagnosis can be made via arteriography. Local treatment must be supplemented by systemic anticoagulation or some other definitive therapy to prevent further embolization.

Venous Disease

Pain is commonly associated with both acute deep venous thrombosis and chronic venous insufficiency. However, differentiating venous from arterial disease is usually not difficult. Careful examination of the pulses is essential because venous disease is not associated with a loss of arterial pulsations. Swelling of the affected extremity is always present in venous disease. Pain associated with acute phlebitis is localized over the affected vein, which may be palpable as a cord. Chronic venous disease is characterized by pigmentation of the medial aspect of the calf with ulcer formation over the medial malleolar area; arterial insufficiency ulcers are more commonly located over the lateral malleolus. Total venous obstruction of an extremity can result in secondary arterial thrombosis and loss of arterial pulsations. This condition, phlegmasia cerulea dolens, occurs only in the most severe cases of acute venous insufficiency and is characterized by pain, swelling, cyanosis, and extensive gangrene.

Musculoskeletal Disorders

Patients with degenerative joint disease involving the hip or knee will experience pain on exertion, particularly in association with weight-bearing. Physical examination reveals pain elicited by the movement of the affected joint. In inflammatory arthritis, synovial effusion or thickening is found.

Neurologic Disorders

Lumbar disk disease is commonly associated with pain on exertion. However, because pain is related to pressure on nerves and not affected by metabolic demand, bedside examination can reproduce the pain syndrome. Sciatic and femoral nerve syndromes have characteristic pain patterns and are often accompanied by specific defects noted on neurologic examination, such as muscle group weakness and loss of reflexes. The presence of intact pulses helps to rule out arterial disease.

Spinal stenosis resulting from hypertrophic bony growth or disk herniation can cause a "pseudoclaudication" syndrome in which compression of the cauda equina or its vascular supply causes lower back and leg pain during activity. Spinal stenosis may be differentiated from aortoiliac occlusion by a careful history, which may reveal that the specific events leading to the production of pain are not as precisely reproducible as one would expect in atherosclerotic vascular disease. Myelography, computerized axial tomography, and arteriography may be needed to confirm the diagnosis.

Neuropathic pains and paresthesias are associated with both vascular and nonvascular disease. A careful history and examination will help sort out the diagnosis. However, particularly in diabetic patients, primary neuropathic and vascular problems may be present together. In these patients the physician must use his or her clinical judgment to determine if extensive evaluation is needed to establish whether correctable vascular or neurologic disease is present.

Erythromelalgia
Erythromelalgia is a rare condition characterized by pain and redness in the feet associated with exposure to heat, exercise, or dependency. On examination, the feet are warm and pulses are intact; occasionally edema is present. Erythromelalgia is of unknown origin and treatment is primarily symptomatic.

CLINICAL COURSE AND PROGNOSIS
The clinical course of atherosclerosis of the lower extremities is surprisingly benign [9,23,26]. Progressive disease requiring arterial reconstruction or amputation develops in less than one-third of patients who have intermittent claudication. However, in diabetics or in patients who continue to smoke cigarettes after the onset of symptoms, progression of disease is more common and the amputation rate is higher.

It is important to recognize that intermittent claudication is usually associated with generalized atherosclerotic vascular disease. As seen in Table 14-5, individuals in whom intermittent claudication develops have a high incidence of generalized cardiovascular morbidity and mortality. Any individual who has intermittent claudication deserves a careful cardiovascular assessment and continued follow-up study.

GENERAL PRINCIPLES OF THERAPY
The intention of either medical or surgical therapy in patients with atherosclerotic vascular disease of the lower extremities is to relieve pain, preserve tissue, and maintain as high a level of physical function as possible [27]. Medical therapy necessitates a common-sense approach that recognizes that

Table 14-5. Cardiovascular Comorbidity in Framingham Study Subjects Developing Intermittent Claudication*

Cardiovascular Disease	101 Men		61 Women	
	No.	%	No.	%
None	51	52	39	64
Coronary heart disease	44	44	21	34
Atheromatous brain infarction	4	4	2	3
Congestive heart failure	11	11	4	7

Source: From N. C. Peabody, W. B. Kannel, and P. M. McNamara. Intermittent claudication: surgical significance. *Arch. Surg.* 109:693, 1974.
* Subjects aged 35 to 76 years. Cardiovascular events not mutually exclusive.

most affected individuals have advanced generalized atherosclerosis. Because hypertension is associated with an increased risk of accelerated vascular impairment, it should always be treated adequately. In addition, hyperlipidemia should be treated, and diabetes, if present, should be controlled. It is unlikely, however, that control of diabetes will prevent progression of vascular disease.

All patients who are obese should be encouraged to lose weight. Although exercise is currently included in the rehabilitation of patients with coronary artery disease, its place in the treatment of intermittent claudication has not been proved. Nonetheless, some data suggest that daily exercise to tolerance can eventually increase maximum walking distance. All patients who smoke must be encouraged to stop. Although this will not improve symptoms, it may prevent progression of atherosclerosis and some secondary features, particularly the development of skin ulcers since nicotine decreases blood flow to the skin.

The use of vasodilator drugs is without proven merit and cannot be recommended. Whatever beneficial effects vasodilation can have on blood flow can be achieved by advising patients to keep their legs warm.

All patients with ischemic leg disease need careful instruction regarding care of skin and nails. The skin should be kept lubricated with lanolin or other mild emollients, and nails should be kept trimmed. Fungal infections should be treated immediately and any other infection given close attention. Foot care is often best administered by a podiatrist or surgeon particularly sensitive to the complications of vascular insufficiency. Patients should be informed that any break in the skin that does not heal rapidly should be brought to the attention of their physician.

Anticoagulants and Antiplatelet Agents
Drugs that affect blood clotting are divided into two classes. Agents that affect the fluid phase coagulant proteins are commonly referred to as anti-

coagulants; agents that inhibit platelet function are called antiplatelet agents. The major anticoagulants are heparin, bishydroxycoumarin (Dicumarol), warfarin (Coumadin, Panwarfarin), and the indanedione derivatives.

Heparin inhibits clotting by accelerating the activity of antithrombin III, a naturally occurring protein inhibitor of activated coagulation factors. It is commonly used for therapy in acute deep venous thrombosis, pulmonary embolization, and in some cases, arterial thrombosis or embolization. Because it must be administered parenterally its chronic use is awkward.

The other anticoagulants are administered orally and thus are suitable for long-term use. All have the same pharmacologic action—to interfere with synthesis of the vitamin K-dependent coagulant proteins, factors II, VII, IX, and X. As is the case with heparin, this effect ultimately prevents fibrinogen conversion to fibrin and interrupts clot formation. Although these agents have been used in patients with advanced atherosclerotic peripheral vascular disease, little evidence exists to support their universal application.

In patients with transient ischemic attacks there is some evidence to suggest a beneficial effect of long-term anticoagulant therapy. The combined results of several studies show that oral anticoagulants reduced the incidence of eventual stroke to 5.6 percent in treated patients, from 15.7 percent in untreated patients; in other studies the results are less impressive [28]. Caution must be exercised in interpreting these results because even the best currently available studies are poorly controlled. Nonetheless, a general trend suggests some efficacy. Long-term use of these agents is generally associated with a significant incidence of major and minor hemorrhage, averaging about 2 and 4 percent, respectively.

Because platelets are an important constituent of arterial thrombi and may be critical in initiating the development of atherosclerosis, much emphasis has been placed on determining the efficacy of antiplatelet agents in the treatment and prevention of atherosclerosis and its associated clinical manifestations [29]. Numerous compounds inhibit platelet function in vivo or in vitro; however, very few agents have been identified that can be easily taken by patients in doses that produce reliable results with minimal side effects.

Aspirin irreversibly inhibits the platelet enzyme cyclooxygenase, blocking the production of thromboxane A_2. Because platelets are anucleate they cannot replace the affected enzyme. The dose of aspirin needed to exert this effect is small; a single daily 160-mg dose (one-half the usual tablet) will inhibit platelet function as determined by bleeding time and platelet aggregation [30]. Because higher concentrations of aspirin can temporarily inhibit endothelial cell PGI_2 synthesis, and perhaps have a thrombogenic effect, the exact dose that affects platelets specifically has not yet been determined. Other nonsteroidal antiinflammatory drugs (ibuprofen, indomethacin) have a similar, but reversible, effect on platelet cyclooxygenase. Dipyridamole and sulfinpyrazone both inhibit platelet function; however, their specific modes of action are not well understood.

Clinical trials of antiplatelet therapy have centered primarily on patients with cerebrovascular disease or myocardial infarction. No good evidence exists to support the chronic use of these agents in patients with peripheral vascular disease. In patients who have had transient ischemic attacks and were treated with aspirin, a number of prospective studies have noted a reduction in the incidence of stroke and an increase in patient survival. Most recently, the Canadian Cooperative Study Group trial demonstrated a significant risk reduction for stroke and death in men receiving 1,300 mg of aspirin a day. Sulfinpyrazone, 800 mg a day, had no effect when taken alone and did not augment the effect of aspirin. No significant risk reduction was noted for women in any of the treatment groups [31].

The ability of aspirin to reduce subsequent cardiovascular mortality after an initial myocardial infarction has been studied extensively. In most trials with aspirin or aspirin and dipyridamole, a favorable trend has been observed; however, no study has produced results that are statistically significant [32].

SURGICAL TREATMENT
Surgical treatment of peripheral vascular disease includes sympathectomy, arterial bypass, or amputation. Sympathectomy results in vasodilatation of cutaneous blood vessels and thus may be helpful in the treatment of patients with rest pain and ischemic ulcers. The effect of sympathectomy on skeletal muscle is minimal; therefore, no improvement will be noted by patients with intermittent claudication. The procedure can be performed via local instillation of alcohol or by direct surgical section. Before considering sympathectomy in any patient, it is important to demonstrate that sympathetic activity is intact. Simple tests include noting the ability of the affected limb to sweat when warmed, or documenting an increase in skin temperature after sympathetic block with local anesthetic.

Bypass Surgery
Arterial bypass surgery in a patient with advanced peripheral vascular disease can result in improved functional capacity and salvage of dangerously ischemic tissue. However, because over two-thirds of affected individuals have stable disease, careful selection of patients for operation is essential. The primary reason for surgical intervention is the presence of significant ischemic symptoms at rest, especially pain and ulceration. Rapid progression of symptoms or intermittent claudication of such severity that the patient suffers intolerable changes in life-style are adequate reasons for surgery. Because patients generally have diffuse disease, the operative procedure is aimed at alleviating the most significant lesions.

Careful arteriographic examination of the circulation in the affected extremity and aortic bifurcation is usually necessary to help plan the procedure and evaluate the extent of collateral flow. Furthermore, the general condition of the patient is also an important consideration; in particular, the location and extent of other sites of atherosclerotic disease must be determined. Severe carotid or coronary artery disease may require prior surgical or medical treatment to improve operative morbidity for intended peripheral vascular surgery. In addition, most surgeons believe that continued cigarette smoking will adversely affect the patency of grafts and therefore insist that persons considered for surgery stop smoking.

Aortoiliac Disease

The favored surgical technique for the amelioration of aortoiliac disease is to replace or bypass the bifurcation with a knitted Dacron graft. This necessitates an intraabdominal approach that can be quite stressful to the patient. Overall mortality for this procedure is between 2.5 and 9.3 percent, and five-year patency rates are between 70 and 90 percent [23,33,34]. Complications include groin infection and aneurysm formation at the site of anastomosis. Return of symptoms is usually the result of progression of disease distal to surgical repair.

In patients too ill to undergo extensive abdominal surgery, an axillofemoral bypass procedure may be attempted. In this procedure a synthetic graft is tunnelled subcutaneously between the axillary artery and the femoral artery. The operative mortality is less than 2 percent and although the thrombosis rate at one year is as high as 40 percent, the graft can be easily thrombectomized, so that patency rates of 76 percent have been reported at five years [23,35]. Femoral-femoral bypass procedures can also be utilized in high-risk patients.

Femoropopliteal Disease and Distal Disease

Surgical repair of disease in the femoropopliteal region usually necessitates the placement of an autogenous saphenous vein graft. If a vein suitable for grafting is not available, synthetic materials can be used. It is difficult to evaluate the published results of these procedures because indications for surgery as well as extent of disease vary. In general, operative mortality ranges from 2 to 7 percent; five-year patency rates vary from 58 to 72 percent [36].

Obstructed vessels of the calf can also be bypassed surgically. Such procedures also involve use of autogenous vein grafts. A successful outcome can prevent the loss of a foot or toes through gangrene.

Amputation

Amputation remains a necessary form of treatment in some patients with advanced atherosclerosis. Gangrene involving the foot or leg or intractable pain are the usual indications for amputation. Arteriography should be performed to ensure that a bypass procedure cannot be attempted. Amputations should involve the least amount of tissue necessary but should be at a level at which an adequate vascular supply will ensure satisfactory healing.

ABDOMINAL AORTIC ANEURYSM

Advanced atherosclerosis is the primary cause of abdominal aortic aneurysms. Complicated atherosclerotic lesions erode into the aortic media directly or obstruct its nutritional supply. Once the media is sufficiently weakened to allow expansion of the vessel, progressive widening becomes inevitable because wall tension increases as the radius increases (LaPlace's law). In general, the greatest incidence of abdominal aneurysm appears to be during the seventh decade. Men are affected six times as often as women. The same risk factors associated with other forms of atherosclerosis apply to the development of aortic aneurysms. The majority of patients with atherosclerotic aneurysms have associated cardiovascular disease.

Dilatation of the abdominal aorta beyond 3 cm is considered aneurysmal. The majority of aneurysms are fusiform in shape though some may be globular. All are filled with laminated thrombus, which only rarely obstructs the lumen. Over 97 percent of abdominal aneurysms end below the renal arteries; distal extension commonly includes the aortic bifurcation and can involve the iliac arteries.

Approximately 40 percent of patients with an abdominal aneurysm will have symptoms at the time of discovery. The most common symptoms include abdominal pain, back pain, pulsation in the abdomen, and discovery of an abdominal mass. On physical examination the most important finding is that of a pulsatile abdominal mass. Aneurysms less than 4.5 cm may be difficult to feel. Because ultrasound examination can provide definitive diagnostic information in almost every instance, any suspicious lesion should be examined by this technique. Angiography is not generally indicated for diagnosis and can actually provide misleading information; actual aneurysm size is difficult to assess by angiography because only the lumen of the aorta is visualized [37].

The natural history of untreated abdominal aneurysms is striking. The five-year survival of affected patients approximates 20 percent, with over half of the patients dying of rupture. In general, the risk of rupture is directly related to the size of the aneurysm. Half of all aneurysms over 6 cm rupture within one year, while 15 to 20 percent of those less than 6 cm will rupture in one year [38].

In light of the high risk of fatal rupture, surgical resection of an abdominal aneurysm seems a highly desirable alternative. All patients with an aneurysm over 6 cm should be considered for elective surgery. An aneurysm between 4 and 5 cm should be carefully followed by serial echo examination and surgery recommended if the growth rate exceeds 1 cm in a year [37].

The surgical procedure necessitates incising the aneurysm longitudinally, removing the aortic contents, and leaving the posterior wall intact. A woven Dacron prosthesis is placed in this cleared bed and sutured into place. The remaining wall is then reapproximated over the graft. In most instances the inferior mesenteric artery is ligated during the procedure.

Operative mortality appears to depend on the general status of the patient, but most importantly on whether the aneurysm has ruptured or is leaking. Currently, operative mortality in good-risk patients should approximate 4 to 8 percent, with many centers reporting mortality rates less than 4 percent. Five-year survival following surgery ranges between 50 and 78 percent. Operative mortality in patients with an expanding aneurysm rises to between 5 to 15 percent, and in patients with a ruptured aneurysm, operative mortality is approximately 50 to 60 percent [37]. Age alone is not a significant risk factor; a number of studies have indicated that immediate surgical mortality in the elderly can be kept to 5 percent by applying the same guidelines for patient selection as are generally used [39].

Acute complications of aneurysm surgery include myocardial infarction, peripheral arterial occlusion, acute renal insufficiency, colonic arterial insufficiency, aortoenteric fistula with gastrointestinal bleeding, and wound infection. Late complications include graft occlusion or stenosis, false aneurysm formation, enteric fistula, and infection.

References

1. Gimbrone, M. A., Jr. Culture of Vascular Endothelium. In T. H. Spaet (Ed.), *Progress in Hemostasis and Thrombosis*. New York: Grune & Stratton, 1976. Vol. III.
2. Moncada, S., and Amezcua, J. L. Prostacyclin, thromboxane A_2 interactions in hemostasis and thrombosis. *Haemostasis* 8:252, 1979.
3. Ross, R., and Glomset, J. S. Atherosclerosis: a problem in the biology of the arterial smooth muscle cell. *Science* 180:1332, 1973.
4. Scher, C. D., et al. The Initiation of Cell Replication by Cationic Polypeptide Hormones. In F. E. Bloom (Ed.), *Peptides: Integrators of Cell and Tissue Function*. New York: Raven Press, 1980.
5. Fischer-Dzoga, K., and Wissler, R. W. Stimulation of proliferation in stationary primary cultures of monkey aortic smooth muscle cells: II. Effect of varying concentrations of hyperlipemic serum and low density lipoproteins of varying dietary fat origins. *Atherosclerosis* 24:515, 1976.
6. Kohn, R. R. Heart and Cardiovascular System. In C. E. Finch and L. Hayflick (Eds.), *Handbook of the Biology of Aging*. New York: Van Nostrand Reinhold, 1977.
7. Dawber, T. R. *The Framingham Study: The Epidemiology of Atherosclerotic Disease*. Cambridge, Mass.: Harvard University Press, 1980.
8. Kannel, W. B., and Shurtleff, D. Cigarettes and the development of intermittent claudication. *Geriatrics* 28:61, 1973.
9. Juergens, J. L., Barker, N. W., and Hines, E. A., Jr. Arteriosclerosis obliterans: review of 520 cases with special reference to pathogenic and prognostic factors. *Circulation* 21:188, 1960.
10. Melton, L. J., III, et al. Incidence and prevalence of clinical peripheral vascular disease in a population-based cohort of diabetic patients. *Diabetes Care* 3:650, 1980.

11. Harker, L. A., Ross, R., and Glomset, J. A.   The role of endothelial cell injury and platelet response in atherogenesis. *Thromb. Haemost.* 39:312, 1978.
12. Wissler, R. W.   Principles of the Pathogenesis of Atherosclerosis. In E. Braunwald (Ed.), *Heart Disease: A Textbook of Cardiovascular Medicine.* Philadelphia: Saunders, 1980.
13. Ross, R., and Glomset, J. A.   The pathogenesis of atherosclerosis. *N. Engl. J. Med.* 295:369, 1976.
14. Minick, C. R., Stemerman, M. B., and Insull, W., Jr.   Role of endothelium and hypercholesterolemia in intimal thickening and lipid accumulation. *Am. J. Pathol.* 95:131, 1979.
15. Kottke, B. A., and Sobbiah, M. T. R.   Pathogenesis of atherosclerosis concepts based on animal models. *Mayo Clin. Proc.* 53:35, 1978.
16. McGill, H. C., Jr.   Atherosclerosis: Problems in pathogenesis. In R. Paoletti and A. M. Gotto (Eds.), *Atherosclerosis Reviews.* New York: Raven Press, 1977. Vol. 2.
17. Stemerman, M. B.   Hemostasis, thrombosis, and atherogenesis. In R. Paoletti and A. M. Gotto (Eds.), *Atherosclerosis Reviews.* New York: Raven Press, 1979. Vol. 7.
18. Moncada, S., et al.   An enzyme isolated from human arteries transforms prostaglandin endoperoxides to an unstable substance that inhibits platelet aggregation. *Nature* 263:663, 1976.
19. Curwen, K. D., Gimbrone, M. A., and Handin, R. I.   In vitro studies of thromboresistance: the role of prostacyclin in platelet adhesion to cultured normal and virally transformed human vascular endothelial cells. *Lab. Invest.* 42:366, 1980.
20. Marcus, A. J.   The role of lipids in platelet function: with particular reference to the arachadonic acid pathway. *J. Lipid Res.* 19:793, 1978.
21. Dembinska-Kiec, A., et al.   The generation of prostacyclin by arteries and by the coronary vascular bed is reduced in experimental atherosclerosis in rabbits. *Prostaglandins* 14:1025, 1977.
22. Ziboh, V. A., et al.   Increased biosynthesis of thromboxane A_2 by diabetic platelets. *Eur. J. Clin. Invest.* 9:223, 1979.
23. Coffman, J. D.   Intermittent claudication and rest pain: physiologic concepts and therapeutic approaches. *Prog. Cardiovasc. Dis.* 22:53, 1979.
24. Juergens, J. L., and Bernatz, P. E.   Atherosclerosis of the Extremities. In J. L. Juergens, J. A. Spittell, and J. F. Fairbairn II (Eds.), *Peripheral Vascular Diseases.* Philadelphia: Saunders, 1980.
25. McKusick, V. A., et al.   Buerger's disease: a distinct clinical and pathological entity. *J.A.M.A.* 181:93, 1962.
26. Imparato, A. M., et al.   Intermittent claudication: Its natural course. *Surgery* 78:795, 1975.
27. Fairbairn, J. F. II, and Juergens, J. L.   Principles of Medical Management. In J. L. Juergens, J. A. Spittell, and J. F. Fairbairn II (Eds.), *Peripheral Vascular Diseases.* Philadelphia: Saunders, 1980.
28. Brust, J. C. M.   Transient ischemic attacks: Natural history and anticoagulation. *Neurology* 27:701, 1977.
29. Schafer, A. I., and Handin, R. I.   The role of platelets in thrombotic and vascular disease. *Prog. Cardiovasc. Dis.* 22:32, 1979.

30. Fuster, V., and Chesebro, J. H. Antithrombotic therapy: role of platelet inhibitor drugs. *Mayo Clin. Proc.* 56:185, 1981.
31. The Canadian Cooperative Study Group. A randomized trial of aspirin and sulfinpyrazone in threatened stroke. *N. Engl. J. Med.* 299:53, 1978.
32. Fuster, V., and Chesebro, J. H. Antithrombotic therapy: management of arterial thromboembolic and atherosclerotic disease. *Mayo Clin. Proc.* 56:265, 1980.
33. Mulcane, R. S., Royster, T. S., and Lynn, R. A. Long-term results of operative therapy for aortoiliac disease. *Arch. Surg.* 113:601, 1978.
34. Malone, J. M., Moore, W. S., and Goldstone, J. The natural history of bilateral femoral bypass grafts for ischemia of the lower extremities. *Arch. Surg.* 110:1300, 1975.
35. Johnson, W. C., Logrefo, F. W., and Vollman, R. W. Is axillo-bilateral femoral graft an effective substitute for aortic-bilateral iliac/femoral graft? An analysis of ten years' experience. *Ann. Surg.* 186:123, 1977.
36. Hansteen, V., et al. Long-term follow up of patients with peripheral arterial obliterans treated with arterial surgery. *Acta Chir. Scand.* 141:725, 1975.
37. Weintraub, A. M., and Gomes, M. N. Clinical Manifestations of Abdominal Aortic Aneurysm and Thoracoabdominal Aneurysm. In J. Lindsay, Jr. and J. W. Hurst (Eds.), *The Aorta.* New York: Grune & Stratton, 1979.
38. Slater, E. E., and Desanctis, R. W. Disease of the Aorta. In E. Braunwald (Ed.), *Heart Disease: A Textbook of Cardiovascular Medicine.* Philadelphia: Saunders, 1980.
39. Baker, W. H., and Munns, J. R. Aneurysmectomy in the aged. *Arch. Surg.* 110:513, 1975.

15. Metabolic Bone Disease

David F. Giansiracusa
Fred G. Kantrowitz

Bone Loss with Aging

Bone in adults is descriptively termed *lamellar* since it consists of an orderly arrangement of parallel and concentric sheets of collagen fibers. Each bone has a densely packed outer layer termed *cortical* or *compact* bone, while the bone within the cortex consists of a loose mesh and is referred to as trabecular bone. The terms *cancellous, medullary,* and *spongy* are used synonymously with *trabecular* [1].

Bone is a dynamic organ that is constantly being remodeled. Although the rates of bone resorption and formation at any given time are fixed relative to each other, these rates vary over the life cycle. Over the life span of the individual, from skeletal development to adolescence, the rate of new bone formation exceeds that of resorption. From adolescence to the mid to late twenties, the two processes are approximately equal. After this period, the rate of bone resorption exceeds the rate of bone formation, resulting in a progressive loss of bone [2].

Resorption occurs throughout adult life in discrete foci. The progressive loss of bone mass is primarily due to endosteal resorption, which is greater than formation of new osteons or bone units.

Endochondral ossification, which creates trabecular bone, ends by age 20 ± 5 years. Trabecular bone loss is associated with a decrease in the thickness of the average trabecula and a decrease in the total number of trabeculae per unit volume of bone [3]. Iliac crest biopsies, which sample trabecular bone, reveal a linear decrease with aging in both men and women. Males lose 27 percent of their trabecular bone mass by age 80; women lose trabecular bone at a linear rate between the ages of 15 and 55. In the menopausal period the rate of bone loss accelerates, and by the age of 90 a woman has lost approximately 43 percent of her trabecular bone mass. In both sexes, the amount of trabecular bone at a given age is a function of the quantity of bone at the time of maximal bone mass and the duration of bone loss [2].

Loss of cortical bone begins by age 45 in women and by age 50 in men. Histologic studies reveal that cortical bone loss occurs at the endosteal surface and is associated with an increase in the number of holes in the compact midportion of the cortex, thus increasing the porosity of cortical bone. In addition to starting earlier in females, cortical bone loss proceeds at a more rapid rate. Women lose 10 percent of their cortical bone mass per decade while men lose 5 percent [4]. These rates do not vary greatly between individuals. The incidence of long bone fractures at various ages correlates with cortical bone loss.

Although the entire skeleton loses mass with aging, the distribution of bone loss is not uniform. The different proportions of trabecular versus corti-

243

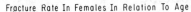

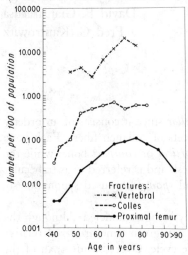

Figure 15-1. Fracture rate in women in relation to age. Vertebral fractures appear earlier and are more frequent than either Colles' or femoral fractures. (From J. Jowsey, Osteoporosis: Idiopathic, Post-Menopausal, and Senile. In C. B. Sledge (Ed.), *Metabolic Diseases of Bone.* Philadelphia: Saunders, 1977.)

cal bone in the various parts of the skeleton contribute to this discrepancy. As stated, trabecular bone loss begins at a younger age than cortical bone loss in both sexes. This results in a relative increase in the ratio of cortical to trabecular bone. At age 15 years, the ratio is 55 : 45 while at 85 it is 70 : 30. Those areas of the skeleton with the highest content of trabecular bone, such as vertebral bodies and bones of the wrist and hip, will lose the greatest amount of their mass. The clinical correlate is the markedly increased incidence of vertebral compression, Colles', and hip fractures with advancing age. Vertebral fractures occur at younger ages and more frequently than either Colles' or femoral fractures [5] (Fig. 15-1).

The following generalizations can be made about bone loss associated with aging: (1) after age 30 to 40, there is a linear fall in the average skeletal mass; (2) skeletal mass in young adults is greater in males than females and is greater in blacks than in whites; (3) bone loss starts earlier in women than men; and (4) in women there is accelerated bone loss after menopause [6].

With aging, various changes in the cellular elements of bone occur. Fibroblast synthesis of matrix precursors diminishes. This is associated with morphologic conversion of fibroblasts to elongated fibrocytes. Cytoplasmic changes occur in fibrocytes and osteocysts; these include disappearance of rough endoplasmic reticulum (REM), simplification of the Golgi complex, and degeneration of mitochondria. Osteocytes deeply positioned in cortical bone undergo necrosis, while cells located in the periosteum retain their ability to respond to trauma even with advancing age. The osteoclasts, specialized multinucleated syncytial cells responsible for bone mineral and matrix removal, retain their function with aging [7].

CHANGES IN CALCIUM ABSORPTION WITH AGE

One factor that may contribute to the age-related decreased bone formation relative to resorption is impaired calcium absorption (Fig. 15-2). Calcium intake correlates with vertebral body mineralization measured by radiodensitometry [8]. Calcium absorption in individuals younger than 65 years of age correlates inversely with dietary calcium intake. This inverse correlation does not occur in individuals over 65 [9]. When faced with a fall in dietary calcium, the aged intestine loses its capacity to increase calcium absorption [10] (Fig. 15-3).

While most studies show no effect of age on serum levels of 25-hydroxy vitamin D_3 (25-OH D_3), some laboratories report slightly lower levels in the elderly. However, levels of 1,25-dihydroxy vitamin D_3 [1,25-$(OH)_2D_3$], the most active metabolite of vitamin D, are decreased. Administration of exogenous 1,25-$(OH)_2D_3$ to elderly individuals results in significant increases of calcium absorption. These findings suggest that a decrease in the baseline level of calcium absorption and the loss of a compensatory increase of intestinal absorption in the setting of low dietary calcium intake in the elderly may be due to impaired renal conversion of 25-OH D_3 to 1,25-$(OH)_2D_3$ [9].

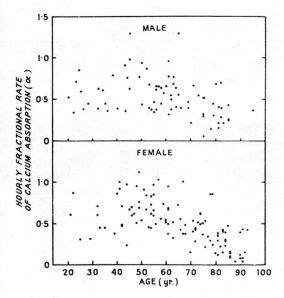

Figure 15-2. Relationship in males and females between hourly rate of calcium absorption (α) and age. (From J. R. Bullamore, et al. Effect of age on calcium absorption. *Lancet* 2:535, 1970.)

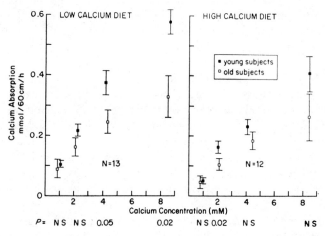

Figure 15-3. Effect of age on calcium absorption. Seven young and six old subjects on the low-calcium diet were studied, and six old and six young subjects on the high-calcium diet were studied. P values are by grouped Student's test. (From P. Ireland and J. S. Fordtran. Effect of dietary calcium and age on jejunal calcium absorption in humans. *J. Clin. Invest.* 52:2672, 1973.)

Terminology of Metabolic Bone Disease

Osteopenia is defined as the presence of less than the normal amount of bone. When this process results from "normal" bone loss associated with aging, it is termed *senile osteopenia. Osteoporosis* is the pathologic state of osteopenia in which bone mass is so reduced that the skeleton loses its integrity and becomes unable to perform its supportive function [11]. Osteoporotic bone histologically is characterized by a reduction in the amount of trabecular bone and, to a lesser degree, of cortical bone. The ratio of mineral to organic matrix is normal. Osteomalacia results from defects in bone mineralization. The amount of unmineralized osteoid is increased relative to the quantity of calcified matrix.

Various techniques are available to quantitate bone mineral content. Photon absorption densitometry is a sensitive indicator of total bone mineral mass. While this technique and radiographs may indicate a decrease in bone mineral content a bone biopsy may be required to differentiate various causes of osteopenia.

Osteoporosis

Clinically, individuals most commonly affected with osteoporosis are postmenopausal white women. Men may be affected later in life [8]. Twenty-nine percent of women and 18 percent of men between the ages of 45 and 79 have osteoporosis [11]. Black women have greater bone masses than white women and are affected less frequently. Women who weigh less than 140 pounds develop osteoporosis more frequently than do heavier individuals. The presence of adipose tissue that stores estrogens and greater physical stresses on bones have been proposed as protective mechanisms [5].

CAUSES

Conceptually, osteoporosis may result from (1) an acceleration of normal bone loss as a function of aging; (2) an abnormally low skeletal mass at skeletal maturity, which decreases at a normal rate; or (3) a combination of the two. Individuals who develop osteoporosis, primarily white women, frequently have abnormally low bone masses prior to the progressive loss with aging [2]. Morphologically, the only significant difference between individuals with normal senile osteopenic bone and those with pathologic osteoporotic bone is the quantity of bone. Thus, patients with osteoporosis may simply be at the extreme end of the spectrum of physiologic senile osteopenia. The rate of bone formation in patients with untreated osteoporosis is normal, while the rate of resorption is increased [5] (Table 15-1). Low bone mass at skeletal maturity and an accelerated rate of bone loss characterize osteoporotic patients as compared to normal individuals.

Various pathophysiologic mechanisms have been proposed to explain the development of osteoporosis. Deficiency in estrogens may contribute to accelerated bone loss after menopause [5]. Estrogen therapy decreases bone resorption by decreasing the responsiveness of bone to parathyroid hormone (PTH). Long-term therapy with estrogen results in a greater decrease in bone resorption than bone formation, thus resulting in a relative slowing of bone loss [12].

As stated previously, calcium malabsorption may contribute to osteoporosis. In a study of subjects with osteoporosis and vertebral compression fractures, 80 percent of those less than 60 years old had calcium absorptions below nor-

Table 15-1. Bone Turnover in Osteoporosis (mean ± SD)*

	Age	N	Formation %	Resorption
Normals	20–44	37	2.3 ± 1.3	4.0 ± 1.4
	45–75	58	2.0 ± 1.4	3.9 ± 1.4
Patients with osteoporosis	20–44	12	2.9 ± 1.7	8.9 ± 3.5
	45–75	143	2.6 ± 1.7	10.5 ± 5.1

Source: From J. Jowsey, Osteoporosis: Idiopathic, Post-Menopausal, and Senile. In C. B. Sledge (Ed.), Metabolic Diseases of Bone. Philadelphia: Saunders, 1977.
* In untreated osteoporotic patients, the rate of bone formation is normal, but the rate of bone resorption is several times greater than normal.

mal as measured by radiocalcium absorption. With advancing age, the differences in calcium absorption between osteoporotic and normal individuals lose significance due to a fall in calcium absorption in normal individuals with advancing age. The difference between calcium intake and calcium output (i.e., net calcium loss) was greater in the osteoporotic patients than in normal individuals. Urinary calcium excretion correlated more closely with calcium absorption than calcium intake.

The use of sensitive assays for immunoreactive parathyroid hormone (iPTH) has identified two groups of osteoporotic individuals, one with elevated and the other with depressed levels. The group with elevated iPTH levels is small and is composed of two subsets: (1) individuals with secondary hyperparathyroidism due to impaired intestinal absorption of calcium and (2) individuals with normocalcemic primary hyperparathyroidism. The larger group of the osteoporotic individuals had normal or low levels of iPTH [13].

Immobilization also contributes to osteoporosis (Fig. 15-4). With disuse, osteoporosis develops primarily in the metaphyseal and subchondral zones. Physical stress such as weight-bearing stimulates bone formation. Studies have demonstrated a reduction in bone loss in a group of postmenopausal women treated with exercise relative to a sedentary control group [14].

Various endocrine disorders may be associated with osteoporosis. Hyper-

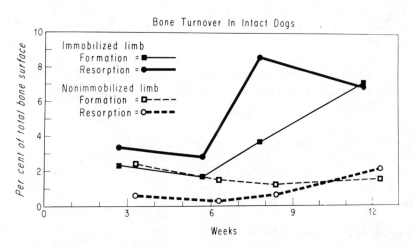

Figure 15-4. Changes in bone resorption and formation in immobilization. One hind limb of an adult dog has been immobilized by a plaster cast. Bone remodeling values measured at 0, 6, 8, and 12 weeks show the marked rise in resorption, which is followed by a delayed rise in formation. (From J. Jowsey, Osteoporosis: Idiopathic, Post-Menopausal, and Senile. In C. B. Sledge, *Metabolic Diseases of Bone.* Philadelphia: Saunders, 1977.)

thyroidism and hyperparathyroidism accelerate bone resorption [5]. Gluco-corticosteroid excess causes osteoporosis by decreasing intestinal calcium absorption, interfering with synthesis of bone matrix and possibly by increasing the catabolism of 1,25-dihydroxycholecalciferol (1,25-dihydroxy vitamin D_3) [11].

DIAGNOSIS

Diffuse demineralization is radiographically apparent after loss of 20 to 60 percent of bone mineral content [11]. Radiographs of peripheral bones may reveal cortical thinning; the non–weight-bearing bones of the upper extremities appear more osteopenic than do radiographs of the weight-bearing lower extremities. In the pelvis and femur, cortical thinning and loss of trabeculae can be seen. Remaining trabeculae correspond to lines of stress. Severe osteoporosis of the skull may appear as patchy or spotty areas of "demineralization." The severity of osteoporosis can be approximated by comparing the cortex of the femur, metatarsal, metacarpal, or phalangeal bones with the total width of the bone. Normally, the sum of the two cortical widths is approximately half the total width of the bone. In osteoporosis, the sum of the cortexes is less than half the total width.

The differential diagnosis of osteoporosis includes diseases that may cause a radiographic appearance of bony demineralization. Bone roentgenograms of patients with hyperthyroidism and hyperparathyroidism, hypercortisolism, osteomalacia, carcinoma metastatic to bone, and plasma cell dyscrasias may appear identical to those of patients with biopsy-proven osteoporosis.

MANAGEMENT

After excluding the previously mentioned disorders, various modalities are available to treat osteoporosis. Treatment with supplemental calcium alone, calcium with vitamin D, and estrogens have all been shown to decrease bone resorption [11] and to slow the rate of bone loss [14]. Estrogens used for several years after menopause, during which time resorption may be particularly accelerated, may slow this process. Studies of the effect of calcium carbonate ($CaCO_3$) and estrogens used individually in postmenopausal women for a two-year period have documented a measurable decrease in bone loss compared with women who have not received treatment [12]. These agents decrease bone loss by retarding the rate of resorption proportionally more than the rate of formation [12]. Prolonged therapy with estrogens does carry inherent risks such as an increase in the incidence of endometrial carcinoma [11]. Fluoride is the one form of therapy that stimulates osteoblastic activity. A recent large, prospective controlled trial compared the efficacy of various combinations of calcium, estrogen, fluoride, and vitamin D in reducing fracture rates in postmenopausal osteoporosis. The fracture rate (per thousand person-years) was 834 in untreated patients, 419 in those given calcium with or without vitamin D, 304 in those given fluoride and calcium with or without vitamin D, 181 in those given estrogen and calcium with or without vitamin D, and 53 in those given fluoride, estrogen, and calcium with or without vitamin D [15].

Depending on the particular setting, treatment may be individualized to the specific patient. In the immediate postmenopausal state, either naturally occurring or secondary to oophorectomy, several years of estrogen therapy may decrease the accelerated rate of bone resorption otherwise occurring in this setting [5]. Malabsorption states can be documented by measurement of 24-hour calcium excretion, which correlates with absorption. A 24-hour urinary calcium excretion of less than 100 mg per total volume (normal, 50–300 mg per total volume in 24 hours) may reflect inefficient calcium absorption. Determination of serum vitamin D levels may document vitamin D deficiency. In a patient with low 24-hour calcium excretion, vitamin D may be given in a dose of 50,000 units orally one to two times a week. Calcium in doses of 1 to 1.5 g of elemental calcium is added to this regimen. The 24-hour urinary calcium should be rechecked after four to six weeks of therapy to avoid hypercalciuria and the potential for calcium urolithiasis.

Exercise is another form of therapy that can be used prophylactically to retard bone loss. As stated previously, mechanical stress of bones such as weight-bearing and muscular exertion is a stimulus for bone formation while immobility accelerates the rate of bone resorption relative to formation. One study evaluated 18 postmenopausal women by treating nine individuals with at least one hour per week of exercise for approximately one year. The total body calcium determination increased in these nine individuals as compared to a decrease that occurred in the nine control individuals [14].

When confronted with a patient with biopsy-documented, severe, symptomatic osteoporosis, combined therapy—fluoride to stimulate new bone formation, calcium, and estrogens if the patient is postmenopausal—may be prescribed. Sodium fluoride (NaFl), 50 mg per day; $CaCO_3$, 1 to 2 g per day; and standard doses of conjugated estrogens is one such regimen [15]. The fluoride and calcium must be given at different times to avoid formation of an insoluble complex of calcium fluoride. Administration of vitamin D, which is associated with substantial risk of hypercalcemia and/or hypercalciuria, does not appear to add substantial benefit to fluoride-containing regimens [15].

COMPLICATIONS
The incidence of fractures, including vertebral body, femoral neck, and Colles' fractures increases with age (see Fig. 15-1). Of approximately one million fractures per year in the United States in women 45 years or older, 70 percent occur in osteoporotic women [11].

Vertebral Fractures
Vertebral compression fractures may lead to a loss of height and cause a dorsal kyphosis. These changes may impair the chest wall mechanics of

breathing and interfere with ventilation. With multiple compression fractures, the lower ribs may come to rest on the patient's anterosuperior iliac spines. In addition to loss of height, such individuals may experience redundant anterior abdominal skin folds, intestinal distention, and constipation. Straining to pass stool may cause new vertebral compression fractures. Lumbar vertebral compression fractures with anterior wedging result in a loss of the normal lordosis. With a loss of the anterior lumbar curvature, the hips and knees are held in several degrees of flexion, which in turn may result in flexion contractures [11].

Osteoporosis, even in the presence of one or more vetrebral compression fractures, is often painless. Vertebral body compression fracture(s) associated with minor trauma may result in the sudden onset of back pain. The pain may occur with a minor fall into a sitting position, which puts great compressive stress on the anterior aspects of the vertebral bodies. Less frequently, the pain has a more gradual onset over several days and is appreciated most on waking in the morning.

Pain associated with vertebral osteoporosis takes two forms. The first is sharp, varying in severity from a mild ache to such intensity that intestinal ileus may develop. This pain is either localized to the site of fracture or may radiate laterally from the midline and around the flanks toward the abdomen. Occasionally, the pain may radiate into the patient's pelvis or legs. Maneuvers that increase intraabdominal pressures such as coughing, sneezing, defecating, and trunk movements may exacerbate the pain. The discomfort usually disappears over two to four weeks of bed rest. Between attacks the patient is generally pain-free. Nerve root and spinal cord compressions are extremely rare [11].

A second form of pain is less well localized and is felt up and down the back, usually several centimeters lateral to one or both sides of the spine. This pain is associated with spasm of the erector spinous muscles. Paraspinous muscle tenderness may be noted on palpation. Discomfort is aggravated by motion, coughing, sneezing, or straining, as well as by sitting. It is relieved by lying flat in bed [11].

Vertebral body compression fractures occur most commonly in the lower thoracic and upper lumbar spine [16] (Fig. 15-5). When viewed on lateral radiographs, the vertebral bodies characteristically display anterior wedging, that is, they are compressed so that the anterior height is less than the posterior height (Fig. 15-6). Fractures occurring in the cervical and upper thoracic vertebral bodies (above T_6) and those at lower sites with posterior vertebral wedging are distinctly unusual for uncomplicated osteoporosis and should suggest the presence of another process such as plasma cell dyscrasias, metastatic tumor, or infection [11]. Vertebral compression fractures may not be detectable on radiographs immediately after the event but may become apparent several weeks later. Fractures may show up as "hot" areas on bone scans several days to a week after the event; these areas are associated with the osteoblastic healing phase.

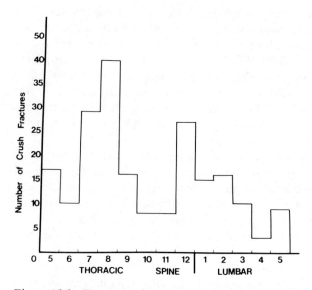

Figure 15-5. Frequency histogram of the sites of vertebral fracture in 58 patients. (From J. C. Gallagher, J. Aaron, A. Horsman, D. H. Marshall, R. Wilkinson, and B. E. C. Nordin. The crush fracture syndrome in postmenopausal women, *Clin. Endocrinol. Metab.* 2:293, 1973.)

Treatment of back pain associated with osteoporotic compression fractures consists of strict bed rest for one to several weeks. It should be emphasized that this means lying flat in bed. Sitting up puts an increased stress on the spine that exceeds even that occurring with standing. Analgesics such as codeine may be necessary. Particular attention should be paid to preventing constipation, which may be aggravated by pain, bed rest, and narcotic analgesics. Application of moist heat and muscle relaxants may decrease paraspinous muscle spasm but should not be prescribed in place of bed rest. With this regimen, the acute pain usually subsides within several weeks. Individuals with severe osteoporosis may suffer repeated vertebral microfractures that may cause persistent pain.

Hip Fractures

Hip fractures are a significant cause of morbidity and mortality in the elderly, especially white women. With progressive bone loss associated with aging, the incidence of hip fracture among white women between 80 and 90 years old approaches 10 percent. The average age of patients with femoral neck fractures is 75 and with intertrochanteric fractures is 78 years [17]. With advancing age, the mortality also increases. The precipitating event in hip fractures in the elderly may be the force of minor trauma or simply vigorous contraction of hip musculature in the presence of osteoporotic bones.

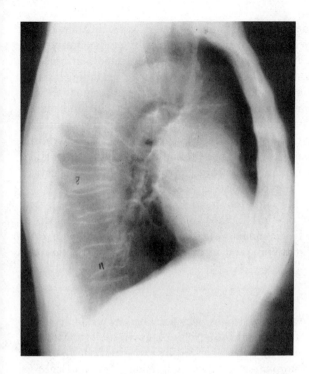

Figure 15-6.   Radiograph of the lateral spine demonstrates the anterior wedging of an osteoporotic vertebral body compression fracture.

The incidence of osteomalacia in patients with fractures thought to be secondary to uncomplicated osteoporosis may be surprisingly high. Histologically documented osteomalacia has been found in 30 percent of femoral fractures in elderly individuals studied in England [18]. Low levels of 25-hydroxy vitamin D_3 have been found more frequently in individuals suffering femoral neck fractures than normal individuals [19].

Because of the enforced immobility, hip fractures in the elderly may result in fatal complications such as mental deterioration, pneumonia, and pulmonary embolism. Prompt stabilization of the patient and surgical fixation are therefore important principles of management. Total hip arthroplasty is the surgical treatment of choice for femoral neck fractures. This procedure minimizes operative time and the duration of immobility, thereby decreasing morbidity from pneumonia and thromboembolic complications. Prosthetic femoral neck and head replacement also avoids complications such as avascular necrosis of the femoral head and delayed union of the fracture site. Intertrochanteric features are surgically managed with internal fixation with a nail and plate [17].

Thromboembolic disease causes significant mortality among elderly individuals who have sustained hip fractures. Of patients who are not anticoagulated, 30 percent develop thrombophlebitis and approximately 10 percent die of pulmonary embolism within three months of the injury [20]. Anticoagulation during and after surgical fixation is an important aspect of management. Although various agents have been used including aspirin, dextran, dipyridamole, and low-dose heparin, only oral anticoagulation with Coumadin has been demonstrated to prevent thrombophlebitis and pulmonary emboli in patients with hip fractures [21]. Prophylactic treatment with Coumadin, maintaining the prothrombin time $1\frac{1}{2}$ to 2 times control during and after surgical fixation of the fracture, is recommended unless the patient has hypertension, active peptic ulcer disease, previous bleeding tendency, or excessive hemorrhage at the fracture or operative site [22].

Rehabilitation of patients with hip fracture includes an active physical therapy program. Chest physical therapy and breathing exercises help to minimize atelectasis and pneumonia. Vigorous muscle-strengthening exercises and appropriate gait training aid in maximizing muscle function and mobility [17].

Paget's Disease of Bone

Paget's disease of bone, osteitis deformans, was described by Sir James Paget in 1877. It is a chronic, focal bone disease of unknown etiology occurring primarily in geriatric patients and characterized by excessive bone resorption followed by accelerated formation of abnormal bone. The incidence of Paget's disease increases progressively after the age of 40, with an overall incidence of approximately three percent. Men and women are affected with equal frequency. It is more common in individuals of English, Australian, and New Zealand ancestry, while it is rare in Africans and Asians. Although the disease may be strikingly prevalent in families, there is no definitive genetic transmission or HLA markers to explain this phenomenon. The recent demonstration of intranuclear structures resembling particles within osteoclasts of patients with Paget's disease provides support for a possible viral etiology [22a].

PATHOPHYSIOLOGY

The pathophysiology of Paget's disease is divided into three stages. However, in an individual patient these stages frequently overlap. The initial phase consists of excessive bone resorption secondary to osteoclastic activity. This is characterized by an increase in the number of large, multinucleated osteoclasts by as much as 10 to 20 times normal [23] (Fig. 15-7).

Parathyroid hormone excess is not responsible for the increased osteoclastic activity. Increased levels of urinary hydroxyproline and the radiographic appearance of focal osteopenia characterize this stage [23].

The second phase of Paget's disease is characterized by a compensatory increase in bone formation. Histologically, as much as 100 percent of bone surfaces may be covered with osteoclasts or osteoblasts in contrast to approximately 2 percent in normal adult bone [5]. The newly formed bone is de-

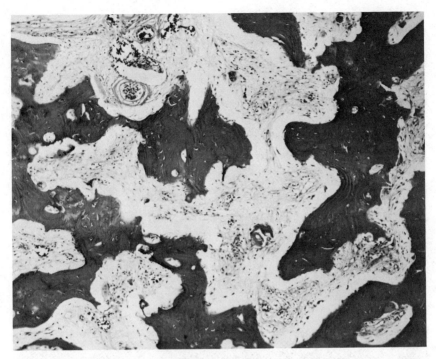

Figure 15-7. A specimen of pagetic bone viewed with the light microscope at 100X magnification demonstrates numerous multinucleated osteoclasts, dilated blood vessels, and increased fibrous stroma.

posited in a chaotic lamellar or so-called mosaic pattern [23] (Fig. 15-8). Each individual section of lamellar bone is normal; however, they are oriented toward one another in a haphazard, rather than parallel or concentric fashion. An elevation of serum alkaline phosphatase reflects the increase in osteoblastic activity.

The final phase is primarily osteoblastic. Radiographic and pathologic studies reveal trabecular thickening with an irregular pattern and in increase in the external size of bone due to periosteal new bone formation [5]. Increased fibrous tissue in the marrow space, increased vascularity, and a decrease in cellular activity can be seen [23].

CLINICAL CHARACTERISTICS
Paget's disease is asymptomatic in over 90 percent of patients and may be detected inadvertently by finding an elevated alkaline phosphatase or characteristic x-ray changes. When pain occurs, it is usually chronic and of an "achy" character. It may be severe, especially during the osteolytic phase. Although exacerbated with weight-bearing, the pain is generally of constant intensity. Abrupt increases in pain rarely occur and suggest the presence of a fracture or development of malignant degeneration [24].

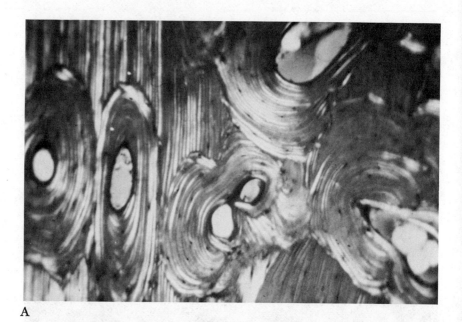

A

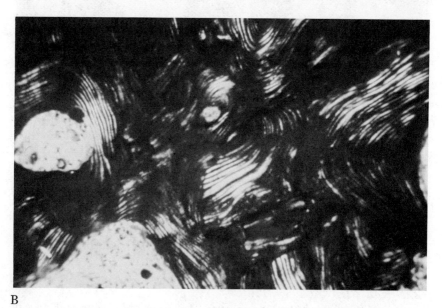

B

Figure 15-8. Polarized microscopic view of (A) normal cortical bone demonstrating orderly parallel and concentric lamellae, and (B) pagetic bone demonstrating haphazard orientation of groups of lamellae to each other. (From F. R. Singer, et al., Paget's Disease of Bone. In L. V. Alvioli and S. M. Krane, *Metabolic Bone Disease*. New York: Academic Press, 1978. Vol. II.)

LOCAL MANIFESTATIONS

Local manifestations of Paget's disease include bone pain, deformities, and fractures; increased temperature of skin overlying affected bone due to increased cutaneous blood flow [25]; facial and dental problems; neurologic impairment; rheumatologic complications; and development of bone tumors (Table 15-2).

The nature of the local manifestations depends on the site of skeletal involvement. The bones involved most commonly, in decreasing order of frequency, are the sacrum, spine, femur, skull, and pelvis. Occasionally, a single bone may be affected, the monostotic pattern, although the polyostotoic pattern is more common [23].

Spine

Paget's disease of the spine most frequently involves the lumbosacral region and affects one or more vertebral bodies. Sudden worsening of chronic back pain is suggestive of a compression fracture. Severe pain may result from spinal cord or nerve root impingement secondary to bony enlargement of the spine, but paraplegia and quadriplegia are rare. Radiologic features of spinal involvement include (1) central vertebral body osteopenia, (2) thickening of vertebral margins and coarsening of central vertical trabeculae, (3) homogeneous increase of vertebral body density, and (4) compression fractures. An increase in the dimensions of the affected vertebral bodies without disruption of the cortexes helps to differentiate this condition from metastatic tumor to the spine [23].

Femur

Involvement of the femur causes pain, lateral bowing, and fractures; osteoarthritis of the knee and hip may result as well. As in other long bones, bone resorption may give the radiographic appearance of an "advancing wedge" of osteopenia (Fig. 15-9). This advancing wedge is the border between normal bone and the osteoclastic phase of Paget's disease. The femur may develop a cystic-appearing lesion on x-ray as a result of the combination of active bone resorption and outward deformity of the cortex secondary to the stress of weight-bearing.

Table 15-2. Local Complications of Paget's Disease

Bone pain	Bone tumors
Deformities	Warmth of skin
Pathologic fractures	Ankylosis of teeth
Neurologic sequelae	Rheumatic sequelae
Deafness	Osteoarthritis
Compression of nerve tissue	Calcific periarthritis
Angioid streaks	Syndrome resembling ankylosing spondylitis

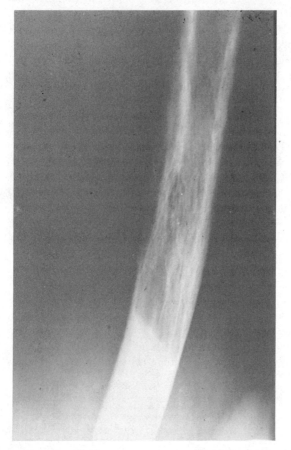

Figure 15-9.   Radiograph of pagetic humerus demonstrates localized osteopenia termed the "advancing wedge."

Skull

Involvement of the skull may cause a variety of problems. Disease in the facial bones may cause localized pain and a "leontiasis ossea" appearance. Maxillary or mandibular involvement may cause ankylosis of the teeth to the jaw, making dental extractions difficult and increasing the risk of osteomyelitis [23]. Involvement of the temporal bone may disrupt the cochlea and cause a sensorineural hearing loss. Eighth cranial nerve compression in the internal auditory canal is rare. Ankylosis of the ossicles, occlusion of the external auditory canal, and chronic otitis media due to eustachion tube obstruction may cause conductive hearing loss. Some form of auditory impairment occurs in 30 to 50 percent of patients with pagetic skull involvement [26].

The calvaria is the most frequent site of skull involvement, manifestations of which include an increase in head size, headaches, posterior neck muscle spasm due to the increased weight of the head, and neurologic complications. The earliest radiologic feature may be a localized, well-demarcated area of osteopenia, termed *osteoporosis circumscripta,* which usually begins in the frontal or occipital areas and may spread to involve the entire calvaria. Other radiographic features include osteoblastic changes with thickening of the inner and outer cranial tables, widening of the diploë, and platybasia, flattening of the base of the skull. Basilar impression by the spine is the result of softening of the calvaria at the base of the skull. Compression of the spinal cord, brain stem, cerebellum, and basilar arteries may occur with this deformity [23]. Skull disease may cause other neurologic abnormalities. With extensive involvement of the calvaria, blood flow from the common carotid arteries is shunted into the external carotid arteries, the so-called cranial steal syndrome [23]. This deprives the brain of blood flow and may cause confusional states, agitation, and even cerebrovascular accidents.

Pelvis

When the pelvis is involved, osteoblastic lesions may resemble those due to a malignancy metastatic to bone, particularly prostatic carcinoma. Several radiologic features help to distinguish these two conditions. In Paget's disease, the pelvic brim or iliopectineal line becomes thickened, the so-called brim sign, which is pathognomonic [27]. The widening of the pubic and ischial rami that occurs in Paget's disease is rare in metastatic bone disease [23].

Involvement of the pelvis may also cause rheumatologic manifestations [24]. When the acetabulum and femoral head are involved, osteoarthritis of the hip may develop. Medial joint space narrowing is very characteristic of a pagetic hip, in contrast to narrowing of the superior aspect of the hip seen in osteoarthritis. Severe involvement of the acetabulum may soften the bone and result in protrusio acetabuli.

Fractures

Fractures occur during the osteolytic phase due to a loss of bone and during the blastic phase due to replacement of normal bone with structurally unsound bone. The vertebral bodies, femur, and tibia are the most common fracture sites. Incomplete cortical fractures, termed *fissure fractures,* occur most frequently on the convex surface of the deformed bones. Fissure fractures may be multiple and are frequently painful. Complete fractures often "start" at the site of a fissure fracture and transect the bone. They are descriptively called "chalkstick" or "banana" fractures, in contrast to the spiral fractures that occur in normal bone [23] (Fig. 15-10). Complete fractures frequently occur in the subtrochanteric portion of the femur. Only 10 percent of femoral fractures occur in the neck, in contrast to the predilection for this site in the osteoporotic population.

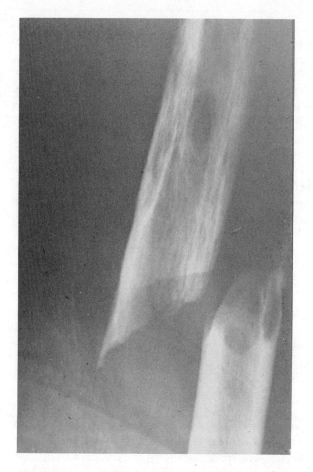

Figure 15-10. Radiograph of a chalkstick fracture through the "advancing wedge" section of a femur involved with Paget's disease.

Tumors

Development of a malignancy in pagetic bone may result in an abrupt increase in the pattern of pain or progressive soft tissue swelling. Although malignant bone tumors, primarily sarcomas, occur approximately 25 times more frequently in patients with Paget's disease of bone than in normal individuals, the overall incidence of sarcomas in these patients is less than one percent [28]. This complication carries a grim prognosis, with only four percent of patients surviving for longer than one year. These tumors always originate in pagetic bone, most frequently in the extremities. Men are affected twice as frequently as women. Osteogenic sarcoma is the most frequent type of tumor.

SYSTEMIC MANIFESTATIONS

The major systemic complications of Paget's disease of bone are hyper- calciuria, hypercalcemia, and high-output congestive heart failure. Hypercal- cemia due to Paget's disease is rare but may become a problem when patients with active disease are immobilized for treatment of fractures. Hypercalciuria is much more common; urinary calculi secondary to hypercalciuria occurred in five percent of 1,300 patients [29].

The major cardiovascular complication is high-output cardiac failure. This often occurs when greater than 35 percent of the skeleton is involved, or when the disease is extremely active. The augmented output is due primarily to an increase in the vascularity of bone. Although pagetic bone contains telangiectatic vessels, functional arteriovenous shunts, previously thought to be a causative factor in the cardiac failure, have not been demonstrated [30].

LABORATORY EVALUATION

Laboratory tests useful in evaluating Paget's disease include 24-hour urinary hydroxyproline excretion and serum alkaline phosphatase, roentgenograms, and radionuclide bone scans.

In general, the levels of bone alkaline phosphate correlate with the extent of pagetic bone disease. The two exceptions are: (1) skull involvement, in which the alkaline phosphatase may be disproportionately elevated; and (2) chronic, generalized Paget's disease, particularly of the pelvis, in which the alkaline phosphatase may be lower than would be expected for the extent of bone disease [23]. Patients with monostotic pagetic involvement may have normal serum alkaline phosphatase levels.

Bone scans may provide information about the stage and activity of Paget's disease. Since radionuclide uptake occurs during bone formation, "hot spots" on bone scans reflect areas of increased osteoblastic activity. Serial bone scans may be useful in monitoring response to therapy [23].

TREATMENT

The goals of therapy for Paget's disease are to relieve pain, maintain skeletal function, and minimize local and systemic complications. Asymptomatic disease does not require treatment. Minimal pain may be improved with analgesics. Nonsteroidal antiinflammatory agents may relieve symptoms secondary to rheumatologic complications. Candidates for specific anti- pagetic medications include patients with (1) severe bone pain, (2) high- output cardiac failure, (3) recurrent renal calculi secondary to hypercalciuria, (4) hypercalcemia due to pagetic bone involvement, (5) anticipated ortho- pedic surgery in an area of pagetic bone, (6) multiple bone fractures, (7) skeletal impingement on nerve tissue, and (8) pagetic involvement that may result in disabling deformities [23] (Table 15-3).

Medical forms of therapy include calcitonin, disodium etidronate, and mithramycin, all of which function to decrease bone resorption.

Table 15-3.   Indications for Specific Antipagetic Therapy

Severe bone pain
High output cardiac failure
Recurrent renal calculi secondary to hypercalciuria
Hypercalcemia due to pagetic bone involvement
Multiple bone fractures
Skeletal impingement of nerve tissue
Anticipated orthopedic surgery on pagetic bone
Pagetic involvement that may result in disabling deformities

Calcitonin

Porcine, salmon, and nonantigenic human calcitonin have all been used to treat Paget's disease. Presently, only salmon calcitonin is available in the United States [23]. Calcitonin's ability to decrease bone resorption is reflected by a fall in urinary hydroxyproline, serum calcium, and phosphatase after a single injection. After several weeks of therapy, the serum alkaline phosphatase level falls. Calcitonin causes a decrease in the number of osteoclasts and reduces their ruffled borders or pseudopods, thus rendering them relatively incapable of resorbing bone. Bone formed after calcitonin therapy has normal structure [31]. Calcitonin may decrease radiographic progression of the disease. It reduces bone pain in as many as 60 percent of patients. Pain relief starts one to two weeks after beginning therapy and reaches a maximum at one to two months. A fall in skin temperature and cardiac output can occur with calcitonin therapy. Auditory dysfunction generally does not improve, nor do the majority of cases of oculomotor and facial nerve palsies or spastic paralyses due to compressive myelopathy [32].

Calcitonin is given as a subcutaneous injection. Various regimens have been proposed, including 100 MRC (Medical Research Council) units daily, 20 MRC units daily, and 50 MRC units three times a week. As little as 50 MRC units given subcutaneously twice weekly has been shown to be effective in decreasing bone turnover [33].

Diphosphonates

Disodium etidronate, or EHDP (disodium ethone-1-hydrosyl-1, 1 diphosphonate) (Didronel), is a diphosphonate used to treat Paget's disease. Diphosphonates are detergents that act by coating hydroxyapatite crystals, making them relatively impervious to the actions of osteoclasts. With therapy, urinary hydroxyproline excretion falls over several weeks, followed by a fall in the serum alkaline phosphatase [34]. The biochemical improvement may persist for months after diphosphonates have been discontinued. A decrease in activity on bone scans also occurs with therapy. Clinical improvement with a decrease in pain is common. In patients with severe Paget's disease, a paradoxical increase in pain may occur. High doses of diphosphonates (20 mg/kg/day) may also lead to pathologic bone fractures, probably secondary to development of defective bone mineralization [35]. EHDP has been used in combination with calcitonin and may result in rapid improvement of bone pain and suppression of bone turnover [23].

Mithramycin
Mithramycin acts as an osteoclast toxin. Therapy results in rapid improvement of bone pain and suppression of bone turnover. Various regimens of intravenous therapy have been proposed, including 15 to 25 μg/kg/day for 10 days, 15 to 25 μg/kg per week, and 15 μg/kg per day for 3 days followed by 10 μg/kg per day for 7 more days [36]. Side effects of mithramycin include nausea, vomiting, and malaise for several days after therapy. Transient hepatitis and elevation in BUN and creatinine may occur [23]. In some patients, impairment of renal function may be persistent. The most serious toxicity of mithramycin is depression of platelets; this has occurred during treatment of malignant disease, at which time the dose of mithramycin may be higher and the bone marrow may be infiltrated with tumor [23].

Surgery
Surgery is occasionally necessary in the treatment of Paget's disease. The most commonly performed procedures are: (1) total hip replacement for osteoarthritis and severe protrusio acetabuli [37], (2) internal fixation of fractures, and (3) decompressive procedures to prevent nervous tissue damage. Severe basilar skull compression may cause cranial nerve palsies, impaired gait, a decrease in mental function, and sphincteric incontinence, and it may require a decompressing suboccipital craniectomy [23]. Basilar impression may also cause hydrocephalus, resulting in a slow deterioration in mental function. Ventriculojugular shunts may improve this condition. In the case of spinal cord radicular nerve compressions, decompressive laminectomy may be useful. Pretreatment with calcitonin or EHDP may prove useful in decreasing bleeding during surgery.

References

1. Jaffe, H. L. Gross and Histologic Structure of Bones. In H. L. Jaffe, *Metabolic, Degenerative, and Inflammatory Diseases of Bones and Joints*. Philadelphia: Lea & Febiger, 1972.
2. Meunier, P., et al. Physiological senile involution and pathological rarefaction of bone. *Clin. Endocrinol. Metab.* 2:239, 1973.
3. Frost, H. M. The spinal osteoporoses: Mechanisms of pathogenesis and pathophysiology. *Clin. Endocrinol. Metab.* 2:257, 1973.
4. Newton-John, H. F., and Morgan, D. B. The loss of bone with age, osteoporosis, and fractures. *Clin. Orthop.* 71:229, 1970.

5. Jowsey, J. Osteoporosis: Idiopathic, Post-Menopausal, and Senile. In C. B. Sledge (Ed.), *Metabolic Diseases of Bone*. Philadelphia: Saunders, 1977.
6. Raisz, L. G. Bone Metabolism and Calcium Regulation. In L. V. Avioli and S. M. Krane (Eds.), *Metabolic Bone Disease*. New York: Academic Press, 1977.
7. Tonna, E. A. Aging of the Skeletal-Dental Systems and Supporting Tissues. In C. E. Finch and L. Hay (Eds.), *The Biology of Aging*. New York: Van Nostrand Reinhold, 1977.
8. Bullamore, J. R., et al. Effect of age on calcium absorption. *Lancet* 2:535, 1970.
9. Gallagher, J. C., et al. Intestinal calcium absorption and serum vitamin D metabolites in normal subjects and osteoporotic patients. *J. Clin. Invest.* 64: 729, 1979.
10. Ireland, P., and Fordtran, J. S. Effect of dietary calcium and age on jejunal calcium absorption in humans. *J. Clin. Invest.* 52:2672, 1973.
11. Avioli, L. V. Osteoporosis: Pathogenesis and Therapy. In L. V. Avioli and S. M. Krane (Eds.), *Metabolic Bone Disease*. New York: Academic Press, 1977.
12. Recker, R. R., Saville, P. D., and Heaney, R. P. Effect of estrogens and calcium carbonate on bone loss in postmenopausal women. *Ann. Intern. Med.* 87:649, 1977.
13. Riggs, B. L., et al. Studies on the pathogenesis and treatment in postmenopausal and senile osteoporosis. *Clin. Endocrinol. Metab.* 2:317, 1973.
14. Aloia, J. F., et al. Prevention of involutional bone loss by exercise. *Ann. Intern. Med.* 89:356, 1978.
15. Riggs, B. L., et al. Effect of the fluoride/calcium regimen on vertebral fracture occurrence in postmenopausal osteoporosis. *N. Engl. J. Med.* 306:446, 1982.
16. Gallagher, J. C., et al. The crush fracture syndrome in postmenopausal women. *Clin. Endocrinol. Metab.* 2:293, 1973.
17. Tronzo, R. G. Fractures of the Hip. In R. G. Tronzo (Ed.), *Surgery of the Hip*. Philadelphia: Lea & Febiger, 1973.
18. Aaron, J. E., et al. Frequency of osteomalacia and osteoporosis in the fractures of the proximal femur. *Lancet* 1:229, 1974.
19. Baker, M. R., et al. Plasma 25-hydroxy vitamin D concentrations in patients with fractures of the femoral neck. *Br. Med. J.* 1:589, 1979.
20. Morris, G. K., and Mitchell, J. R. A. Can death from venous thromboembolism be prevented in elderly patients with hip fractures? *Am. Heart J.* 95:139, 1978.
21. Morris, G. K., and Mitchell, J. R. A. Warfarin sodium in prevention of deep venous thrombosis and pulmonary embolism in patients with fractured neck of femur. *Lancet* 2:869, 1979.
22. Amstutz, L. D. Total Hip Replacement. In R. G. Tronzo (Ed.), *Surgery of the Hip*. Philadelphia: Lea & Febiger, 1973.
22a. Proceedings of the Kroc Foundation Conference on Paget's Disease of Bone. *Arthritis Rheum.* 23:1073, 1980.
23. Singer, F. R. *Paget's Disease of Bone*. New York: Plenum Medical Books, 1977.

24. Franck, W. A., et al. Rheumatic manifestations of Paget's disease of bone. *Am. J. Med.* 56:592, 1974.
25. Heistad, D. D., et al. Regulation of blood flow in Paget's disease of bone. *J. Clin. Invest.* 55:69, 1975.
26. Sparrow, N. A., and Duvall, A. J. III. Hearing loss and Paget's disease. *J. Laryngol.* 81:601, 1967.
27. Marshall, T. R., and Ling, J. T. The brim sign, a new sign found in Paget's disease (osteitis deformans) of the pelvis. *Am. J. Roentgenol. Radium Ther. Nucl. Med.* 90:1267, 1963.
28. Ross, F. G. M., Middlemiss, J. H., and Fitton, J. M. Paget's Sarcoma in Bone—A Radiological Study. In C. H. G. Price and F. G. M. Ross (Eds.), *Bone—Certain Aspects of Neoplasia.* London: Buttersworth, 1973.
29. Nagant de Deuxchaisnes, C., and Krane, S. M. Paget's disease of bone: clinical and metabolic observations. *Medicine* 43:233, 1964.
30. Rhodes, B. A., et al. Absence of anatomic arteriovenous shunts in Paget's disease of bone. *N. Engl. J. Med.* 287:686, 1972.
31. Woodhouse, N. J. Y., et al. Human calcitonin in the treatment of Paget's bone disease. *Lancet* 1:1139, 1971.
32. DeRose, J., et al. Response of Paget's disease to porcine and salmon calcitonins. *Am. J. Med.* 56:858, 1974.
33. Singer, F. R., Rude, R. K., and Mills, B. G. Studies in the Treatment and Etiology of Paget's Disease of Bone. In I. MacIntyre (Ed.), *International Symposium on Human Calcitonin and Paget's Disease,* Ciba Foundation Symposium. Amsterdam: Excerpta Medica, 1977.
34. Altman, R. D., et al. Influence of disodium etidronate on clinical and laboratory manifestations of Paget's disease of bone (osteitis deformans). *N. Engl. J. Med.* 289:1379, 1973.
35. Kantrowitz, F. G., Byrne, M. H., Krane, S. M. Clinical and metabolic effects of the diphosphonate EHDP in Paget's disease of bone. *Clin. Res.* 23:445A, 1975.
36. Russell, A. S., et al. Long term effectiveness of low dose mithramycin for Paget's disease of bone. *Arthritis Rheum.* 22:215, 1975.
37. Stauffer, R. N., and Sim, F. H. Total hip arthroplasty in Paget's disease of the hip. *J. Bone Joint Surg.* 58A:476, 1976.

16. Rheumatic Disease

David F. Giansiracusa

Fred G. Kantrowitz

Erythrocyte Sedimentation Rate

The erythrocyte sedimentation rate (ESR), an easily performed laboratory test used to evaluate the presence of various diseases and to monitor their activity [1], measures the settling of red blood cells suspended in anticoagulated blood in a vertically positioned tube of specific dimensions for a 60-minute period. Normal values depend on the dimensions of the tube used [2]. Generally quoted normal ESR values in millimeters per hour by the Westergren method are less than 15 for men and less than 25 for women; by the Wintrobe method, they are 0 to 6.5 for men and 0 to 16 for women.

The sedimentation rate is affected predominantly by red blood corpuscle rouleau formation, which, by increasing the size of the particle and weight relative to the surface area, accelerates the rate of red corpuscle fall. Large, asymmetric plasma molecules facilitate rouleau formation. Fibrinogen is the predominant plasma protein responsible for this, while alpha and gamma globulins contribute to lesser degrees. Elevated ESRs may reflect the presence of a malignancy, infection, systemic rheumatic disease, paraproteinemia, or renal failure [3].

The effects of aging must be considered when interpreting the ESR. Several studies have examined ESRs in healthy individuals of various ages and indicate a linear increase with each advancing decade [4]. A study of 1,457 healthy men and 1,021 women with the Westergren method revealed a constant increase in men of 0.85 mm per hour and in women of 0.53 mm per hour every five years until age 50 [5]. After menopause, the ESR increased 2.8 mm per hour every five years [6]. Thus, for individuals older than 65, an ESR up to 40 mm per hour with the Westergren method may be normal for the patient's age.

Possible explanations for the increased ESR seen in elderly individuals include the presence of an occult disease process, an increase in the production or a decrease in the catabolism of asymmetric plasma proteins.

Antinuclear Antibodies

Antinuclear antibodies (ANA) are immunoglobulins predominantly of the IgG class directed against various nuclear constituents, including deoxyribonucleic acid (DNA), ribonucleic acid (RNA), and nucleoprotein [7]. The homogeneous or diffuse pattern reflects antibody to deoxyribonuclear protein (DNP) and occurs in approximately 98 percent of patients with systemic lupus erythematosus (SLE). The diffuse pattern also occurs in individuals with other systemic rheumatic diseases and chronic active hepatitis.

The peripheral or rim pattern is seen when antibody to double-stranded

267

DNA and occasionally to single-stranded DNA is present. Patients with active SLE frequently have high-titer antinuclear antibodies (ANAs) with a peripheral pattern that may change to a lower-titer homogeneous pattern during remissions. Although antibodies to single-stranded DNA may occur in various diseases, such as rheumatoid arthritis, scleroderma, and chronic active hepatitis, antibodies in significant titer to double-stranded or native DNA are specific for SLE [8].

The speckled pattern of immunofluorescence frequently reflects antibody to an extractable nuclear antigen (ENA) that is composed of ribonuclear protein (RNP) and the Sm antigen. This pattern is seen in patients with Sjögren's syndrome, rheumatoid arthritis, SLE, progressive systemic sclerosis, and mixed connective tissue disease (MCTD). Antibody to the Sm antigen component of ENA occurs with SLE. The nucleolar pattern reflects antibody to nucleolar ribonucleoprotein. It occurs most commonly in patients with progressive systemic sclerosis but is also seen in patients with systemic lupus erythematosus and Sjögren's syndrome.

In addition to these disease states, antibodies to nuclear constituents occur with relatively high frequency in normal elderly individuals. In one study antinuclear antibodies were found in 3 percent of normal individuals 16 to 59 years of age and in 16 percent of individuals 60 to 91 years of age [9].

ANAs occurring as a "normal" function of age typically have a homogeneous or diffuse immunofluorescent pattern and occur in low titer (less than 1 : 16) [10]. They are directed against nucleic acid-histone; antibodies to purified deoxyribonucleic acid do not occur simply as a function of aging.

In summary, antinuclear antibodies in low titer may occur in normal elderly individuals and in patients with systemic rheumatic diseases. High-titer ANAs with peripheral (or rim), speckled, or nucleolar patterns occur in the setting of various systemic rheumatic disease and would be an extremely unusual finding in a normal elderly person.

Rheumatoid Factor

Rheumatoid factor is an antibody, usually IgM and rarely IgG or IgA, that reacts with IgG. These antibodies occur (1) in 70 to 80 percent of individuals with rheumatoid arthritis; (2) with lesser frequency in other systemic rheumatic diseases such as systemic lupus erythematosus; (3) with infectious diseases such as tuberculosis, leprosy, leishmoniasis, syphilis, and subacute bacterial endocarditis; (4) with chronic inflammatory processes of unknown etiology such as sarcoidosis and interstitial pulmonary fibrosis; and (5) with hematologic and oncologic diseases such as multiple myeloma and macroglobulinemic states [11].

Rheumatoid factors occur with increasing frequency with advancing age. Using the latex fixation method, they were found in 1 to 3 percent of individuals less than 65 and in 16 percent of a group of 325 people between the ages of 65 to 103. In over half of these 16 percent, the titer was 1 : 80 or less. In a fifth of those with positive rheumatoid factor, the titer was greater than 1 : 160 [12]. Other studies have found rheumatoid factor activity in approximately 25 percent of healthy individuals older than 70 years of age [13].

Gamma Globulins

Various changes of B and T lymphocyte function with advancing age may alter gamma globulin concentrations in elderly individuals. Several studies reveal that after the fourth decade, concentrations of IgG and IgM decrease while IgA levels remain constant [14,15].

Benign monoclonal gammopathies occur in approximately 3 percent of healthy individuals older than 70 and in as many as 19 percent of healthy individuals over 90 [16]. Monoclonal immunoglobulinemia is the presence in the serum and/or urine of a homogeneous globulin composed of immunoglobulin molecules or fragments produced in excess by a clone of immunocytes. A characteristic M spike in the gamma globulin area noted on protein electrophoresis of the serum and urine can identify the specific immunoglobulin class. Immunoelectrophoresis using monovalent anti–heavy-chain and anti–light-chain sera can then be performed to identify specific fragments [16].

Monoclonal immunoglobulin disorders may be due to a variety of benign and malignant conditions. Malignant immunocytopathies include multiple myeloma, Waldenström's macroglobulinemia, amyloidosis, and heavy-chain diseases. Monoclonal immunoglobulin elevation can also occur in association with various conditions such as carcinomatosis, hepatic cirrhosis, diseases of suspected autoimmune origin, and chronic inflammatory diseases [16].

The clinician may be confronted with distinguishing a benign from a malignant gammopathy. Several features indicative of a malignant immunocytopathy help to make this distinction [16]. These include: (1) a serum M component IgG concentration equal to or greater than 2 gm/dl or concentration of IgM or IgA M component equal to or greater than 1 g/dl; (2) the presence of Bence Jones proteinuria; (3) a progressive increase in the serum paraprotein over time; (4) a marked decrease in the synthesis of normal immunoglobulins; (5) serum hyperviscosity; (6) marrow plasmacytosis greater than 20 percent, with an increase in the number of immature and atypical cells; (7) a decrease in the number of peripheral blood B lymphocytes; and (8) the presence of hypoalbuminemia [16].

Recommendations for evaluation and follow-up study of individuals found to have a monoclonal immunoglobulin elevation include: (1) evaluation for covert carcinomatosis and malignant immunocytic disease with yearly bone marrow examinations; (2) serum and urine electrophoresis every three months for the first year, then repeated at six-month intervals; and (3) determinations of hemoglobin, white blood count, platelet count, serum iron, and total iron-binding capacity every six months [16].

Amyloid and Amyloid Arthropathy

This section reviews the biochemical and immunologic properties of amyloid fibrils and the circulating plasma precursors, the relationship between amyloid protein precursors and deposition of amyloid material in tissues, and concludes with a discussion of amyloid arthropathy.

Amyloidosis has been classified into six categories: (1) amyloidosis associated with plasma cell dyscrasias; (2) secondary amyloidosis that occurs in the setting of a chronic infectious, inflammatory, or malignant process; (3) primary amyloidosis in which no predisposing illness can be identified; (4) heredofamilial amyloidosis, including familial Mediterranean fever; (5) localized amyloidosis; and (6) amyloid deposition occurring with advancing age [17].

The biochemical composition of the amyloid fibril in primary amyloidosis and that associated with plasma cell dyscrasias, called the AL protein, differs from fibrils occurring in other forms of amyloidosis. The AL protein is composed of kappa or lambda immunoglobulin light chains or fragments. The fibrils found in secondary amyloidosis are composed of AA protein, an alpha globulin with a molecular weight of 8,400 daltons that has no structural relationship to immunoglobulin [18].

A plasma protein called SAA, an alpha globulin, has been identified as a precursor of the AA protein [19]. The SAA protein is found in low concentrations in normal individuals. It is elevated in individuals with secondary amyloidosis and, to a lesser degree, in patients with primary amyloidosis and amyloidosis associated with plasma cell dyscrasias.

The concentration of SAA protein also increases with aging, most strikingly after the age of 70 [20] (Fig. 16-1). The observation that some normal individuals older than 70 have normal levels of SAA suggests that the aging process itself may not be responsible for the elevated concentration of SAA protein, but rather that the protein may be a marker of an occult inflammatory or neoplastic disease.

Elevated SAA protein concentrations that are associated with advancing age are paralleled by an increased incidence of amyloid deposition in the brain, heart, and pancreatic Langerhans islets. Cardiac deposits were found in approximately 40 percent of individuals older than 60. In the brain, localized amyloid deposits were found in small cerebral blood vessels or plaques in 50 to 65 percent of individuals older than 60 years. Aortic amyloid deposits, found most frequently at the base of well-developed atheromatous plaques in the area of degenerated inner media, were found in 40 to 50 percent of individuals older than 60 years [21].

Amyloid can also form deposits in the structures of joints, resulting in an arthropathy that may resemble rheumatoid arthritis [22]. Less frequently, amyloid deposits cause joint complaints secondary to bone involvement. Deposits in the marrow space of bones of large joints, most frequently the

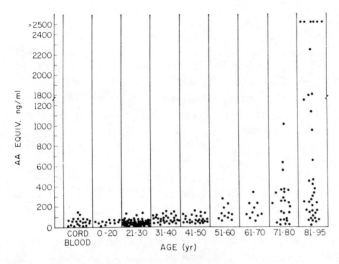

Figure 16-1. Concentration of SAA in a healthy population in relation to age. (From C. J. Rosenthal and E. C. Franklin. Variation with age and disease of amyloid A-related serum component. *J. Clin. Invest.* 55:746, 1975.)

hip, may form tumefactions, resulting in bone fractures and swelling of the involved joints [23].

Classic multiple myeloma is the underlying disorder found most frequently in amyloid arthropathy, although cases have been reported in association with Waldenström's macroglobulinemia. Although a number of individuals reported in the literature with amyloid arthropathy were thought to have primary amyloidosis, these diagnoses were often made in the absence of bone marrow examination or immunoelectrophoretic evaluation of serum and urine for identification of M spikes. Thus, plasma cell dyscrasias were not definitely ruled out [22].

Amyloid joint involvement occurs most often in the sixth decade of life. The clinical features may be similar to those of rheumatoid arthritis and include morning stiffness, painful joint swelling, and synovial thickening, most commonly in the shoulders, knees, wrists, metacarpophalanges (MCPs), proximal interphalanges (PIPs), elbows, and hips [23]. The involvement is usually of large as well as small joints, including temporomandibular and acromioclavicular joints. Flexion contractures are frequent. Subcutaneous nodules, frequently over the olecranon, occur in 70 percent of individuals. Concurrent or antecedent carpal tunnel syndrome occurs in one-third of patients. The prominent shoulder swelling has been described as the "padded shoulder sign." Dorsal synovial thickening of the wrist may have a gritty or nodular feeling on palpation. Although involved joints may be slightly tender, joint inflammation, evidenced by warmth, erythema, and marked tenderness, is conspicuously lacking.

Laboratory studies reveal a monoclonal light chain or M component in the serum or urine in almost all individuals, with kappa chains occurring eight times more frequently than lambda light chains. Bence Jones proteinuria is found in over two-thirds of those tested.

Radiographic features of amyloid arthropathy include osteolytic lesions, which may be the result of amyloid deposits or myelomatous aggregates. Generalized osteopenia and periarticular soft tissue swelling are common findings. Joint effusions are radiographically apparent in approximately 25 percent of individuals.

Synovial fluid from involved joints tends to be viscous and yellow or xanthochromic. The mean white blood count (WBC) is 1,000 with a range of several hundred to 10,000. The cells are most commonly mononuclear, but a predominance of neutrophils has also been described. Amyloid deposits in fragments of synovial membrane or as free fibrils are frequently found in aspirated synovial fluid samples when they are stained and viewed under polarized light. Immunoelectrophoresis of the synovial fluid frequently results in identification of immunoglobulin light chains similar to those found in the serum.

Histologic examination of articular tissues frequently reveals amyloid deposits that are located in the synovial layer superficial to or mixed with the synovial lining cells. Articular cartilage and periarticular tissue, including the joint capsule, tendons, ligaments, and bones, may contain amyloid deposits. Cellular reaction to these deposits is minimal.

The natural history of these patients is dependent on the underlying plasma cell dyscrasia. Articular improvement frequently occurs associated with corticosteroid and cytotoxic therapy for the underlying disease.

Changes Associated with Aging of Articular Cartilage

Articular cartilage is formed from mesenchymal cells derived from embryonic mesoderm and is composed of collagen fibers, produced by chondrocytes, embedded in a matrix or ground substance. Each collagen macromolecule consists of three tropocollagen fibers or alpha chains, each of approximately 1,000 amino acid sequences wrapped together in an alpha helix structure [24]. Chondrocytes also synthesize the ground substance of articular cartilage, proteoglycans, which are composed of glycosaminoglycans. The highly viscous and strongly hydrophilic properties of proteoglycans provide articular cartilage with resiliency to compression and with lubrication that lessens friction between articular surfaces [25].

Normal articular cartilage is devoid of blood vessels, lymphatics, and nerves. Chondrocytes derive their nourishment by diffusion through articular cartilage from the synovial fluid and to a lesser extent from subchondral blood vessels. During the developmental stages of articular cartilage (through adolescence), the collagen content increases while the water, hexosamine, chondroitin sulfate, ash, and sialoprotein content decreases [26].

As the person ages after reaching 30, there are no demonstrable changes in articular cartilage in the content of total hexosamine, water, and ash; in the concentration of chondroitin sulfate and keratan sulfate; and in the degree of chondroitin sulfate polymerization [24,27].

Osteoarthritis
HISTOLOGIC, BIOCHEMICAL, AND METABOLIC CHANGES OF CARTILAGE

The histologic changes of osteoarthritis are similar to those that occur with aging, that is, loss of superficial, tangential layers of cartilage and an increase in the number of chondrocytes occurring in clones or islands within the cartilage matrix. Other changes occurring specifically in osteoarthritic cartilage include progressive loss of proteoglycan content and extension of vertical clefts into subchondral bone. The defects in the cartilage and subchondral bone formed by these clefts cause scar and reactive bone formation and result in the radiographic appearance of subchondral sclerosis and heterotopic bone formation. The exposed bone becomes sclerotic, and subchondral cysts develop that may be due to small fractures in the trabecular bone or to synovial fluid forced into bone through cartilage defects. The new cartilage that proliferates in the areas of erosions and over marginal ostephytes is mechanically inferior to the normal articular cartilage [26].

Biochemical changes occurring in osteoarthritic cartilage include a decrease in proteoglycan content that is proportional to the severity of the disease and an increase in the content of chondroitin-4-sulfate relative to keratan sulfate [26]. This is in contrast to normal aging cartilage, in which the concentration of chondroitin-4-sulfate and keratan sulfate do not change [27]. There is also a decrease in proteoglycan chain length in osteoarthritis. Studies of proteoglycan synthesis is osteoarthritic cartilage initially reveals a doubling of synthetic rate compared with normal cartilage. As the osteoarthritis progresses in severity, the rate of proteoglycan synthesis markedly declines [26]. Chondrocyte DNA synthesis as measured by ^{3}H thymidine incorporation is increased, as is collagen synthesis. Chondrocytes in osteoarthritic cartilage produce normal type II $(\alpha_1 (II))_3$ collagen as well as type I $(\alpha_1 (I)_2)\alpha_2$, which normally occurs in skin and bone [26].

BIOCHEMICAL AND MECHANICAL PATHOGENESIS

Recognition of the biochemical and histologic features of osteoarthritic joints aids in understanding the pathophysiology of osteoarthritis. Bleeding, occurring with subchondral bone damage or intrasynovial hemorrhage, is associated with high cytoplasmic quantities of iron pigment in chondrocytes. As chondrocytes phagocytize the iron, lysosomal enzymes are released that degrade cartilage. Repeated articular bleeding decreases metachromatic staining, reflecting loss of proteoglycans, and results in superficial and deep cartilage erosions [26]. Depletion of glycosaminoglycans before fibrillation of the cartilage suggests that degradation of proteoglycans by proteolytic enzymes such as cathepsin may be the initiating process [28]. The levels of cathepsin D are increased in osteoarthritic cartilage [29]. Immunofluorescent studies localize cathepsin D in the chondrocyte lysosomes and in the area of chondrocyte surfaces. Low–molecular weight proteases, which at a neutral pH digest proteoglycans, may also be present in cartilage. Phagocytosis of particles of abraded cartilage may also cause the release of lysosomal proteases and collagenases.

Normal articular cartilage is resistant to sheer forces due to the low coefficient of friction. With impact, articular cartilage and subchondral bone deform in a manner that maximizes the surface area of contact between the two articular surfaces, thereby distributing the load over the greatest area possible [30]. Repeated impact-loading of joints causes rapid cartilage wear, an increase in the coefficient of friction of the articular surfaces, exposure of subchondral bone, and development of microfractures. With healing, the subchondral bone remodels and loses its ability to absorb stress. This subjects the articular cartilage to increased mechanical stresses and results in progression of cartilage damage. A cycle is thus established of trauma or abnormal physical stresses and proteolytic enzymes damaging articular cartilage and subchondral bone, and disrupting the properties of the joint that protect it from physical stresses. The enzymatic damage to cartilage stimulates chondrocyte synthesis of abnormal proteoglycans and articular collagen. The cartilage synthesized in an attempt to repair the damage is inferior to normal articular cartilage with respect to both the collagen and the ground matrix components [30].

CLINICAL FEATURES

Osteoarthritis is a progressive disorder commonly occurring in later life that is characterized clinically by pain, deformity, and limitation of joint motion. The pathologic features of affected joints include cartilage destruction, subchondral sclerosis and bone cyst formation, and osteophytic new bone and cartilage proliferation at joint margins [27]. Degenerative changes at autopsy examination of weight-bearing joints can be demonstrated as occurring as early as the second decade and can be found in 90 percent of individuals by age 40. Radiographic changes may be seen in weight-bearing joints in 85 percent of individuals by age 75, only 30 percent of whom are symptomatic. A disparity between the individual's symptoms and the radiographic extent of the disease is common [31]. The cardinal clinical feature of osteoarthritis is pain, which early in the disease occurs with motion, particularly with weight-bearing, and is relieved with rest. As the disease progresses, the pain may occur with minimal motion and at rest, may be troublesome at night, awaken the individual from sleep, and is often of aching quality and poorly localized. Stiffness for several minutes after inactivity and on awakening may occur, but it is not of the duration seen in patients with rheumatoid arthritis. Progressive loss of range of motion occurs on the basis of joint surface incongruity, muscle spasm, tendon and joint capsule contractures, and osteophytes [31].

Women tend to be affected more commonly than men with severe osteo-arthritis of the knee. Obese women over 50 with varus deformities of the knee are at high risk of developing osteoarthritis of the knee. Patients with osteoarthritis of the knee may complain of a "crunching" sound or sensation with movement and of joint instability. Examination may reveal crepitus on palpation of the joint during motion, limited active and passive ranges of motion, irregular enlargement of the joint due to cartilage and bony pro-liferation, quadriceps atrophy, instability due to laxity of the collateral liga-ments, and knee effusion. Synovial fluid is noninflammatory with less than 2,000 WBC, and shows a predominance of mononuclear white blood cells and a good mucin clot. Occasionally, cartilage fragments can be seen on synovial fluid analysis. Radiographic studies routinely include anteroposterior (AP) and lateral views. Special studies include the AP view during weight-bearing to evaluate the degree of joint space narrowing, reflecting cartilage loss, as well as the degree of genu varus or valgus deformity. Tunnel views with the knee flexed expose the intercondylar notch and are useful to evaluate intraarticular loose bodies and spurs [31].

Osteoarthritis of the hip is more common in men than in women. Al-though true hip pain is usually appreciated in the groin or inner aspect of the thigh, it may be referred to the buttocks, down the front of the thigh to the knee, or in a sciatic distribution. Low back pain results from an in-crease in lumbar lordosis that compensates for flexion contractures at the hips. Osteophytes, joint space narrowing, subchondral sclerosis, and cysts occur predominantly on the superior, i.e., weight-bearing, aspect of the hip joint.

The prominent symptom of osteoarthritis of the spine is pain. This may be due to soft tissue reaction of the periosteum, paraspinous ligaments, joint capsule, or to paraspinous muscle spasms. Paresthesias and reflex motor changes may occur secondary to radicular irritation. Changes that may im-pinge on neural foramina and cause nerve root compression include osteo-phytes, lateral disc protrusion, and apophyseal joint subluxation. Since the diameter of the spinal canal is smaller in the cervical area than elsewhere in the spine, neurologic abnormalities due to spinal cord compression most commonly occur with osteoarthritis of the cervical spine [31].

Anterior osteophytes are particularly common in the thoracic vertebrae but may extend the entire length of the spine. Radiographic features of osteo-arthritis, in addition to anterior osteophytes, include narrowing of inter-vertebral disks, which is most severe in the lower cervical and lower lumbar regions, with sclerosis of adjacent vertebral body borders, lateral and pos-terior vertebral osteophytes, joint space narrowing with vertebral body sclero-sis of posterior apophyseal joints, and subluxation of apophyseal joints. Al-though osteophytes are generally asymptomatic, severe cases of exostosis with fusion of vertebral body osteophytes has been termed "ankylosing verte-bral hyperostosis of the aged," a condition with little pain but marked limi-tation of motion [31].

Primary osteoarthritis of the hands involves distal and proximal inter-phalangeal joints of the fingers, the carpometacarpal joint of the thumb, and the first metatarsophalangeal joint of the foot. Women are affected about 10 times as frequently as men. Features of this condition include the develop-ment of cartilaginous and bony enlargement, usually of multiple distal interphalangeal (DIP) joints (Heberden's nodes) and PIP joints (Bou-chard's nodes). These changes may cause flexion contractures and medial or lateral deviation of the distal phalanx. Involvement of the carpometacarpal joint of the thumb may cause pain. Prominence at the base of the thumb gives it a squared appearance. Involvement of the first metatarsophalangeal joint of the foot usually results in progressive swelling and pain, especially with tight-fitting shoes. Attacks of inflammation of the bursa over the me-dial aspect of this joint may mimic acute podagra (gout).

Although Heberden's and Bouchard's nodes and arthritis usually develop gradually with little pain, they occasionally develop rapidly and may be associated with erythma, swelling, tenderness, pain, and distal finger pares-thesias. The acute onset of Heberden's and Bouchard's nodes associated with inflammatory and degenerative changes of the DIP and PIP joints, first MCP and IP joints is termed *inflammatory osteoarthritis* and occurs almost exclusively in elderly women [32].

Secondary osteoarthritis develops in the setting of joint damage caused by an identifiable condition, including structural abnormalities (congenital hip dysplasia, slipped capital femoral epiphysis) or avascular necrosis of a joint secondary to Legg-Perthes disease, or in association with steroids, systemic lupus erythematosus, sickle cell anemia, liver disease, Caisson's disease, Gaucher's disease, or trauma. Metabolic diseases associated with cartilage damage, including hemochromatosis, Wilson's disease, ochronosis, Morquio's syndrome, gout, hypophosphatasia, hemophilia with repeated intraarticular hemorrhage, and inflammatory arthritides such as rheumatoid and septic arthritis, also result in osteoarthritis as a final common pathway. Occupa-tional demands and neurologic abnormalities that subject joints to severe mechanical stresses may cause osteoarthritis, including involvement at atypi-cal locations such as the elbows of coal miners, and the shoulders of weight lifters.

MANAGEMENT

Treatment of osteoarthritis includes measures to prevent cartilage injury and to delay the progression of joint damage. Once osteoarthritis is established, the major objectives of therapy are relief of pain and preservation of joint motion. Preventive measures include medical treatment of metabolic dis-orders that predispose to cartilage damage and correction of abnormal mechanical stresses on the joints such as leg length discrepancy, postural abnormalities, meniscal tears, and ligamentous laxity. Maintenance of ideal body weight, appropriate conditioning of the neuromuscular apparatus, avoidance of excessive fatigue during exercise, and use of mechanical assistive devices such as canes or walkers help to minimize mechanical injury to joints.

Medical management of pain associated with osteoarthritis includes the use of appropriate rest, antiinflammatory agents, analgesics, and local steroid injections. Rest as therapy to relieve pain may be divided into two components: rest for the entire body to avoid generalized fatigue, and rest for a particular part of the body in the form of splints or braces. Rest coupled with physical measures such as application of moist heat, massage, and traction may relieve painful muscle spasm.

Medications that provide pain relief include aspirin and other nonsteroidal antiinflammatory drugs [33] and a variety of nonnarcotic analgesics, including acetaminophen (Tylenol) and proxyphene hydrochloride (Darvon). Since osteoarthritis requires prolonged therapy, use of narcotic analgesics, which may be associated with addiction and toxicity, should be avoided. A variety of nonsteroidal antiinflammatory drugs (NSAIDs) are available, including aspirin, various nonacetylated salicylate preparations, naproxen, ibuprofen, sulindac, tolmetin, fenoprofen, meclofenamate sodium, and indomethacin. These agents should be taken with food or antacid to minimize gastrointestinal side effects. In the older patient who cannot tolerate acetylsalicylic acid or enteric-coated aspirin, naproxen (250- or 375-mg tablets) or sulindac (150- or 200-mg tablets) may be given on a twice-a-day schedule and are generally well tolerated.

The nonacetylated salicylate preparations, including salsalate (Disalcid), magnesium choline trisalicylate (Trilisate), and choline salicylate (Arthropan) are well tolerated and have the advantage, unlike other NSAIDs, of not impairing platelet function and not precipitating a reaction in patients who, when treated with aspirin, develop urticaria and angioedema and occasionally nasal polyps and bronchial asthma. Because of the tremendous individual variability of patient response to the NSAIDs, failure to achieve benefit and/or development of adverse reactions to one NSAID does not mean that a particular patient will fail to respond or will fail to tolerate another NSAID. A regimen consisting of a NSAID alone, of a nonnarcotic analgesic alone, or the combination of a NSAID with a pure analgesic may be tailored to the individualized needs of the particular patient. The combined use of an NSAID with an analgesic or the use of two different analgesic agents may provide additive analgesia without additive toxicity.

In the osteoarthritic patient whose problems are localized to a single joint, intraarticular injection of a depot steroid preparation (approximately 40 mg of depot methylprednisolone or its equivalent) mixed with 1 ml of 1% lidocaine may provide relief for weeks to months. Because intraarticular steroids impair the normal synthetic activity of chondrocytes, as a rule, steroid injections into a given joint should be performed no more than two to three times and at no shorter intervals than two to three months.

Physical therapy plays an important role in achieving and maintaining joint motion and muscle strength. Flexion contractures at the hips and knees and quadriceps weakness and atrophy are particularly disabling. A program of physical therapy designed specifically to treat these musculoskeletal problems is an essential component of management of the patient with osteoarthritis.

Surgical intervention may be useful, particularly for the correction of deformities such as flexion contractures and for relief of pain [25,34]. Surgical procedures such as removal of intraarticular loose bodies and repair of a torn meniscus may improve joint function dramatically. The patient with severe pain occurring particularly at night or severe impairment of joint function of the hip or knee is a candidate for total joint replacements.

Pseudogout–Calcium Pyrophosphate Dihydrate Crystal Deposition Disease

Deposition of calcium pyrophosphate dihydrate (CPPD) in articular cartilage increases with advancing age and is associated with various clinical presentations of arthritis. Articular chondrocalcinosis, the radiographic finding of abnormal deposition of calcium salts in hyaline and fibrocartilage, increases in incidence with advancing age and by the ninth decade is found in 25 to 30 percent of individuals [35].

A definite diagnosis of CPPD deposition requires either identification of calcium pyrophosphate dihydrate crystals, $Ca_2P_2O_7 \cdot 2H_2O$, in synovial fluid or biopsy specimens or arthritic cartilage, or the presence of typical polyarticular chondrocalcinosis together with identification of weakly positive birefringent crystals on compensated polarized microscopic examination of synovial fluid [36].

The arthritis associated with articular chondrocalcinosis is variable and six categories—types A through F—have been defined [37]. Type A is an acute monoarticular or oligoarticular arthritis that is termed *pseudogout* because it resembles an acute attack of gout. This occurs in approximately 25 percent of patients with CPPD deposition disease and is characterized by acute or subacute attacks of inflammation, usually in one appendicular joint, that last from one to four days. The attack may spread to surrounding joints and involve multiple contiguous joints at a given time, resulting in a "cluster" attack. The knee is the most frequently involved joint, being affected in 50 percent of attacks; the ankles, wrists, elbows, and small joints of the hands and feet are involved less frequently. Between attacks, the individual is asymptomatic. Identification of crystals is necessary to establish the diagnosis of an acute pseudogout attack. Various physiologic stresses such as medical illnesses, surgery, and trauma may precipitate an attack.

Type B, or *pseudorheumatoid arthritis,* occurs in approximately five percent of individuals with CPPD deposition disease. Attacks last several weeks to months and multiple joint involvement with synovial thickening, pitting edema, and limited range of motion secondary to flexion contractures and pain may mimic rheumatoid arthritis.

Type C and D presentations have been termed *pseudoosteoarthritis.* These occur in approximately 50 percent of individuals with CPPD crystal deposition disease. Progressive degeneration of multiple joints, commonly in a bilateral and symmetric pattern, is seen clinically and radiographically. Women are affected more commonly than men. The knee is the most common joint involved, but other affected joints include the wrist, MCP, hip, shoulder, elbow, and ankle joints, all of which are seldom involved in classic osteoarthritis. Individuals with superimposed acute attacks of pseudogout are said to have type C; those without the acute episodes have type D.

Type E, the *lanthanic* or asymptomatic form, and type F, the *pseudoneuropathic* form comprise the final two clinical presentations. In type E, individuals have radiographic articular cartilage calcification without symptoms. Individuals with type F have severe destructive changes characteristic of a neuropathic or Charcot's joint in the presence of articular chondrocalcinosis without having identifiable sensory abnormalities [38].

The radiologic features of CPPD crystal deposition disease are varied. CPPD crystal deposition in fibrocartilage of the menisci, radioulnar joint, triangular cartilage of the wrist, symphysis pubis, and annulus fibrosus of the intervertebral disks appears as dense punctuate calcifications. Crystal deposition in hyaline cartilage appears as fine, linear calcifications paralleling the subchondral bone of the femoral chondyles and head of the humerus. Crystal deposition in the synovial lining may create an irregular appearance of radiodense foci similar to calcifications seen in synovial chondromatosis. Joint capsule calcifications may occur in the hips, shoulders, elbows, and small joints of the hands. Occasionally CPPD crystal deposition occurs in the Achilles, triceps, quadriceps, and supraspinatus tendons and in connective tissue of the hip adductors [39]. Hook-like or tear drop osteophytes at the distal metacarpal heads are characteristic of patients with CPPD crystal deposition disease. Patients with appendicular chondrocalcinosis have been demonstrated to have an increased incidence of ankylosing hyperostosis of the spine [39].

Biopsies performed during acute attacks of pseudogout reveal proliferation of the lining cells of the synovial membrane, vascular congestion, fibrinous exudate overlying the synovial membrane, and rhomboid-shaped, weakly positive birefringent crystals in the synovial membrane, connective tissue, fibrin exudate, and synovial and tissue-based leukocytes. In the chronic forms of CPPD arthropathy, the synovium and underlying connective tissue appear fibrotic, with infiltration of mononuclear cells and presence of foreign body granulomas. Giant cells are seen in areas of CPPD crystal deposits. In severe cases the cartilage is replaced by granulation tissue [40]. These fibrotic changes most likely contribute to the flexion contractures seen in the sub-acute and chronic forms of CPPD-associated arthropathy.

Familial CPPD disease has been described in populations in Chile, Holland, and Czechoslovakia. In the last group, absence of male-to-male transmission suggests X-linked genetics, and the finding of more severe phenotypic expression at a younger age in the homozygote suggests that an enzymatic defect is a possible etiology. In the Chilean and Dutch populations, male-to-male transmission is consistent with autosomal genetics [41].

Various metabolic diseases have been associated with CPPD disease, including hyperparathyroidism, hemochromatosis, hypothyroidism, gout, hypophosphatasia and Wilson's disease [42]. Patients with CPPD arthropathy should be evaluated for evidence of hyperparathyroidism and hypothyroidism, and a family history for pseudogout or other forms of CPPD arthropathy obtained. Laboratory investigation should include determinations of serum calcium and phosphorus and tests of thyroid function. Serum iron and total iron-binding capacity (TIBC) are a simple screen for hemochromatosis.

An understanding of the pathophysiology of CPPD disease clarifies its association with various metabolic disorders. An acute attack is initiated when CPPD crystals residing in articular cartilage or joint tissues are shed into the synovial fluid. There they are coated with IgG and phagocytized by polymorphonuclear leukocytes and monocytes, which then release a low–molecular weight chemotactic factor that recruits additional inflammatory cells. As the leukocytes attempt to phagocytize the CPPD crystals, they release destructive lysosomal enzymes, including collagenases and elastases [37]. The result of these processes is joint inflammation and articular cartilage damage.

Calcium ions, Ca^{++}, and pyrophosphonate, P_2O_7-4, are in equilibrium with the crystalline form of calcium pyrophosphate dihydrate, $Ca_2P_2O_7 2H_2O$. Patients with hypophosphatasia have a deficiency in alkaline phosphatase, a pyrophosphatase. As a result, high concentrations of pyrophosphate accumulate, which facilitates formation of the CPPD crystal. Individuals with hyperparathyroidism have elevated Ca^{++} levels, which also facilitate the formation of CPPD crystals. A fall in serum calcium in a patient with hyperparathyroidism, either as a result of medical management or resection of parathyroid tissue, may precipitate an acute attack of pseudogout by disturbing the equilibrium between the crystalline and ionic forms of calcium pyrophosphate. Crystals may then be shed into the synovial fluid. The precipitation of pseudogout attacks by surgery is also consistent with this pathophysiologic mechanism, since a significant (approximately 10 percent) fall in serum Ca^{++} occurs after abdominal and thoracic surgical procedures. An additional precipitating factor in patients with hyperparathyroidism is the collapse of subchondral bone, which causes "shedding" of crystals into the synovial fluid. Degenerated cartilage may elaborate inorganic pyrophosphate. This may be the explanation for the increased incidence of chondrocalcinosis and CPPD arthropathies in the elderly, a population with prevalent osteoarthritis, and is consistent with the experimental observation of elevated concentrations of synovial fluid inorganic pyrophosphate, which is elaborated by osteoarthritic articular cartilage but not by normal adult cartilage [37].

The finding of inflammatory synovial fluid with intraleukocytic calcium pyrophosphate dihydrate crystals does not necessarily indicate that the crystals initiated and are the only cause of the joint inflammation. Any inflammatory arthritis, including pyogenic arthritis and acute gout, is associated with a leukocytic response. If calcium pyrophosphate is present in the articular cartilage, the lysosomal enzymes released by the leukocytes may leach the crystals out of the cartilage. Because of this mechanism of lysosomal "enzymatic strip mining," patients with CPPD arthritis must be evaluated for septic arthritis with Gram's stain and culture of the synovial fluid [37].

TREATMENT

Treatment of pseudogout and other forms of CPPD crystal arthropathies includes management of any associated underlying disorder and administration of antiinflammatory medications. An attack of pseudogout treated with an oral NSAID (e.g., ibuprofen, 1,600 to 2,400 mg in three or four divided doses a day; naproxen, 250 to 375 mg twice a day; or sulindac, 150 to 200 mg twice a day) will generally respond within three to four days. Joint aspiration and intraarticular injection of 40 mg of a depot prednisone preparation or its equivalent usually provides relief of signs and symptoms within one to two days [43]. The patients with the more subacute and chronic forms of CPPD arthropathy such as pseudorheumatoid arthritis and the pseudoosteoarthritic forms are generally treated, as are patients with osteoarthritis (see the section on management of osteoarthritis, p. 276).

Rheumatoid Arthritis

Rheumatoid arthritis (RA) is a chronic, systemic disease of unknown etiology affecting diarthrodial joints and associated with multiple extraarticular manifestations. The arthritis tends to be symmetric in distribution and frequently involves the wrist, MCP, PIP, metatarsophalangeal (MTP), knee, elbow, ankle, shoulder, and hip joints. Morning stiffness is a common complaint. Objective signs of synovitis are frequently found on examination and joint destruction may be demonstrated radiographically with joint space narrowing and marginal erosions. Synovial fluids are characteristically inflammatory.

Extraarticular manifestations tend to occur in rheumatoid factor–positive patients who have severe arthritis. Subcutaneous nodules, pericarditis, pleuritis, interstitial lung disease, peripheral neuropathies, anemia, Sjögren's syndrome, and vasculitis may accompany the articular disease [44,45]. The natural history varies from a several-month period of arthritis followed by complete remission, to chronic, active multi-system disease.

Although rheumatoid arthritis occurs most commonly in individuals between the ages of 20 and 60, approximately 10 percent of patients experience the onset of their disease after age 60. In one group of elderly patients, the arthritis affected men more often than women and was characterized by an acute onset with a predilection of large joints. These patients had a high frequency of remission within the first year [46]. In a group of 110 patients with onset of rheumatoid arthritis between the ages of 60 and 86, 74 percent had disease identical to rheumatoid arthritis occurring in younger patients [47]. However, the remaining 26 percent (29 patients) experienced remission within 12 to 18 months of onset compared to the usual remission rate of 5 to 10 percent in published series.

The characteristics of this group of 29 patients included the sudden onset of polyarticular arthritis, usually over a one- or two-day period, and severe constitutional symptoms, including anorexia, weight loss, malaise, depression, and severe morning stiffness that lasted as long as four to five hours. All had elevated erythrocyte sedimentation rates with a mean of 95 mm per hour for men and 75 mm per hour for women. Men comprised over half of the 29 individuals. Proximal joint involvement, including shoulders and neck, occurred in about half. In 6 of the 29, manifestations of pain and stiffness of the neck, shoulders, and buttock area suggested a diagnosis of polymyalgia rheumatica until more distal synovitis developed.

All 29 patients had positive rheumatoid factors that varied in titer from 1/32 to 1/5,120. All had radiographic periarticular osteopenia and 7 of 26 developed erosions. The association of acute onset with good prognosis in this group is similar to the pattern seen in younger populations. This group of elderly individuals is of particular interest since all experienced complete remissions, even those who had disease activity for longer than 12 months. This study of RA in the elderly also revealed that gold therapy was well tolerated and may be prescribed as it is when the disease occurs in a younger patient population. Steroids were used in 12 of the 29 patients for severe systemic symptoms. Prednisone in a dose of 5 to 10 mg per day was prescribed for 10 and was never administered in excess of 20 mg on a daily basis. In all patients, it was possible to eventually discontinue the steroids [47].

MANAGEMENT

Although the basic therapeutic principles and modalities used to treat rheumatoid arthritis in younger patients apply to the patient in whom rheumatoid arthritis develops in later years of life, several aspects of treatment of the elderly rheumatoid patient deserve particular attention. First, due to coexisting medical problems such as renal impairment, congestive heart failure, subclinical gastritis, and/or osteopenia, the elderly patient may be more susceptible to the toxicities and side effects of aspirin, other nonsteroidal antiinflammatory agents, and steroids than are younger patients. Differences in drug metabolism and, in the case of aspirin, the decreased ability to perceive tinnitus in the elderly may also predispose them to adverse drug reactions. The elderly patient may also have a greater tendency for the development of muscle weakness and atrophy, flexion contractures, and progressive bone loss than the younger patient, who may have a stronger musculoskeletal system at the onset of arthritis. For these reasons particular attention must be paid to physical therapy, including range of motion and strengthening exercises, to the appropriate use of joint splints, to the appropriate use of supplemental dietary calcium and vitamin D, and to avoidance of immobilization whenever possible. In the elderly patient whose rheumatoid arthritis is characterized by severe stiffness, constitutional symptoms, and particularly proliferative synovitis, treatment with low-dose steroids (5–10 mg of prednisone a day) used in addition to NSAIDs, may be particularly beneficial.

Systemic Lupus Erythematosus

Systemic lupus erythematosus (SLE) is a chronic, multisystem, inflammatory disease characterized by abnormalities in the immune system. Evidence of disordered humoral immunity includes circulating autoantibodies to nuclear and cytoplasmic antigens, lymphocytes, platelets, red blood cells, and various clotting factors as well as the identification of nuclear antigen, immunoglobulin, and complement deposition in small blood vessels [48]. Clinical manifestations include polyarthralgias/polyarthritis, alopecia, mucosal ulcerations, Raynaud's phenomena, skin rashes, fevers, glomerulonephritis, pleuritis, parenchymal lung disease, pericarditis, myocarditis, myositis, peritonitis, cerebritis, meningitis, peripheral neuritis, leukopenia, hemolytic anemia, and thrombocytopenia [49,50].

Although SLE occurs most commonly during adolescence and young adulthood and decreases in incidence and prevalence after age 45, idiopathic SLE may occur at any age. Between 4 and 10 percent of patients with SLE develop their disease after age 50 [51]. The percentage of men in whom SLE develops after the age of 50 is higher than in the younger group. In those with onset after age 50 to 60, 12.5 percent are men, whereas in younger populations of SLE patients males comprise approximately 5 percent [52]. The onset of SLE in the elderly does not differ significantly from that in younger patients. In the older age group, however, initial symptoms can be confused with those seen in other rheumatic diseases. Myalgias, weight loss, and fatigue may suggest polymyalgia rheumatica. The presentation of arthritis without associated symptoms may suggest rheumatoid arthritis.

The incidence of various manifestations of SLE varies with age of onset [53]. Individuals in whom SLE develops after age 50 have a higher incidence of pneumonitis, pulmonary fibrosis, discoid lupus, and photosensitivity than do younger individuals. Skin rash, alopecia, arthralgias, myalgias, serositis, renal disease, and renal biopsy findings are similar in both groups. Manifestations occurring less frequently in individuals with onset after age 50 include oral ulcers, Raynaud's phenomena, cutaneous vasculitis, thrombocytopenia, hemolytic anemia, leukopenia, neuropsychiatric manifestations, and hypocomplementemia [53,54].

SLE in elderly individuals in general requires less steroids and azathioprine to suppress the disease [54]. This implies that SLE with onset after age 50 to 60 is a milder disease and is more responsive to therapy than is SLE in younger individuals [55]. However, the authors of one study concluded that, like the mode of onset, the prognosis for those developing SLE after age 50 is the same as that for patients developing SLE at a younger age [52].

DRUG-INDUCED LUPUS

A number of medications associated with the development of lupus-like syndromes are administered to elderly individuals. These include procainamide, hydralazine, isoniazid, diphenylhydantoin, propylthiouracil, chlorpromazine, and, less frequently, practolol, methylthiouracil, methimazole, and penicillamine [56]. Positive antinuclear antibodies occur most frequently with administration of procainamide [57], hydralazine, and anticonvulsant therapy and less frequently with chlorpromazine, isoniazid, and alpha-methyldopa. As many as 50 percent of individuals in a prospective study treated for six months with procainamide developed antinuclear antibodies without symptoms of SLE. Positive lupus erythematosus tests and antibodies to denatured DNA and to deoxyribonucleoprotein (anti-DNP) but not to native DNA occur in one-third to one-half of individuals treated with procainamide for longer than six weeks [57].

The diagnosis of drug-induced lupus is made based on the same clinical features as idiopathic SLE. Clinical signs and symptoms may disappear within days to weeks while antinuclear antibodies may remain positive for months to years after the offending drug has been stopped. Rechallenge with the drug results in prompt reappearance of the signs and symptoms [56].

The relationship between drug use and development of lupus-like features may take three forms. Antinuclear antibodies without clinical symptoms of lupus erythematosus may develop. This type of reaction is not associated with production of lymphocytotoxins, Coombs positivity, or antibodies to native or double-stranded DNA. A second type of reaction is characterized by the development of antinuclear antibodies and symptoms of lupus erythematosus. Exacerbation of preexisting SLE with drug administration is the third type of reaction [58], in which sulfonamides are a frequent offender.

The incidence of clinical features of lupus differs in drug-induced lupus as compared with idiopathic SLE. In the former, pleuropulmonic manifestations such as pleuritic pain, pleural effusions, and pneumonitis occur with greater frequency and severity and may be more recalcitrant to therapy [56].

Constrictive pericarditis and cardiac tamponade have both been reported with procainamide-induced lupus [59]. Renal and central nervous system (CNS) involvement, febrile episodes, dermal manifestations, and hematologic manifestations are much less common in drug-induced SLE than in idiopathic SLE. Antibodies to native or double-stranded DNA do not occur in high titer in drug-induced lupus except when hydralazine is the drug administered [60]. Although hypocomplementemia is a feature of idiopathic SLE, it rarely occurs in drug-induced lupus.

TREATMENT OF SYSTEMIC AND DRUG-INDUCED LUPUS

Other than discontinuing the offending drug, if possible, in cases of documented drug-induced lupus syndromes, the management of idiopathic SLE in the elderly patient and of drug-induced lupus does not differ appreciably from the management of idiopathic SLE in younger patients [50]. Aspirin and other nonsteroidal antiinflammatory agents are helpful in controlling arthralgias, arthritis, myalgias, serositis, fevers, and malaises. Topical steroid preparations are efficacious for skin rashes and mucosal ulcerations. Sun screens should be used in patients with sun sensitivity. Hydroxychloroquine (Plaquenil) may be helpful, particularly for the management of skin and articular manifestations. The occurrences of hemolytic anemia, thrombocytopenia, severe renal disease, pericarditis, pleuritis, peritonitis, fevers, and neurologic manifestations may be indications for the use of steroids alone or in combination with cytotoxic agents in both the elderly patient and in the younger patient with lupus erythematosus.

Sjögren's Syndrome

Histologic changes of the salivary glands with aging include fatty degeneration and fibrosis of the parenchyma and lymphocytic infiltration, occasionally causing glandular enlargement [61]. Salivary secretions diminish with advancing age and are associated with loss of filiform papillae on the dorsum of the tongue, resulting in a smooth, glazed appearance. Lacrimal secretions also decrease, causing complaints of dry eyes. Vaginal dryness and dyspareunia may occur in elderly postmenopausal women as the vaginal epithelium becomes thin and dry in the absence of significant levels of circulating estrogens. These various complaints may suggest the presence of Sjögren's syndrome, a specific entity with characteristic clinical and pathologic features.

Sjögren's syndrome is composed of keratoconjunctivitis sicca (dry eyes) and xerostomia (dry mouth) and is often associated with rheumatoid arthritis or another systemic rheumatic disease [62]. Ocular complaints related to lacrimal gland dysfunction are common in patients with Sjögren's syndrome, occurring in over 90 percent. A burning sensation of the eyes or inability to produce tears results from inadequate lacrimal secretion of the aqueous portion of tears. A sensation of a foreign body or dust in the eyes and of a film covering the eyes and obscuring vision may result from production of an abnormal lacrimal mucus component [63].

Oral manifestations are related to inadequate salivary gland secretions and mechanical problems secondary to salivary gland infiltration. Dryness of the mouth and lips with development of fissures and ulcers on lips, tongue, and buccal mucosa, and loss of sense of taste may occur. Difficulty with mastication and swallowing result from inability to produce adequate saliva to form a bolus of food. Rampant dental caries may also occur due to inadequate salivary gland secretions.

Swelling of the salivary glands, particularly the parotids, occurs as a result of lymphocytic infiltration. Discrete episodes of swelling occur in approximately two-thirds of patients while chronic, progressive swelling, which is usually symmetric, is seen in about one-third of patients [62]. Although salivary gland swelling may be painful, this finding, especially in the setting of fever, raises the concern of a complication of Sjögren's such as suppurative parotitis or development of a lymphoreticular malignancy. The differential diagnosis of parotid swelling is large and includes viral, fungal, and bacterial infections; tuberculosis; sarcoidosis; deficiency of vitamins C, B_6, or A; iodide ingestion, hyperlipidemias types III, IV, and/or V; diabetes mellitus; cirrhosis; and primary or metastatic neoplasms [62].

Since the symptoms of Sjögren's syndrome may be found in many healthy elderly individuals, definite criteria have been developed to establish the diagnosis. These include objective evidence of keratoconjunctivitis sicca or xerostomia and characteristic histopathologic findings on biopsy of minor salivary glands [63]. Various tests to document keratoconjunctivitis sicca include the Schirmer's test, which measures tear production with filter paper placed at the intercanthous of the lower eyelid, measurement of tear lysozyme, and conjunctival and corneal staining. Clinically, the Schirmer's test is performed as a screening examination, but since tear production decreases with age, the test lacks specificity [64]. Conjunctival and corneal staining with rose bengal or fluorescein and viewed with a slit lamp can be performed as a more specific examination. The stain collects in areas of devitalized and epithelialized corneal and conjunctival tissue and reflects damage occurring as a result of lacrimal dysfunction. Evaluation of salivary gland function includes determination of salivary flow rates, technetium salivary gland radionuclide scans, and sialography [65].

Biopsy of minor salivary glands of the lower lip is done for histopathologic documentation. This procedure has evolved due to complications from parotid gland biopsies such as fistula formation and facial nerve damage and from the recognition that the minor salivary glands are involved in Sjögren's syndrome [65]. Major changes include parenchymal acinar atrophy, fibrous and adipose tissue replacement, lymphocytic infiltration, hyperplasia and proliferation of intraglandular ductal lining cells, and epimyoepithelial islands, the most specific of the histologic findings for Sjögren's. The severity of histologic changes correlates well with severity of sicca symptoms [63].

Even though clinical and diagnostic features emphasize lacrimal and salivary gland involvement, Sjögren's syndrome is a systemic disease [62]. In addition to eye and oral involvement, the skin, respiratory tract, genito-urinary tract, and gastrointestinal systems may be affected. Clinically, manifestations include dryness of the skin with lack of sweating, nonthrombo-cytopenic hyperglobulinemic purpura, nasal dryness, chronic nonproductive cough, pleurisy and pleural effusions, atelectasis, pulmonary fibrosis, dys-pareunia, hyposthenuria, and proximal renal tubular acidosis with its sequelae (osteomalacia secondary to urinary phosphate wasting, hypoka-lemia, and nephrocalcinosis), dysphagia and abnormal esophageal motility, liver function abnormalities, pancreatitis, and peripheral neuropathies. Histo-logic studies reveal lymphocytic infiltration in the affected organs. Raynaud's phenomena is also associated with Sjögren's syndrome, as are the presence of multiple circulating antibodies to tissue constituents, including antibodies to thyroglobulin, gastric parietal cells, and salivary ductal cells. Hypergamma-globulinemia, especially IgG, is common. Antinuclear antibodies occur in one- to two-thirds and IgM rheumatoid factor in about two-thirds of patients with documented Sjögren's syndrome. Beta$_2$ microglobulin, believed to be a product of lymphocytes and consisting of polypeptide chains homologous to immunoglobulin, is found in serum, salivary gland secretions, and urine [62] and reflects the degree of lymphocytic infiltration in these organs and the general activity of the disease. Elevated concentrations of immunoglobulin G and of IgM rheumatoid factors are also found in salivary gland secretions. Erythrocyte sedimentation rates are frequently elevated. An increased inci-dence of anergy associated with impaired lymphocyte transformation to phytohemagglutinin in vitro is another immunologic abnormality seen in patients with Sjögren's syndrome. In the peripheral blood, B lymphocytes are increased while T lymphocytes are decreased [63].

The immunologic features and the animal model of Sjögren's syndrome, the F_1 hybrid population of the New Zealand black/white (NZB/NZW) mice, provide evidence that Sjögren's syndrome results from a deficiency in suppressor T cell lymphocytes, leading to excessive B lymphocyte activity [66,67].

The natural history of patients with Sjögren's syndrome is now appreciated as a spectrum, ranging from benign lymphocytic infiltration of various exocrine glands to lymphocyte infiltration of viscera described as pseudo-lymphoma to frank lymphoproliferative malignancies or hyperviscosity syn-dromes [68] (Fig. 16-2). In a given patient, however, the disease usually does not evolve through all three stages. Striking elevation in the concen-tration of β_2 microglobulin may reflect lymphocytic proliferation and signal the development of a lymphoproliferative malignancy [69]. A progressive increase in IgM levels may signal the development of a macroglobulinemic

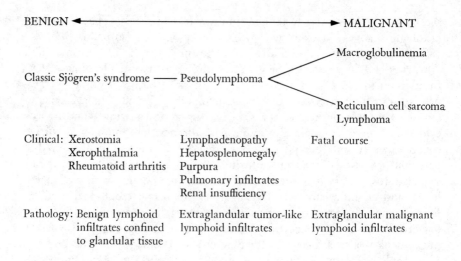

BENIGN ◀—————————————————————————▶ MALIGNANT

Classic Sjögren's syndrome ——— Pseudolymphoma ⟨ Macroglobulinemia

Reticulum cell sarcoma
Lymphoma

Clinical: Xerostomia   Lymphadenopathy   Fatal course
         Xerophthalmia   Hepatosplenomegaly
         Rheumatoid arthritis Purpura
                            Pulmonary infiltrates
                            Renal insufficiency

Pathology: Benign lymphoid   Extraglandular tumor-like   Extraglandular malignant
          infiltrates confined lymphoid infiltrates   lymphoid infiltrates
          to glandular tissue

Figure 16-2. The spectrum of benign to malignant lymphoproliferation in Sjögren's syndrome, with pertinent clinical and histologic features noted. (From N. A. Cummings, et al.   Sjögren's syndrome—newer aspects of research, diagnosis, and therapy. *Ann. Intern. Med.* 75:937, 1971.)

hyperviscosity syndrome. Several features of patients with Sjögren's syndrome identify them as being at risk to develop lymphoproliferative malignancies. These include parotid enlargement, lymphadenopathy, and splenomegaly, as well as an increased frequency of the HLA-Dw3 antigen that appears to serve as a marker of patients with Sjögren's syndrome without rheumatoid arthritis [70].

TREATMENT

Treatment of patients with Sjögren's syndrome includes supplementation of the inadequate exocrine gland secretions and management of complications. The treatment of lacrimal gland insufficiency includes the use of methylcellulose or polyvinylpyrol-based tears. Various maneuvers to retard loss of tears, such as the use of shielding eyeglasses and humidification of the environment, are useful. Infectious conjunctivitis should be treated aggressively. Oral symptoms can be treated with secretagogues including sugarless chewing gum and Slippery Elm lozenges. Meticulous dental care must be observed, including brushing and flossing after meals and frequent visits to a dentist and dental hygienist. Patients treated with cyclophosphamide for lymphoproliferative complications have noted improvement in their sicca symptoms, but cytotoxic therapy is not indicated for uncomplicated Sjögren's syndrome.

Polymyalgia Rheumatica

Polymyalgia rheumatica (PMR) is a specific clinical entity consisting of proximal muscle aching and stiffness that occurs in individuals over the age of 50, with peak incidence in the mid-60s. It occurs twice as frequently in women as in men, almost exclusively in white populations, and is associated with an elevated erythrocyte sedimentation rate [71].

The onset of myalgias often starts with the posterior neck muscles and spreads to the shoulder and pelvic girdles. Initially, the distribution may be unilateral but most frequently becomes symmetric and affects muscles of both the shoulders and hips. The onset of myalgias may be either insidious or abrupt. Exercise may aggravate the discomfort. Morning stiffness may last about an hour, sometimes suggesting rheumatoid arthritis in the differential diagnosis. The stiffness may be so severe that getting out of a bed or chair becomes very difficult. Myalgias at night may interfere with sleeping. Fatigue, lethargy, anorexia, weight loss, malaise, apathy, and depression are commonly associated symptoms.

Objective abnormalities may include limited range of motion of the shoulders and hips secondary to muscle discomfort. Muscles of the shoulder and pelvic girdles and posterior neck may be tender to palpation. Although the individual may make poor effort on strength testing due to discomfort, true muscle weakness is not part of the clinical picture of polymyalgia rheumatica. Knee effusions have been described [72].

Laboratory studies reveal an elevated erythrocyte sedimentation rate, usually greater than 50. A normochromic anemia, elevated α_2 globulins, and hypoalbuminemia are associated findings. Muscle enzymes, electromyograms, and muscle biopsies are normal in contrast to polymyositis and dermatomyositis [73]. Joint scans may be positive in the areas of the shoulders and hips in some individuals with PMR [74]. Abnormal liver function tests occur as reflected by increased bromsulphalein (BSP) retention and elevation of alkaline phosphatase [75].

The differential diagnosis of PMR includes virus-induced myalgias, rheumatoid arthritis, polymyositis, and hypothyroidism. Viral infections are characteristically of less than one month's duration and are associated with fever and normal sedimentation rates. In PMR the ESR is elevated and fever is unusual unless giant cell arteritis is present. In rheumatoid arthritis, initial symptoms may include upper arm myalgias and morning stiffness that may be indistinguishable from PMR [71]. Knee effusions described in PMR make this "differential" even more difficult, as can the finding of a positive rheumatoid factor in the elderly patient with PMR. With time, the development of a peripheral synovitis, nodules, and radiographic changes, such as periarticular osteopenia and marginal erosions, help establish the diagnosis of rheumatoid arthritis. Polymyositis can be distinguished from PMR on the basis of weakness, abnormal muscle enzymes, electromyograms, and muscle biopsies.

The myalgias of PMR characteristically improve dramatically when the patient is given low-dose steroids (10 mg per day of prednisone), usually within 12 hours to four days. Decrease in the sedimentation rate occurs within days, while the associated anemia improves over a few weeks. Most commonly, polymyalgia rheumatica runs approximately a two-year course, although disease activity may persist for several years.

TREATMENT

The goal of therapy for polymyalgia rheumatica in the absence of giant cell arteritis is to relieve symptoms until the disease has run its natural course. Nonsteroidal antiinflammatory drugs such as antiinflammatory doses of aspirin, 8 to 14 tablets in four divided daily doses; ibuprofen, 1,600 to 2,400 mg in three or four divided doses; naproxen, 250 to 375 mg twice a day; or sulindac, 150 to 200 mg twice a day, may significantly relieve muscle stiffness and pain. If PMR symptoms do not respond to a two- to four-week trial of nonsteroidal antiinflammatory drug therapy, systemic steroids in a dose of 5 to 15 mg of prednisone a day usually provide rapid improvement, often within 12 to 24 hours, of the musculoskeletal symptoms. After approximately one month of steroid therapy, the dose may be reduced as the symptoms permit. The erythrocyte sedimentation rate usually decreases to normal while the patient is treated with even low doses of steroids. If, however, the sedimentation rate remains markedly elevated, i.e., greater than 60 to 70 mm per hour by the Westergren method, after four to six weeks of steroid therapy, the possibility that the patient may also have occult giant cell arteritis must be considered.

Giant Cell Arteritis

Giant cell arteritis (GCA) is a form of vasculitis of unknown etiology, occurring most frequently in individuals in their seventh decade. The clinical symptoms in any given patient may include those of polymyalgia rheumatica as well as symptoms secondary to vascular inflammation [76]. The most frequent age of onset is between 65 and 73 years of age, with a range of 48 to over 90 years of age [73]. Although giant cell arteritis occurs almost exclusively in white individuals and with a 2 : 1 predominance of women to men, nonwhite patients have been reported with biopsy-documented GCA. The onset and character of the myalgias associated with giant cell arteritis may be indistinguishable from the symptoms occurring with only PMR. PMR symptoms have been noted in 40 to 60 percent of individuals with giant cell arteritis. Of patients presenting with PMR symptoms alone, 40 percent have characteristic histologic features of giant cell arteritis on temporal artery biopsies [76]. Low-grade fevers are present in about half of the individuals with GCA and may be the initial manifestation of this disease. For this reason, temporal artery biopsy is recommended as part of the evaluation of fever of unexplained origin in an elderly individual [77].

In addition to PMR symptoms, patients with giant cell arteritis may have constitutional symptoms, including fever, malaise, weight loss, fatigue, and apathy, as well as symptoms due to vasculitic lesions. The most commonly involved vessels are the branches of arteries originating from the aortic arch, although almost any artery may be involved. Pathologic examinations at postmortem from patients dying of GCA reveal frequent involvement of superficial temporal, vertebral, ophthalmic, and posterior ciliary arteries, with the internal carotid, external carotid, and central retinal arteries being involved less frequently [78]. Classic symptoms include headache, claudication of muscles of mastication, scalp pain and tenderness, and visual disturbances.

Headache occurs in 44 to 98 percent of individuals with GCA and is the initial symptom in 30 to 45 percent [79]. These may be localized over the arteries of the scalp, but the type and location are variable. A significant historic feature is either a change in the pattern or severity of old headaches or the onset of new headaches. Visual disturbances include ptosis, diplopia, transient or permanent visual impairment, and complete blindness. Visual impairment and blindness are most commonly due to involvement of the posterior ciliary arteries and branches of the ophthalmic artery and less commonly to central retinal artery involvement. Visual symptoms usually occur several weeks or months after other symptoms such as myalgias or headaches have developed. Transient visual disturbances frequently precede the development of blindness, but the sudden onset of blindness may be the first visual symptom. Although complete blindness usually does not improve with corticosteroid therapy, lesser degrees of visual impairment improve in about 15 percent. Visual impairment due to involvement of the posterior circulation has been reported but is a much less frequent cause than ciliary and ophthalmic artery vasculitis. Other symptoms of vasculitis include the aortic arch syndrome, with claudication of upper extremities, renal artery vasculitis, brain stem strokes due to vasculitis of the posterior circulation, and aortic aneurysm dissections and ruptures [80].

Physical findings in patients with giant cell arteritis include impairment of visual acuity. Funduscopic examination may reveal fundic hemorrhages, cotton wool patches, and pallor and edema of the optic disk. Arterial examination may reveal tenderness, dilatation of the involved arteries, diminished pulses, and bruits distal to the vasculitic lesions. Although palpation of the superficial temporal arteries may reveal tenderness, warmth, firm nodules, or diminished pulses, in approximately half of patients the temporal arteries are normal on examination [76]. Palpation of occipital arteries may elicit tenderness. Other findings include evidence of synovitis, primarily of the knee.

Lesions occur in arteries with elastic fibers in the vessel walls. The pathologic features of giant cell arteritis include inflammation of the internal elastic lamina, thrombosis at the site of vessel inflammation, necrosis of the arterial wall, granuloma formation, and infiltration of histiocytic giant cells, lymphocytes, plasma cells, and fibroblasts. Polymorphonucleocyte (PMN) infiltration is minimal [76,78].

Vascular involvement tends to be segmental. Skip lesions are found in 28 percent of patients with some foci of vasculitis as short as 330 μ in length [81]. The need to examine temporal artery specimens of several centimeters in length with multiple sections thus becomes clear. For this reason angiography has been performed to localize involved segments of the temporal artery for biopsy. Although angiography is a sensitive method for localizing arterial narrowing, the angiographic patterns demonstrated are not specific for giant cell arteritis and may be caused by other processes such as atherosclerosis [82].

The major laboratory abnormality is elevation of the erythrocyte sedimentation rate. ESRs greater than 100 mm per hour are common in patients with untreated GCA. Rare cases of biopsy-proven GCA have been reported, however, with normal or near-normal sedimentation rates. Mild normochromic or hypochromic anemias are common. White blood cell counts may be normal or moderately elevated. Platelet counts are normal or elevated. ANA and rheumatoid factors are negative. Fibrinogen and α_2 globulins are elevated and albumin is depressed. Immunoglobulin levels are occasionally elevated. Liver function abnormalities occur in approximately one-third of patients. Alkaline phosphatase elevations are most frequently found, but serum glutamic-oxaloacetic transaminase (SGOT) and prothrombin elevations may also occur. Joint imaging may reveal increased uptake of radionucleotide in the hips and shoulders [74]. Synovial fluids may be mildly inflammatory, with WBC ranging from 1,000 to 8,000 with a differential of 50 percent PMN and poor mucin clots. Synovial biopsies may reveal nonspecific synovial proliferation and lymphocytic infiltration [72]. Muscle biopsies of individuals with GCA and polymyalgia are normal.

TREATMENT

The goal of treatment of GCA is to suppress the vasculitis and thereby prevent the sequelae. Once a diagnosis is suspected clinically, prednisone should be started immediately at a dose of 40 to 60 mg per day. A several-centimeter temporal artery biopsy should be obtained and examined with multiple sections. The histology of the vasculitic lesions is not altered significantly by several days of high-dose steroid therapy, which should be maintained until the sedimentation rate plateaus or returns to normal and all reversible symptoms disappear. This generally takes two to four weeks. At that time, the dose of prednisone may be tapered off gradually by approximately 10 percent every two to three weeks while the ESR and symptoms are followed closely. If the ESR rises or arteritic symptoms recur with steroid tapering, the dose must be increased. Patients are at risk to develop arteritic sequelae as long as their ESRs are elevated.

Although GCA is generally a self-limited disease, the authors of a study of giant cell arteritis over a seven-year period found that, due to either symptomatic relapses or elevation in the sedimentation rate, many of the 34 patients with biopsy-proven cases required steroids for longer than two years [83]. These authors saw a typical patient with GCA whose disease recurred 10 years after the original diagnosis of giant cell arteritis was made clinically and confirmed by a positive temporal artery biopsy. The patient's initial episode of giant cell arteritis had responded to a year of prednisone therapy, and she had been asymptomatic with normal ESR for the subsequent nine years before her recurrence, which was also documented by temporal artery biopsy.

References

1. Marquis, D. The Blood. In J. B. Miale (Ed.), *Laboratory Medicine* (5th ed.). St. Louis: Mosby, 1977.
2. Fischel, E. E. The Erythrocyte Sedimentation Rate. In A. S. Cohen (Ed.), *Laboratory Diagnostic Procedures in Rheumatic Disease* (2nd ed.). Boston: Little, Brown, 1975.
3. Zacharski, L. R., and Kyle, R. A. Significance of extreme elevations of erythrocyte sedimentation rate. *J.A.M.A.* 202:264, 1967.
4. Hayes, G. S., and Stinson, I. N. Erythrocyte sedimentation rate and age. *Arch. Ophthalmol.* 94:939, 1976.
5. Boyd, R. V., and Hoffbrand, B. I. Erythrocyte sedimentation rate in elderly hospital inpatients. *Br. Med. J.* 1:901, 1966.
6. Bottiger, L. E., and Svedberg, C. A. Normal erythrocyte sedimentation rate and age. *Br. Med. J.* 2:85, 1967.
7. Notmann, D. D., Kurata, N., Tan, E. M. Profiles of antinuclear antibodies in systemic rheumatic diseases. *Ann. Intern. Med.* 83:464, 1975.
8. Kredich, N. M., Skyler, J. S., and Foote, L. J. Antibodies to native DNA in systemic lupus erythematosus. *Arch. Intern. Med.* 131:639, 1973.
9. Svec, K. H., and Viet, B. C. Age-related anti-nuclear factors: immunologic characteristics and associated clinical aspects. *Arthritis Rheum.* 10:509, 1967.
10. Ritchie, R. F. The clinical significance of titered antinuclear antibodies. *Arthritis Rheum.* 10:544, 1967.
11. Christian, C. L. Rheumatoid Factors. In A. S. Cohen (Ed.), *Laboratory Diagnostic Procedures in Rheumatic Disease* (2nd ed.). Boston: Little, Brown, 1975.
12. Cammarata, R. J., Rodnan, G. P., and Fennell, R. H. Serum anti-gamma-globulin and anti-nuclear factors in the aged. *J.A.M.A.* 199:115, 1967.
13. Litwin, S. D., and Singer, J. M. Studies of the incidence and significance of anti-gamma globulin factors in the aging. *Arthritis Rheum.* 8:538, 1965.
14. Rowe, D. S. Standardization of Quantitative Measurements of Human Immunoglobulins G, A, M. In E. Merler (Ed.), *Immunoglobulins: Biologic Aspects and Clinical Uses*. Washington, D.C.: National Academy of Sciences, 1970.

15. Buckley, C. E., and Dorsey, F. C. The effect of aging on human serum immunoglobulin concentration. *J. Immunol.* 105:964, 1970.
16. Zawadski, Z. A., and Edwards, G. A. Clinical significance of monoclonal immunoglobulinemia, *Bull. Rheum. Dis.* 25:810, 1974–1975.
17. Cohen, A. S. Studies of amyloidosis. *Arthritis Rheum.* 20:S76, 1977.
18. Natvig, J. B., and Anders, R. F. Characterization of four different immunochemical classes of amyloid fibril proteins. *Clin. Rheum. Dis.* 3:589, 1977.
19. Benson, M. D., and Cohen, A. S. Serum amyloid A protein in amyloidosis, rheumatic, and neoplastic diseases. *Arthritis Rheum.* 22:36, 1979.
20. Rosenthal, C. J., and Franklin, E. C. Variation with age and disease of amyloid A-related serum component. *J. Clin. Invest.* 55:746, 1975.
21. Kyle, R. A., and Bayrd, E. D. Amyloidosis: review of 236 cases. *Medicine* 54:271, 1975.
22. Cohen, A. S., and Canoso, J. Rheumatological aspects of amyloid disease. *Clin. Rheum. Dis.* 1:149, 1975.
23. Wiernik, P. H. Amyloid joint disease. *Medicine* 51:465, 1972.
24. McDevitt, C. A. Biochemistry of articular cartilage: nature of proteoglycans and collagen of articular cartilage and their role in aging and in osteoarthritis. *Ann. Rheum. Dis.* 32:364, 1973.
25. Pearson, C. M., et al. Diagnosis and treatment of erosive rheumatoid arthritis and other forms of joint destruction. *Ann. Intern. Med.* 82:241, 1975.
26. Mankin, H. J. The reaction of articular cartilage to injury and osteoarthritis. *N. Engl. J. Med.* 291:1285–1292, 1335–1340, 1974.
27. Bollet, A. J. An essay on the biology of osteoarthritis. *Arthritis Rheum.* 12:152, 1969.
28. Mankin, H. J., et al. Biochemical and metabolic abnormalities in articular cartilage from osteoarthritic human hips: II. Correlation of morphology with biochemical and metabolic data. *J. Bone Joint Surg.* 53A:523, 1971.
29. Howell, D. S. Degradative enzymes in osteoarthritic human articular cartilage. *Arthritis Rheum.* 18:167, 1975.
30. Radin, E. L. Mechanical aspects of osteoarthritis. *Bull. Rheum. Dis.* 26:862, 1975–1976.
31. Moskowitz, R. W. Clinical and Laboratory Findings in Osteoarthritis. In D. J. McCarty (Ed.), *Arthritis and Allied Conditions* (9th ed.). Philadelphia: Lea & Febiger, 1979.
32. Ehrlich, G. E. Inflammatory osteoarthritis: I. The clinical syndrome. *J. Chronic Dis.* 25:317, 1972.
33. Hasloch, I. Medical treatment of osteoarthritis. *Clin. Rheum. Dis.* 2:615, 1976.
34. Moskowitz, R. W. Treatment of Osteoarthritis. In D. J. McCarty (Ed.), *Arthritis and Allied Conditions* (9th ed.). Philadelphia: Lea & Febiger, 1979.
35. Ellman, M. H., and Levin, B. Chondrocalcinosis in elderly persons. *Arthritis Rheum.* 18:43, 1975.
36. McCarty, D. J. Calcium pyrophosphate dihydrate crystal deposition disease: nomenclature and diagnostic criteria. *Ann. Intern. Med.* 87:240, 1977.
37. McCarty, D. J. CPPD crystal deposition disease—1975. *Arthritis Rheum.* 19:275, 1976.

38. Jacobelli, S., et al. Calcium pyrophosphate dihydrate crystal deposition in neuropathic joints. Four cases of polyarticular involvement. *Ann. Intern. Med.* 79:340, 1973.

39. Genant, H. K. Roentgenographic aspects of calcium pyrophosphate dihydrate crystal deposition disease (pseudogout). *Arthritis Rheum.* 19:307, 1976.

40. Reginato, A. M., et al. Polyarticular and familial chondrocalcinosis. *Arthritis Rheum.* 13:197, 1970.

41. Van der Korst, J. K., Geerards, J., and Driessens, F. C. M. A hereditary type of idiopathic articular chondrocalcinosis: survey of a pedigree. *Am. J. Med.* 56:307, 1974.

42. Hamilton, E. B. D. Diseases associated with CPPD deposition disease. *Arthritis Rheum.* 19:353, 1976.

43. O'Duffy, J. D. Clinical studies of acute pseudogout attacks. *Arthritis Rheum.* 19:349, 1976.

44. Williams, R. C. The Clinical Picture of Rheumatoid Arthritis. In D. J. McCarty (Ed.), *Arthritis and Allied Conditions* (9th ed.). Philadelphia: Lea & Febiger, 1979.

45. Decker, J. L., and Plotz, P. H. Extra-Articular Rheumatoid Disease. In D. J. McCarty (Ed.), *Arthritis and Allied Conditions* (9th ed.). Philadelphia: Lea & Febiger, 1979.

46. Ehrlich, G. E., Katz, W. A., and Cohen, S. H. Rheumatoid arthritis in the elderly. *Geriatrics* 25:103, 1970.

47. Corrigan, A. B., et al. Benign rheumatoid arthritis of the aged. *Br. Med. J.* 1:444, 1974.

48. Brunner, C. N., and Davis, J. S. Immune mechanisms in the pathogenesis of systemic lupus erythematosus. *Bull. Rheum. Dis.* 26:854, 1975–1976.

49. Decker, J. L., et al. Systemic lupus erythematosus, contrasts and comparisons. *Ann. Intern. Med.* 82:391, 1975.

50. Fries, J. F., and Holman, H. R. *Systemic Lupus Erythematosus.* Philadelphia: Saunders, 1975.

51. Estes, D., and Christian, C. L. Natural history of systemic lupus erythematosus. *Medicine* 50:85, 1971.

52. Dimant, J., et al. Systemic lupus erythematosus in the older age group: computer analysis. *J. Am. Geriatr. Soc.* 27:58, 1979.

53. Baker, S. B., et al. Late onset systemic lupus erythematosus. *Am. J. Med.* 66:727, 1979.

54. Foad, B. S. I., Sheon, R. P., and Kirsner, A. B. Systemic lupus erythematosus in the elderly. *Arch. Intern. Med.* 130:743, 1972.

55. Urowitz, M. B. SLE subsets: divide and conquer. *J. Rheum.* 4:332, 1977.

56. Lee, S. L., and Chase, P. H. Drug-induced systemic lupus erythematosus: a critical review. *Semin. Arthritis Rheum.* 5:83, 1975.

57. Molina, J., et al. Procainamide-induced serologic changes in asymptomatic patients. *Arthritis Rheum.* 12:608, 1969.

58. Stahl, N. I., and Klippel, J. H. Recognizing drug-induced lupus syndromes. *Drug Ther.* Pp. 80–88, September, 1978.

59. Sunder, S. K., and Shah, A. Constrictive pericarditis in procainamide-induced lupus erythematosus syndrome. *Am. J. Cardiol.* 36:960, 1975.

60. Hahn, B. H., et al. Immune responses to hydralazine and nuclear antigens in hydralazine induced lupus erythematosus. *Ann. Intern. Med.* 76:365, 1972.

61. Bauer, W. H.   Old age in human parotid glands with special reference to peculiar cells in uncommon salivary gland tumors. *J. Dent. Res.* 29:686, 1950.

62. Shearn, M. A.   *Sjogren's Syndrome, Problems in Internal Medicine*. Philadelphia: Saunders, 1971. Vol. II.

63. Bloch, K. J., et al.   Sjogren's syndrome. *Medicine* 44:187, 1965.

64. Van Bijsterveld, O. P.   Diagnostic tests in the sicca syndrome. *Arch. Ophthalmol.* 82:10, 1969.

65. Greenspan, J. S., et al.   The histopathology of Sjogren's syndrome in labial salivary gland biopsies. *Oral Surg. Oral Med. Oral Pathol.* 37:217, 1974.

66. Recent clinical and experimental developments in Sjogren's syndrome, Medical Staff Conference, University of California, San Francisco. *West. J. Med.* 122:50, 1975.

67. Berry, H., Bacon, P. A., and Davis, J. D.   Cell-mediated immunity in Sjogren's syndrome. *Ann. Rheum. Dis.* 31:298, 1972.

68. Cummings, N. A., et al.   Sjogren's syndrome—newer aspects of research, diagnosis, and therapy. *Ann. Intern. Med.* 75:937, 1971.

69. Michalski, J. P., et al.   Beta$_2$ microglobulin and lymphocytic infiltration in Sjogren's syndrome. *N. Engl. J. Med.* 293:1228, 1975.

70. Moutsopoulos, H. M., et al.   Sjogren's syndrome (sicca syndrome): current issues. *Ann. Intern. Med.* 92(Part I):212, 1980.

71. Anderson, L. G., and Bayles, T. B.   Polymyalgia rheumatica. *DM* January, 1974.

72. Bruk, M. I.   Articular and vascular manifestations of polymyalgia rheumatica. *Ann. Rheum. Dis.* 26:103, 1967.

73. Hunder, G. G., and Allen, G. L.   Giant cell arteries: a review. *Bull. Rheum. Dis.* 29:980, 1978–1979.

74. O'Duffy, J. D., Wahner, H. W., and Hunder, G. G.   Joint imaging in polymyalgia rheumatica. *Mayo Clin. Proc.* 51:519, 1976.

75. Long, R., and James, O.   Polymyalgia rheumatica and liver disease. *Lancet* 1:77, 1974.

76. Fauchald, P., Rygvold, O., and Øystese, B.   Temporal arteritis and polymyalgia rheumatica: clinical and biopsy findings. *Ann. Intern. Med.* 77:845, 1972.

77. Ghose, M. K., Shensa, S., and Lerner, P. I.   Arteritis of the aged (giant cell arteritis) and fever of unexplained origin. *Am. J. Med.* 60:429, 1976.

78. Wilkinson, I. M. S., and Russel, R. W. R.   Arteritis of the head and neck in giant cell arteritis: a pathologic study to show the pattern of arterial involvement. *Arch. Neurol.* 27:378, 1972.

79. Hamilton, C. R., Shelley, W. M., and Tumulty, P. A.   Giant cell arteritis: including temporal arteritis and polymyalgia rheumatica. *Medicine* 50:1, 1971.

80. Klein, R. G., et al.   Large artery involvement in giant cell (temporal) arteritis. *Ann. Intern. Med.* 83:806, 1975.

81. Klein, R. G., et al.   Skip lesions in temporal arteritis. *Mayo Clin. Proc.* 51:504, 1976.

82. Layfer, L. F., et al.   Temporal arteriography: analysis of 21 cases and a review of the literature. *Arthritis Rheum.* 21:780, 1978.

83. Beevers, D. G., Harpur, J. E., and Turk, K. A. D.   Giant cell arteritis—the need for prolonged treatment. *J. Chronic Dis.* 26:571, 1973.

17. Gastrointestinal System

Kenneth L. Minaker

John W. Rowe

Functional and pathologic gastrointestinal abnormalities are common in the elderly; 20 percent of geriatric deaths are caused by gastrointestinal illnesses [1]. Studies of community-dwelling elderly show that even when nutritional supplements and vitamins are excluded, 42 percent of nonprescription drugs are gastrointestinal medications. Nearly 27 percent of geriatric medical admissions are due to gastrointestinal disease [2]. The incidence of gastrointestinal malignancy is second only to skin cancer, and its mortality is second only to cancer of the lung.

Diagnostic difficulties are particularly common in geriatric gastroenterology. One-half of patients referred for gastroenterologic consultation who are examined carefully and followed for one year will have no identifiable pathologic explanation for their complaints [3]. The long "silent period" of many gastrointestinal diseases compounds the notorious underreporting and late presentation of illness characteristic of the geriatric population. Invasive and noninvasive techniques requiring patient cooperation are more difficult and uncomfortable for the less mobile elderly patient. However, since the prevalence of gastrointestinal malignancy increases progressively with age and forms 30 to 40 percent of all malignancies of very old patients, accurate diagnosis of any significant symptom is clearly crucial in the elderly population. The aged patient is thus often in the unfavorable position of being overinvestigated with uncomfortable techniques for fear of missing a malignant lesion. The proper approach to diagnosis and therapy of gastrointestinal disease is based on individualization of the problems presented. In general, each case should receive the least investigation leading to specific diagnosis. Therapy should be based on awareness of the good potential life expectancy of otherwise healthy old individuals.

Oral Cavity
PHYSIOLOGY
Normal aging affects oral function minimally. Since our Western diet is soft and refined, tooth wear generally does not cause significant dental loss. The finding that caries and periodontal disease are virtually nonexistent in some elderly populations outside Western countries suggests that dental loss is likely to be disease-related. The normal changes with age, including reduction in dentine production, shrinkage and fibrosis of root pulp, gingival retraction, and loss of bone density in the alveolar ridge, all contribute to the increased vulnerability of the elderly to dental disease.

The normal reductions in taste and smell with age interfere minimally with nutrition but certainly minimize enjoyment of food. The number of tongue papillae and taste buds decrease with normal aging. Clinical studies have shown increased taste thresholds for individual amino acids, salt, and

297

sugars. Older people clearly have more difficulty recognizing common smells and flavors, and it appears that food odor is the main gustatory factor that decreases [4]. The net effect is that bitter tastes predominate and more concentrated sugar is required to experience a sweet taste. Mucous and parotid gland secretion show age-related declines but can only be considered to be partial contributors to xerostomia in the elderly. Oral mucosal changes with advancing age are mainly due to loss of submucosal elastic tissue. The tongue may develop a lobular appearance and papillary loss may be marginal or diffusely distributed. The most frequent change is appearance of sublingual varicosities on the ventral surface of the tongue in 50 percent of the over-65 population.

PATHOLOGY
In our Western civilization dental caries affect 99 percent of our population. This is largely a dietary problem, with sticky carbohydrate-containing foods provoking proliferation of acid-producing bacteria in plaque, in peridontal pockets, and dental crevices. With advancing age the bacteriology of the accumulated plaque and calculus changes; the usual mixture of fusospirochetal organisms remains stable, but the gram-negative anaerobic rods are increasingly replaced by gram-positive facultative cocci. The two processes contribute to the startling loss of secondary dentition in our community; 50 percent of all Americans are edentulous by the age of 65 and 80 percent by the age of 75. Fully 50 percent of the elderly population experience painful traumatic lesions of the oral cavity due to dental fractures and maladjusted or malfitting plates. These changes may be ulcerative; atrophic, such as lichen planus; or hyperplastic, such as leukoplakia. Our soft diet conveniently permits adequate nutrition in the presence of impaired dentition, but the potential for illness of a local and general nature dictates appropriate dental referral for geriatric patients.

Once teeth are lost the alveolar ridge loses height rapidly (50 percent over three years), which makes denture-fitting an ongoing necessity. Denture comfort becomes a decreasing reality as there is less purchase for plates. Mandibular bony integrity is impaired in the edentulous jaw. Fully 20 percent of edentulous mandibular fractures result in nonunion, likely due to the combination of osteoporosis and more general architectural changes. The facial collapse consequent to alveolar bony loss causes muscular incompetence and predisposes to angular cheilitis, which is commonly complicated by monilial infection. This mechanical cause for angular cheilitis is more prevalent than iron or riboflavin deficiency.

Monilial infections are now being recognized, with iron deficiency, as common causes of red, beefy tongues. The classic flat surface of the tongue in pernicious anemia remains as a clue to that specific geriatric disease. Enlargement of the tongue is commonly seen in the aged. This may be compensatory for or related to loss of teeth in several ways. The tongue may have increased masticatory function and hypertrophy or it may passively have enlarged because of the increased space afforded it by dental loss [5].

Dry mouth is a complaint of 20 percent of elders. The major contributors are obstructing nasal disease that causes mouth breathing, anticholinergics or drugs that cause volume depletion, and the normal decrease in salivary gland secretion with age. Salivary gland duct obstruction commonly associated with infection is an important cause of impaired salivary secretion. Middle-aged and elderly women may develop Sjögren's syndrome, which in full form consists of keratoconjunctivitis sicca, salivary gland enlargement, xerostomia, and seronegative peripheral polyarthritis. Awareness of the frequent partial expression of this syndrome will lead to its inclusion in the differential diagnosis of dry mouth. The consequences of xerostomia are disturbed taste sensation, increased vulnerability of the oral mucosa, and decreased clearance of bacteria prominent in causing caries. Severely dehydrated elderly patients may develop acute bacterial parotitis, often due to *Staphylococcus aureus*.

Malignancies of the oral cavity are 90 percent squamous cell carcinomas and are statistically associated with smoking and alcohol use. The peak incidence of these lesions is in the seventh decade. Inspection of lower lip, back of tongue, gingiva, and floor of mouth will cover the major sites of occurrence. Lesions may present as ulcers in high-wear areas and hypertrophic masses in sheltered areas.

MANAGEMENT
The initial approach to therapy is clarification of whether the symptoms are due to aging or disease. If illness is the cause, has it been the result of a more systemic disease (i.e., acute leukemia predisposing to oral infections) or purely local factors (i.e., poorly fitting dentures causing mucosal ulceration)?

Maintenance dental care includes salvage or rebuilding of remaining dentition and temporary denture refitting as needed. Oral carcinoma requires careful assessment, therapy, and follow-up study, as the illness is potentially deforming and painful and may involve vital structures. Xerostomias should be viewed as a syndrome requiring specific differential diagnosis. The results of trauma and infection are seen more rapidly in the dry mouth and preventive and early measures are useful.

Esophagus
PHYSIOLOGY
Esophageal function is essentially preserved during normal aging. The major change consists of smooth muscle weakness with normal vagal enervation [6]. On esophageal manometry the only change with age is a decreased amplitude of peristalsis, with no increased prevalence of clinically important motility abnormalities. No clear physiologic changes can be identified as being responsible for the increased prevalence of hiatus hernia with age.

PATHOLOGY

Esophageal dysfunction is common in the elderly and is usually secondary to diseases of the nervous system that cause neuromuscular incoordination. Parkinson's disease, amyotrophic lateral sclerosis, pseudobulbar palsy, peripheral neuropathy, diabetes mellitus, and stroke are the most prevalent disorders. The common radiologic picture on cinesophagoscopy reveals absent or reduced peristalsis, tertiary contractions, delay in esophageal emptying, and esophageal dilatation. The motility pattern is similar to that seen in diffuse esophageal spasm. In contrast to that disorder, however, the patients with esophageal dysfunction are usually asymptomatic. Symptoms, when present, will include aspiration, painless dysphagia, which is often more for solids than liquids, and progressive protein-calorie malnutrition.

The differential diagnosis of dysphagia does not change dramatically with advanced age, but there is some variation in the underlying diseases. Esophageal spasm, esophageal webs, and classic achalasia are unusual in the elderly. Zenker's diverticulum and neuromuscular disease should be given priority in interpretation of upper esophageal dysphagia in elderly men. Vascular dysphagia due to dilatation or aneurysm of the aorta and osteophytic disease of the cervical spine causing dysphagia are uniquely geriatric.

In cancer of the esophagus, the most common cause of progressive dysphagia in the elderly, 50 percent of the lumen must be stenotic before symptoms appear. Squamous cell carcinoma is common above the diaphragm and adenocarcinoma predominates at the esophagogastric junction. Eight percent are found in the cervical region, 25 percent are upper thoracic, 17 percent are lower thoracic and 50 percent are found at the esophagogastric junction.

Hiatus hernia is common in the elderly, demonstrable in 60 percent of patients over the age of 60. Fortunately, it is rarely symptomatic, and symptoms, when present, can usually be controlled.

MANAGEMENT

For the geriatric patient who has often accumulated several illnesses that may affect the esophagus, adequate diagnosis requires several types of relatively complex studies. Barium swallow studies should be supplemented by cinesophagograms and fiberoptic esophagoscopy when symptoms are progressive or associated with weight loss or bleeding. Hiatus hernia symptoms are responsive to weight reduction; reduction in size of meals, particularly before recumbency; and elevation of the head of the bed. Foaming agents taken after meals create a bubble of antacid in the less dependent areas of the stomach and esophagus, which is helpful in reducing peptic symptoms. Antacid regimens are otherwise similar to those for duodenal ulceration.

Esophageal malignancy commonly yields a dismal 10 percent five-year survival with any mode of therapy, and the debate over the best mode of therapy continues. Treatment that aggressively attempts to control the spread of disease tends to lead to a poorer quality of survival. The best survival rates are reported when combined staged surgical and radiotherapeutic approaches are used. For individuals who are unsuitable surgical risks (up to 75 percent of this largely geriatric population), fluoroscopically guided dilatation and placement of a fashioned tube through the lesion can provide excellent palliation with a minimum of discomfort or hospitalization time. Palliative radiation can be added. Individualization of therapy is crucial here and depends on the patient's preferences, site and pathologic type of tumor, and the locally available surgical and radiotherapeutic expertise [7].

Stomach and Duodenum

PHYSIOLOGY

The impaired secretory capacity of the aged stomach is well documented. With advancing age, maximal stimulated gastric acid decreases 5 mEq per hour per decade in men and slightly less in women. Enough acid is present, however, to facilitate recurrence and progression of established acid-peptic disease. In asymptomatic patients, serum gastrin levels increase with advancing age and are associated with the presence of antiparietal cell antibodies. Hyposecretion of intrinsic factor may lead to vitamin B_{12} malabsorption. The increasing prevalence of atrophic gastritis with age strongly suggests that aging increases susceptibility to the disease. The prevalence is reported to be between 28 and 96 percent in the elderly population (the secretory abnormalities of aging may be related to some degree to the existence of gastritis). Long-term studies show that atrophic gastritis tends to persist, and superficial gastritis progresses slowly to atrophic gastritis. No age differences are observed in pathologic appearance [8]. Gastric motility may be somewhat impaired in the elderly, but the influence of age on gastric emptying has not been well defined. Gastritis certainly causes delayed gastric emptying.

PATHOLOGY

Peptic disease and peptic ulceration of the stomach and duodenum will be considered together because of similar pathophysiology. Peptic gastric ulcer is more likely to occur at advanced ages and carries a graver prognosis than duodenal ulcer disease, with more than two-thirds of ulcer deaths being caused by gastric ulcers. The 10 : 1 ratio of duodenal : gastric ulcer in the young becomes 2 : 1 in the elderly. Sex incidence ratio remains unchanged in old age with a male predominance of 2 : 1. Atypical presentation is likely, with unusual pain or unphysiologic but disturbing symptomatology. Contrasting with this is the occurrence of catastrophic complications such as hemorrhage or perforation with little forewarning. Fully one-half of gastric ulcer fatalities occur in patients with symptoms of less than one month's duration. Giant benign gastric ulcerations (ulcers with diameters larger than 3 cm) have their peak incidence in the seventh decade, later than that of the common smaller ulcers.

Anatomically, gastric ulcers in the elderly occur more proximally, with 40 percent occurring in a juxtacardia or posterior wall location; in younger patients 85 percent are found within 9 cm of the pylorus. In the long term over 50 percent of individuals will have recurrent disease. Etiologic factors such as salicylate ingestion may be more common in the elderly because of a high prevalence of arthritic disease in that age group.

While the prevalence of duodenal ulcer does not increase with age, the morbidity and mortality associated with complications is increased. As many as 20 percent of patients hospitalized with peptic ulcer disease are elderly. It is well established that peptic ulcer is a disease of middle age. Since current views on the natural history of peptic ulcer suggest a varying course of over 15 to 20 years from initial symptoms, the risk period for complications or recurrent symptomatology clearly extends into the geriatric age. range. While estimates vary, up to half of patients initially come to physicians with their first peptic ulcer symptoms after age 60. Clinical features vary with advancing age. The elderly patient more commonly presents late in the course of the disease or with a complication but with surprisingly little prior symptomatology. Although pain is often present, it is poorly localized with unusual radiation, and response to food is atypical. Other organs or organ systems may be recruited and provoke the presenting complaint. For example, a patient may present with angina due to anemia from chronic low-grade blood loss.

Of the rarer causes of peptic ulceration, 20 percent of cases of Zollinger-Ellison syndrome occur in patients older than 60 and 2 percent in those older than 70. Presentation and course of this illness are not strongly influenced by age.

Bleeding is the most common complication of peptic ulcer of any type and is more common in the elderly [9]. In addition, if bleeding is the first symptom, recurrence increases with age, reaching a recurrence rate of 7 percent yearly over the age of 70 years. Emergency surgery for bleeding carries a 20 percent mortality in the elderly (much higher than in the younger age group) because of a combination of factors, including delayed presentation and diagnosis and physiologically and pathologically limited reserves to surgical stress. Prognostic factors for likelihood of recurrent bleeding and indications for surgery do not change with age.

Perforation as a complication of peptic ulcer disease occurs three times as commonly (10 to 20 percent of cases) in the elderly as it does in the younger age group, and it represents the second major complication. The mortality rate from perforation is clearly higher. One factor contributing to this excess morbidity and mortality is the delay in diagnosis fostered by the unusual presentation of the "acute abdomen" in the elderly. There may be minimal past history, poorly localized symptoms, and few signs of peritonitis.

Persistingly painful ulcer disease is uncommon in the elderly and a rare indication for hospitalization or surgery. Finally, gastric outlet obstruction may present in an unusual way in the elderly, with the secondary metabolic or catabolic disturbances leading to atypical presentation. The surgical approach to the latter two conditions is unchanged with advancing age.

CANCER OF THE STOMACH
Cancer of the stomach has a peak incidence in the eighth and ninth decades. Vague symptomatology and delay in diagnosis lead to advanced illness at presentation. The five-year survival of 15 percent has not increased significantly in 40 years. Atrophic gastritis, which is prevalent with advancing age, increases the stomach cancer risk 20-fold. Pernicious anemia is likewise associated with an increased risk. Poor prognostic indicators at laparotomy include lymph node involvement and more aggressive pathologic classification. Complications are similar to those with peptic ulceration.

GASTRITIS
Erosive gastritis causes as much upper gastrointestinal bleeding in the elderly as duodenal ulceration and is second only to gastric ulcer as a source of bleeding. The use of multiple medicines, known to provoke gastritis, is common because of the accumulation of illness with advancing age. Salicylates, phenylbutazone, indomethacin, steroids, and nonsteroidal antiinflammatory agents are commonly used for geriatric medical illnesses.

MANAGEMENT OF DISEASES OF THE STOMACH AND DUODENUM
Once a clear diagnosis is established, treatment for peptic ulcer disease must be modified for the elderly patient. Medical therapy in the elderly has several caveats. Anticholinergic agents in the elderly are prone to cause complications outside of the gastrointestinal tract and should be discouraged. The use of carbenoxolone may cause symptoms related to sodium retention and hypokalemia. Gastric irradiation involving divided doses of 1,600 rads may be a useful adjunct in high-risk circumstances in that it is 50 percent efficacious and noninvasive. Renal shielding is important to prevent radiation nephritis.

Cimetidine is enjoying popularity in the treatment of peptic ulcer disease. Of the short-term side effects of this agent, one, confusion, is almost completely a geriatric syndrome. One factor clearly demonstrated is the reduced plasma clearance of this agent with advancing age. Dosage modification is indicated in the elderly, but at present clear, safe guidelines do not exist.

It is of interest to note that 42 percent of all nonprescription drugs used by the elderly are gastrointestinal medications [10], and a careful drug history is required before any therapy is begun. A standard regimen for the elderly with peptic ulcer disease includes a regular diet and avoidance of foods known to reproduce symptoms. Use of frequent around-the-clock antacids

(30-ml doses) or cimetidine in reduced doses four times a day promotes ulcer healing. Known irritant medications, smoking, and alcohol are best avoided. Surgical management of the elderly patient follows the same general principles as those used for patients of any age but risk-benefit analysis requires closer scrutiny. Since more catastrophic complications are the rule in the elderly, nonemergency surgery is commonly contemplated. Gastric malignancy in the elderly may be cured by gastrectomy if discovered early, but most surgical procedures for this illness are deemed palliative. Chemotherapy in the form of 5-fluorouracil with or without a nitroso-urea compound seem most useful at the present time. The elderly are more sensitive to the bone marrow suppression of these agents, thus further limiting their marginal effectiveness.

Small Intestine
PHYSIOLOGY
Small intestine weight decreases with advancing age. Jejunal biopsies in healthy elderly patients with normal fat, xylose, iron, and folate absorption reveal significant reduction in mucosal surface area. Other structural abnormalities include a reduction in the number of Peyer's patches and in lymphatic follicles within individual patches.

With gastric acid decreasing, the sterility of the upper gastrointestinal tract is threatened, and the elderly harbor fewer anaerobic lactobacilli and larger numbers of coliforms than younger patients [11]. Blood supply to the gut does not alter with aging, dispelling the notion that chronic ischemia influences aging-related gut function.

Absorption of nutrients in the small intestine of elderly individuals is in general preserved. Deficits do exist and when complicated by poor intake predispose to deficiency syndromes. With advancing age D-xylose (a sugar absorbed from the proximal jejunum and duodenum) ingestion results in lower peak blood levels. The gut absorption of this agent appears definitely diminished after the age of 80 [12]. Fat absorption is moderately decreased in the elderly, although there is no evidence to suggest that this is clinically important.

Iron transport, and the increased iron transport noted across the intestinal lumen in iron deficiency, is preserved in normal aging [13]. Calcium absorption decreases steadily with aging and is related directly to decreasing values of 1,25-dihydroxy vitamin D_3 [14]. Serum levels of vitamins C and B_{12} decrease gradually with aging. Marginal lack of intrinsic factor is a postulated cause of vitamin B_{12} malabsorption, but there is little evidence to suggest that these lower levels are significant or that they predispose to the development of specific deficiency syndromes.

PATHOLOGY

Malabsorption presents either as steatorrhea or with chronic diarrhea, anemia, and bone pains. Several diagnoses predominate in the differential diagnosis of this condition in the elderly.

Celiac disease may present at an advanced age even though it is often a lifelong illness. Slow or incomplete recovery characterizes the elderly individual's response. However, consideration should be given to the existence of a complicating lymphoma in such slow-to-respond cases. Pancreatic insufficiency from benign or malignant disease should be considered next, with abdominal pain a major clue to the presence of malignancy [15].

A distinctive geriatric syndrome of malabsorption caused by bacterial overgrowth in solitary or multiple duodenal or jejunal diverticula seems clearly defined. Small bowel biopsy is normal, and radiographic examination fails to show a malabsorption pattern. The clinical presentation is one of general debility rather than specifically diarrhea or steatorrhea. Also known in the elderly is malabsorption secondary to bacterial overgrowth in the absence of an anatomic blind pouch. Diagnosis is supported by 14_C-glycocholate breath testing; the therapeutic response to a broad-spectrum antibiotic is excellent [16].

The final major cause of malabsorption in the elderly is the postgastrectomy syndrome. Gastrectomy is associated with mild fat and protein malabsorption and iron malabsorption, and vitamin B_{12} deficiency may develop after many years.

MANAGEMENT

In spite of the vast array of illnesses potentially responsible for small bowel dysfunction, there are a limited number of major causes for malabsorption in the elderly as outlined. The approach to diagnosis is identical at all ages, with perhaps an earlier trial of tetracycline therapy to assess the possibility of the presence of bacterial overgrowth in the elderly patient.

Liver and Biliary Tract
PHYSIOLOGY

In individuals who die of unrelated illnesses, the liver does not change in size or weight with age [17]. Light microscopy shows a mild increase in hepatic fibrous tissue. Hepatic blood flow shows a 1.5 percent fall per year, resulting in a 50 percent reduction in blood flow from maturity to advanced old age. Giant parenchymal cells with multiple nucleoli appear. The intracellular organelles also show changes. The Golgi apparatus size decreases with age. Mitochondria decrease in number but morphologically increase in size and have increased density of cristae. There appear to be more lysosomes. There are a large number of reports in the literature concerning the hepatic enzyme systems of numerous intrahepatic enzymes in mammals, the majority showing no change with aging, some an increase, and some a decrease [18]. The overall pattern is a decrease in the inducible microsomal enzymes involved in redox mechanisms and an increase in hydrolytic enzymes. This is compatible with the electron microscopy findings already discussed relating to numbers and morphology of intracellular organelles. Standard liver function studies including bromsulphalein (BSP) retention do not change with age [19]. Serum albumin falls slightly with age, influencing some hormone and drug-binding characteristics.

PATHOLOGY

Jaundice in the elderly patient is an ominous sign. The most common cause of progressive jaundice in the elderly is cancer, with pancreatic neoplasm accounting for half of all cases. Jaundice caused by viral hepatitis carries a mortality rate approaching 25 percent. Other diagnostic considerations include choledocholithiasis, or drug-related jaundice (which is equal in rate of occurrence to viral hepatitis in the elderly) [20].

For numerous reasons the elderly are susceptible to chemical hepatotoxicity. They are frequent recipients of hepatotoxic drugs, commonly receive combinations of agents, and are likely to have reduced clearance of drugs. Common patterns of toxicity seen in the elderly include a hepatitis-like reaction, intrahepatic cholestasis, and a mixed pattern. Examples of drugs causing a hepatitis-like reaction are antidepressants (monoamino-oxidase inhibitors), anticonvulsants (carbamazepine, Dilantin), antituberculosis drugs (rifampin, isoniazid), and antirheumatic drugs (gold, allopurinol, acetaminophen). The incidence and severity of isoniazid hepatitis increases with age, and age strongly influences the choice and use of this drug for antituberculosis prophylaxis.

The intrahepatic cholestasis pattern of liver injury may be caused by chlorpromazine, antidepressants, oral hypoglycemic agents (sulfonylureas), benzodiazepines, thiazides, phenylbutazone, antithyroid drugs (propylthiouracil), and sulfonamides. The mixed pathology is seen with antituberculosis drugs, sulfonamides, oral antidiabetic drugs, methyldopa, and erythromycin estolate [21].

While alcoholic hepatitis is usually a disease of early middle age, it is certainly reported in the elderly. The development of cirrhosis of the liver may be the major predisposing factor in the United States for the development of hepatoma. Of individuals with biopsy-proven hepatoma, 66 percent have preexisting cirrhosis of the liver associated with alcohol intake [22]. Although the incidence of alcoholic hepatitis and cirrhosis of the liver peaks in early middle age, between 30 and 60 percent of hepatoma patients are over the age of 60, making it a geriatric illness. Males outnumber females with this disease by a 3 : 1 ratio. Symptoms of abdominal discomfort (62%), weight loss (34%), and abdominal swelling (30%) are the common presenting symptoms. The majority will have hepatomegaly (75%) and ascites (30%) at the time of diagnosis. Most will have abnormal liver function studies (SGOT is increased in 88 percent; alkaline phosphatase in 78 percent). Alphafeto-protein levels are elevated in 74 percent, and in most series hepatitis-associated antigen is rarely found to be positive. Various paraneoplastic syndromes such as polycythemia, thrombocytosis, hypoglycemia, hypercalcemia, and fever may cloud the presentation and delay diagnosis. Median survival with this illness is about six months from diagnosis.

Recent studies of age-related factors that contribute to the supersaturation of bile with cholesterol may help to explain the increased prevalence of cholelithiasis from 10 to 20 percent at age 55 to 65 years to 35 to 40 percent after age 70 years.

The morbidity and mortality of complicated biliary tract disease increases with aging. Again, delayed diagnosis and intercurrent disease are largely responsible.

The presence of common bile duct stones increases progressively with age, with some series reporting a fourfold greater incidence in older patients. Adverse sequelae of this are so frequent that therapy is promptly indicated. One form of acute cholecystitis is uniquely geriatric. This is acute emphysematous cholecystitis in which gas-producing organisms such as *Clostridium welchii*, anaerobic streptococci, *Escherichia coli*, *S. aureus*, *Pseudomonas*, and *Klebsiella* have been implicated. The course is more toxic and associated with more severe pain than uncomplicated cholecystitis.

Carcinoma of the gallbladder is three times more common in patients over the age of 70 and is a disease of elderly women. It is usually associated with chronic calculous cholecystitis. Its rarity precludes its use as an indication for prophylactic cholecystectomy, except when gallbladder calcification is present. In patients in this situation there is a 25 percent incidence of carcinoma.

MANAGEMENT

The principles of therapy for alcoholic, viral, and drug-induced hepatitis do not change with advancing age. The aims are to remove the offending agents, nutritionally support the patient, and anticipate and correct any signs of hepatic failure.

Hepatobiliary malignancy is not managed differently with advancing age, but associated medical illness often dictates less aggressive surgical approaches. Chemotherapy using 5-fluorouracil or adriamycin requires decreased dosage with advancing age due to decreased marrow reserve in the elderly.

Principles of surgery are equally well applied to symptomatic biliary tract disease at young and old ages. As older individuals are more likely to have concomitant disease, vigilant perioperative care is needed to maintain the accepted mortality rate of one percent for the procedure. The preoperative stabilization of medical conditions moves the elderly individual from a disproportionately high-risk group into a risk group equal to young patients.

New forms of therapy presently under investigation promise alternatives to present methods. Chenodeoxycholic acid and several related compounds promote dissolution of gallstones. Recurrent disease and intolerance to the agent may be limiting factors in its general use, however. Endoscopic papillotomy is promising and is well tolerated by the elderly [23]; restenosis and morbidity rates in larger series have been low. Removal or spontaneous passage of stones is the rule.

Pancreas
PHYSIOLOGY
Pancreatic size increases or remains unchanged with aging. Structurally, duct ectasia is common and follows hyperplastic change in ductules. Various microscopic changes occur, including islet cell atrophy and amyloid and adipose infiltration. There is no reduction in volume of pancreatic fluid or its content of trypsin, amylase, or bicarbonate with aging. Since 90 percent of pancreatic function must be impaired before significant fat malabsorption occurs, clinically important maldigestion of fat does not occur as a consequence of normal aging.

PATHOLOGY
The incidence of pancreatitis increases with advancing age. Biliary tract disease, hypothermia, carbon monoxide poisoning, and steroid and thiazide therapy are all more common in the elderly and may be contributory causes of pancreatitis. Atypical location of pain, frequently altered mental function, and higher morbidity characterize elderly patients with pancreatitis. The differential diagnosis of abdominal pain and hyperamylasemia is more difficult with advancing age because of the increased prevalence of illnesses well known to cause hyperamylasemia, such as dissecting abdominal aortic aneurysm and acute arterial and venous obstruction. Assessment of amylase clearance helps to differentiate from macroamylasemia but not the other conditions. Pancreatitis in the very elderly is often painless, further confusing the clinical picture.

The incidence of pancreatic carcinoma is increasing steadily and has become the fourth most common death-causing cancer in the United States for males [24]. Peak incidence is in the sixth decade with a 3 : 1 male-to-female incidence ratio. Diagnosis is notoriously difficult, leading in all age groups to late advanced presentation. Recently developed diagnostic modalities such as retrograde pancreatography and computerized tomography may permit earlier diagnosis of this cancer. The paraneoplastic syndrome of psychosis or depression as the initial presentation of pancreatic malignancy may be a diagnostic clue in a previously stable geriatric patient.

MANAGEMENT
The management of pancreatitis aside from pain management is unchanged with advancing age. Analgesic effectiveness increases with advancing age,

necessitating a reduction in doses of major analgesics. A careful search for common bile duct stones is indicated.

Pancreatic malignancy carries a less than 5 percent five-year survival, but where operation is possible survival increases modestly to 15 percent at five years.

Large Bowel
PHYSIOLOGY
The large bowel has active resorptive (water, chloride, sodium) and secretory (mucus, potassium, bicarbonate) functions. In addition, food residues and bacteria are compacted and stored temporarily before evacuation. Alterations in gut flora occur in the elderly, as discussed previously. Transit time analysis of radiopaque markers in healthy elderly subjects reveals that the first marker is always excreted in three days and 80 percent have passed by five days [25]. The transit time from cecum to rectum is short, with most of the delay in evacuation occurring below the sigmoid colon. These transit times are no different than those seen in healthy, young, normal individuals. Normal stool frequency is between 3 and 20 stools per week. The reflex action in defecation involves a voluntary response to anal canal relaxation that occurs when the rectum is distended by fecal material. Study has shown that elderly individuals have normal sensibility to balloon distention of the rectum.

PATHOLOGY
Ischemic Colitis
Narrowings of major intestinal arteries by atheroma become significant in the geriatric age group. Once two vessels are blocked or severely compromised, the large bowel mucosa is vulnerable to any further insult. This may include digoxin overdose (intestinal vasospasm and increased oxygen demands), heart failure (compromised perfusion), or polycythemia (stasis). Three distinct clinical pictures can result, depending on the acuteness of the obstruction. They include transient abdominal ischemia, slow development of ischemic stricture, and gangrenous colitis. The first two appear clinically as food avoidance, postprandial abdominal pain, and rectal bleeding with normal rectal mucosa. If a segment is totally infarcted, an intraabdominal catastrophe results. More often spontaneous resolution occurs, with subsequent development of a long, smooth stricture in the watershed area of arterial blood supply at the splenic flexure.

Ulcerative Colitis
The demonstration of a second peak in the incidence of ulcerative colitis at age 60 establishes a bimodal age distribution to this disease [26]. Retrospective studies suggest a more rapid appearance of significant symptoms, less systemic involvement, and lower relapse rates in the elderly. Therapeutic principles are unchanged with advancing age.

Angiodysplasia

When conventional methodology, short of angiography, has failed to disclose the source of colonic bleeding, the most likely cause is venous ectasia. These lesions are felt at present to be degenerative immature venules and capillaries [27]. Similar lesions occur in association with aortic stenosis. These lesions occur almost exclusively in the elderly, are usually in the right colon, and are best identified by angiography during acute hemorrhage. The usual presentation is with recurrent bright red or maroon-colored rectal bleeding, but massive or occult bleeding may also be present. Colonoscopy may visualize the lesion, but the most specific diagnostic test is angiography. Therapy is surgical removal of the involved colonic segment.

Diverticular Disease

Several surveys of asymptomatic healthy volunteers indicate a progressive development of colonic diverticula with advancing age, with prevalence rates of 18 percent at ages 40 to 59, 29 percent at ages 60 to 79, and 42 percent above age 80. There is a female preponderance in a ratio of approximately 1.5 : 1. Most patients with radiologically confirmed diverticula are asymptomatic. The risk of hemorrhagic complications appears to be increased in the elderly (particularly those who are hypertensive). Management both at the time and prophylactically is as in the younger age groups—high-residue diets (bran) or Metamucil. Peridiverticular abscess requires close in-hospital observation, bowel rest, and antibiotics (since the elderly seem to have less capacity to avoid free peritonitis). Pneumaturia should lead to the suspicion of diverticular disease in the otherwise healthy geriatric patient.

Appendicitis

With advancing age there is a decreased amount of lymphoid tissue in the appendix. Obliteration of the lumen is common. Appendicitis is more complicated in the elderly, with a higher incidence of perforation and less than 20 percent of these patients able to leave the hospital in the usual five postoperative days. The classic principles of atypical pain, delay in presentation, and intercurrent disease in the geriatric patient are of major importance in the diagnosis of appendicitis in the elderly. There is a strong relation between delay in presentation and perforation, with a 60 percent rate of perforation seen after a less than 48-hour delay and a 90 percent perforation rate for those delaying greater than 48 hours [28]. Nonoperative management of appendicitis, which may be necessary in some compromised elderly patients, requires bowel rest, antibiotics for aerobic gram-negative rods and anaerobic bacteria, as well as carefully planned interval appendectomy.

A rare variant of appendicitis, appendicitis occurring in a femoral hernia, occurs almost exclusively in postmenopausal women and should be included in the differential diagnosis of inflammatory right groin masses in such patients. Appendiceal abscesses complicate 3 percent of cases of acute appendicitis. Although death is unusual, 28 percent will have significant complications perioperatively and extended hospital stays. Interval appendectomy after medical treatment of abscess is associated with a 19 percent complication rate; if the appendectomy is not performed (usually because of serious associated illness) less than 10 percent are likely to have recurrent symptomatology.

Incidental appendectomy should be avoided in the elderly. In individuals over the age of 65, 100 incidental appendectomies need to be done to avoid a single case of appendicitis in the remaining lifetime of the individual. The common confounding differential diagnoses in younger individuals, such as ectopic pregnancy, salpingitis, and ruptured ovarian cysts, are less relevant in the elderly. Because of the relative rarity of death from appendicitis, 3.5 percent, it would take 3,000 incidental appendectomies to save a single elderly person's life [29].

Overall the mortality from appendicitis in the elderly has fallen dramatically from 54 percent in 1928 gradually and progressively to 3.5 percent in 1978, which is a more dramatic improvement than improvement in anesthetic risk alone would allow. This suggests an improvement in the natural history of this disorder.

Constipation

Constipation and laxative use become more prevalent as one ages. Between 40 and 60 percent of elders use laxatives regularly, largely on a self-administered basis. Many individuals who take laxatives regularly do not consider themselves constipated but wish to maintain a preconceived idea of regular bowel function. Of those who claim to be constipated, 25 percent have normal bowel transit times [25]. Clearly, physiologic bowel function is perceived as abnormal and is manipulated by self-prescribed agents. The cost of this routine in the United States has been estimated at $130 million per year. Bills for cathartics in chronic-care hospitals often approach 15 percent of their drug budget.

The elderly become constipated for the same reasons as the younger population. The main reason for the increased prevalence in the elderly is that multiple etiologies contribute to overcome normal physiologic habit. Some of the factors provoking constipation include the following.

1. Insufficient dietary fiber
2. Inactivity
3. Anxiety or depression
4. Drugs
5. Inadequate fluid intake
6. Laxative abuse
7. Poor muscle power
8. Dementia

9. Anal disease
10. Neurologic disease
11. Others: carcinoma, hypothyroidism, diverticulitis, strictures, hypercalcemia, hypokalemia

Some of the drugs causing constipation are: narcotic analgesics, anticholinergics, narcotic-containing cough medicines, iron, phenothiazines, tricyclic antidepressants, antiparkinsonian agents, and any drug leading to oversedation and, thus, neglect of the call to stool [30]. In long-term care facilities as many as two-thirds of the patients consume one or more drugs on this list.

One cause of constipation that demands consideration is carcinoma of the colon. This concern prompts investigation of any change in bowel habits, particularly constipation. A primary care physician caring for 3,000 people with a typical age range is likely to encounter one case of colorectal carcinoma every 16 months in his geriatric patients. Aggressive investigation is indicated in high-risk cases, especially in the presence of weight loss or bleeding. Additional risk factors include previous colon, endometrial, or bladder cancer; immunodeficiency states; inflammatory bowel disease; previous sporadic polyps; and Gardner's or familial polyposis syndromes. The minimum relevant investigation in a newly identified constipated patient would be a hematocrit, rectal examination, sigmoidoscopy, and three stools for occult blood testing.

Therapy for constipation has not received much physician interest. Many agents are available, and it is evident from institutional surveys that no clear prescribing practices exist. The regimen popularly suggested now includes a two-level therapeutic prescription of bulk laxative followed by an irritative cathartic should this first agent not be satisfactory. Bulk laxatives such as bran are easily introduced into the daily diet at doses of 5 g twice a day. Metamucil can be considered an equivalently efficacious agent. One of the senna derivatives can be an effective second agent should bulk laxatives fail.

The institution and continued administration of these agents must be considered carefully and reviewed in the context of encouraging a general plan of management. This should include educating the patient in normal bowel habits, making modifications in diet, recommending an increase in activity, encouraging him or her to heed the call to stool, and minimizing or eliminating painful local conditions or contributing drugs.

Complicated constipation may present as spurious diarrhea and usually requires more aggressive acute and chronic therapy. The atonic megacolon of the neglected, chronically constipated patient requires vigorous local therapy in the form of enemas to clear the colon of residue and a comprehensive plan of therapy. No clear guidelines exist regarding types and frequencies of enemas or strong cathartics. Perforation of the rectum with enema nipples may not be immediately reported and will obviously worsen the presenting difficulty.

Fecal Incontinence

Fecal incontinence, a socially isolating disease of predominantly institutionalized demented geriatric patients, may be caused by local anal disease, fecal impaction, or neurologic disorder. Occasional cases may result from diarrheal illnesses or laxative abuse. Clearly, senile dementia of the Alzheimer's type or obvious neurologic disorder is almost always present. Studies have shown that neurologically intact, fecally incontinent patients often demonstrate intense rectal contractions that are not observed in continent subjects and that are reminiscent of the findings in patients with uninhibited neurogenic bladder and urinary incontinence [31].

Therapy for this disturbing problem is difficult. Once fecal impaction and proximal or local pathology have been excluded by specific studies, the best form of therapy is a low-residue diet, pharmacologic induction of constipation, and periodic planned evacuation. Other modalities such as operant conditioning or rigorous bowel habit training may be useful in patients with more resistant cases.

Carcinoma of the Colon

Digestive malignancies are the most common internal malignancies in old age. The incidence for such disease increases in individuals in their late eighties, where it accounts for 30 percent (male) and 40 percent (female) of all cancers. Its mortality is second only to lung cancer. Of all digestive malignancies, 50 percent are adenocarcinomas of the colon. Pathologic studies have indicated less distant disease in the elderly, thus usually allowing local symptoms and prolonged course to dominate the clinical picture.

Symptoms provoked by the primary tumor are unchanged across the age spectrum. Confounds are introduced by the presence of concomitant benign disease that could also explain the same symptomatology, leading to both patient delay in reporting and physician delay in appropriate investigation.

Metabolic or nonmetastatic manifestations of cancer may dominate the clinical picture in the elderly and lead to the oft-quoted "altered presentation." Nonspecific vague symptomatology often includes loss of drive and interest, anorexia, weight loss, weakness, malaise, failing mobility, and tendency to fall. The more typical presentations are rectal bleeding, alteration in stool habit from a previously stable routine, and intraabdominal catastrophies resulting from obstruction and perforation.

The general trend to conservative care for senescent patients with malignancy is based, in part, on their shorter life expectancy. In some cases it is more desirable to preserve function and quality of life with disease rather than to invoke disturbing or disfiguring radical therapy. Although leading to increased cure rates, radical surgery or radiotherapy also invokes significant morbidity. Concomitant illness may preclude investigation and therapy and indeed may hasten or be totally responsible for the elderly patient's demise. Each case must be weighed carefully. This is crucially important when one considers the extended life expectancy of otherwise healthy elders.

Palliative care principles apply equally well to young and old patients, but it must be realized that the older patient may have less family support, more complex social isolation, and increased nursing care needs.

Acute Abdominal Pain

A particularly frustrating picture is presented to the clinician assessing acute abdominal pain in the elderly. History is often lacking because of organic brain disease, confusion, or the absence of family to provide history. Co-existence of several diseases (multiple pathology) further complicates the picture.

The expected abdominal signs may be minimal to absent. Retroperitoneal and intrathoracic disease may present with abdominal pain. The most common cause of surgical abdominal pain in the elderly is cholecystitis. Intestinal obstruction is the second most common acute abdominal pain requiring surgical investigation. Half of these are caused by hernias, followed by adhesions and malignancy. In the large bowel, malignancy and colonic volvulus are most likely to cause acute pain. The third most common cause of acute abdominal pain is appendicitis, and the increased difficulties with this diagnosis have been discussed [32].

Gallstone ileus is another unique female geriatric illness. Acute pancreatitis is the most common nonsurgical cause of abdominal pain in the elderly.

Acute mesenteric infarction is almost limited to the geriatric population. Its presentation is variable and often quickly associated with altered mental function and vascular instability, leading to disastrous results. In addition to abdominal pain, hyperperistalsis, bloody stool, and pseudoobstructive pattern on x-ray are part of the clinical presentation. This illness may be the most common cause of fatal acute abdominal crises in the geriatric population.

References

1. McKeown, F. *Pathology of the Aged.* London: Butterworth, 1965.
2. Geboes, K., and Bossaert, H. Gastrointestinal disorders in old age. *Age Ageing* 6:197, 1977.
3. Sklar, M., Kirsner, J. B., and Palmer, W. L. Symposium on medical problems of the aged; gastrointestinal disease in the aged. *Med. Clin. North Am.* 40:223, 1956.
4. U.S. DHEW. Special Report on Aging, 1979. NIH Pub. No. 79–1907. Washington, D.C.: U.S. Government Printing Office, 1979. P. 16.
5. Klein, D. R. Oral soft tissue changes in geriatric patients. *Bull. N.Y. Acad. Med.* 56:724, 1980.
6. Hollis, J. B., and Castell, D. O. Esophageal function in elderly men. *Ann. Intern. Med.* 80:371, 1974.
7. Cancer of the esophagus: three different views. *Hosp. Pract.* P. 63, October, 1976.
8. Siurala, M., et al. Prevalence of gastritis in a rural population. *Scand. J. Gastroenterology* 3:211, 1968.

9. Narayanan, M., and Steinheber, F. V.   The changing face of peptic ulcer in the elderly. *Med. Clin. North Am.* 60:1159, 1976.
10. Law, R., and Chalmers, C.   Medicines and elderly people: a general practice survey. *Br. Med. J.* 1:565, 1976.
11. Gorbach, S. L., et al.   Studies of intestinal microflora. *Gastroenterology* 53: 845, 1967.
12. Guth, P. H.   Physiologic alterations in small bowel function with age: The absorption of D-xylose. *Am. J. Dig. Dis.* 13:567, 1968.
13. Marx, J. J.   Normal iron absorption and decreased red cell iron uptake in the aged. *Blood* 53:204, 1979.
14. Gallagher, J. C., et al.   Intestinal calcium absorption and serum vitamin D metabolites in normal subjects and osteoporotic patients. *J. Clin. Invest.* 64: 129, 1979.
15. Price, H. L., Gazzard, B. G., and Dawson, A. M.   Steatorrhoea in the elderly. *Br. Med. J.* 1:1582, 1977.
16. Bayless, T. M.   Malabsorption in the elderly. *Hosp. Pract.* P. 57, August, 1979.
17. Morgan, Z., and Feldman, M.   The liver, biliary tract and pancreas in the aged: an anatomic and laboratory evaluation. *J. Am. Geriatr. Assoc.* 5:59, 1967.
18. Hyams, D. E.   The Liver and Biliary System. In J. C. Brocklehurst (Ed.), *Textbook of Geriatric Medicine and Gerontology* (2nd ed.). New York: Churchill-Livingstone, 1978.
19. Koff, R. S., et al.   Absence of an age effect on sulfobromopthalein retention in healthy men. *Gastroenterology* 65:300, 1973.
20. Huete-Armyo, A., Exton-Smith, A. N.   Causes and diagnosis of jaundice in the elderly. *Br. Med. J.* 1:1113, 1962.
21. Hyams, D. E.   Gastrointestinal problems in the old. II. *Br. Med. J.* 1:150, 1974.
22. Al-Sarraf, M., et al.   Primary liver cancer. *Cancer* 33:574, 1974.
23. Seigel, J.   Endoscopic management of choledocholithiasis and papillary stenosis. *Surg. Gynecol. Obstet.* 148:747, 1979.
24. Cancer statistics, 1979.   *CA* P. 811. January/February, 1979.
25. Eastwood, H. D. H.   Bowel transit studies in the elderly. Radiopaque markers in the investigation of constipation. *Gerontol. Clin.* 14:154, 1972.
26. Evans, J. G., and Acheson, E. D.   An epidemiologic study of ulcerative colitis and regional enteritis in the Oxford area. *Gut* 6:311, 1965.
27. Stewart, W. B., Gathright, J. B., and Ray, J. E.   Vascular ectasias of the colon. *Surg. Gynecol. Obstet.* 148:670, 1979.
28. Owens, B. J., and Hamit, H. F.   Appendicitis in the elderly. *Ann. Surg.* 187: 392, 1978.
29. Nockerts, S. R., Detmer, D. E., and Fryback, D. G.   Incidental appendectomy in the elderly? No. *Surgery* 88:301, 1980.
30. Hutchinson, B.   Constipation in the elderly. *Can. Fam. Physician* 24:1018, 1978.
31. Brocklehurst, J. C.   Bowel management in the neurologically disabled. The problems of old age. *Proc. R. Soc. Med.* 65:66, 1972.
32. Steinheber, F. V.   Interpretation of gastrointestinal symptoms in the elderly. *Med. Clin. North Am.* 60:1141, 1976.

18. Nutrition

Vernon R. Young

This chapter will review, in a general way, how the aging process in the adult free of significant clinical disease might bring about changes in the utilization of nutrients. In addition, a brief account will be given of the current estimates of the requirements for nutrients in older adults. The significant increase in numbers of elderly persons in the United States and technically developed nations makes it especially important to explore these aspects of metabolism and nutrition in human subjects. Unfortunately, there has been little detailed scientific inquiry in this field. Of the approximately 50 essential nutrients in human nutrition, few have received investigation with specific reference to their metabolism and requirements during advancing old age in humans [1].

Nutrient Categories and Function

A consideration of the utilization of nutrients during aging involves an adequate understanding of the biochemical and physiologic pathways that are involved in nutrient function. At the organ and cellular levels, glucose and fatty acids, or their precursors and products, as well as amino acids in excess of tissue needs, are the quantitatively important energy-yielding substrates. In relation to energy requirements, there is no specific dietary requirement for these compounds and the need can be met from either the carbohydrate, fat, and/or protein components of the diet.

Lipid contributes a significant proportion of the total dietary energy intake. There is a specific need for essential fatty acids that are involved in the maintenance of membrane composition, fluidity, and function, and they also serve as precursors of a class of "local" hormones, the prostaglandins and thromboxanes. These hormones exhibit diverse actions involving, for example, gastric secretion, blood platelet function, and nervous system activity. Carbohydrate intake provides a ready source of energy to support cellular activities. Excess ingested carbohydrates are easily converted to triglyceride for energy storage in fat depots. The need for dietary protein consists of two components—the requirement for essential (indispensable) amino acids and also a utilizable nontoxic source of nitrogen (nonspecific)—for synthesis of the nonessential (dispensable) amino acids. The major quantitative function of dietary protein in the adult is to furnish substrate for maintenance of tissue and organ protein synthesis. In addition, amino acids participate in the synthesis of the purine and pyrimidine moieties of nucleic acids and in the formation of neurotransmitters and other metabolically active molecules such as porphyrins, creatinine, and peptide hormones.

The metabolic functions of vitamins are diverse. B-complex vitamins serve as cofactors and coenzymes that are associated with many of the enzyme systems involved in carbohydrate, lipid, protein, and nucleic acid metabolism. Others, particularly the lipid-soluble vitamins, fulfill specific functions of key metabolic importance such as the glycosylation of proteins (vitamin A), calcium transport and utilization (vitamin D), prothrombin production (vitamin K), and antioxidation (vitamin E).

Of substantial gerontologic importance is the organ- or site-dependence of the conversion of some of the vitamins to their active forms. For example, conversion of vitamin D to its active form depends on the coordinated activities of the liver and kidney and also on hormonal factors and the concentration of phosphate ions in kidney cells. Thus, changes in specific cells or organs during senescence might easily alter the metabolism of, and possibly the quantitative need for, vitamins.

Biochemical and Physiologic Changes During Aging of Possible Nutritional Significance

Numerous biochemical and physiologic changes of potential nutritional importance occur with aging. At the molecular, subcellular, and cellular levels, alterations include changes in the DNA concentration and gene dosage of ribosomal RNA in various tissues, ultrastructural changes in the mitochondria and in the degree of cross-linking in collagen, and tissue accumulation of pigmented inclusion bodies. The composition of cell and subcellular membrane changes during senescence include changes in the binding sites for hormones and complex changes in the activities of enzymes. In some organs, such as the kidney and central nervous system, there is a reduction in the number of cells with advancing age [2].

Many organs and organ systems show alterations in function with advancing age that may have a direct influence on the utilization of nutrients. Variables associated with the maintenance of internal environment under resting conditions, such as fasting blood glucose, show little or no consistent age-related change. However, there is a marked decline in maximal organ performance and the rate at which these functions return to resting levels after stimulation is reduced by aging. Whether these alterations extend to an altered capacity to regulate the nutrient supply to cells following changes in nutrient intake is not known, but it does have important practical implications with respect to the frequency and levels of nutrient intake necessary for maintenance of adequate nutritional status in the aged individual. The importance of such effects is underlined by the finding that the nocturnal rise in urinary calcium excretion in postmenopausal women was greater than that observed in premenopausal women [3].

Gastrointestinal Tract and Nutrient Utilization

IMPORTANCE OF THE GASTROINTESTINAL TRACT

The central importance of the gastrointestinal tract in nutrient utilization relates, in part, to the fact that the level and nature of food ingested may be modulated by gastrointestinal function; for example, cancer in the gastrointestinal tract may result in obstruction, reduced food and nutrient intake, and anorexia. Furthermore, loss of teeth or frequent constipation have been suggested as important causes for altered dietary habits and food choices. It has been stated, and often assumed, that intestinal malabsorption is one of the major causes of malnutrition in the elderly. Based on an interview survey, Werner and Hambraeus [4] found, as summarized in Table 18-1, that symptoms of intestinal distress were higher in the elderly than in the young, but there was little difference betewn middle-aged and older people. From these findings it appears that the main changes occurred before the age of 50 and that they were not a characteristic of advanced old age per se.

The nutritional state of the host can also affect the biochemical and functional status of the gastrointestinal tract. Food or nutrient restriction leads to profound changes in the gastrointestinal tract, which may precipitate a reduction in absorption of other nutrients, exacerbating the effects of specific dietary inadequacies on the overall nutritional status of the host.

Finally, due to the rapid turnover and high metabolic activity of the cells of the gastrointestinal mucosa, there is a considerable flux of nutrients within the gastrointestinal tract, and this organ plays an important role in the economy of nutrient utilization. For example, the rate of the endogenous protein entry into the intestinal tract may account for about one-quarter of total body nitrogen turnover [5]. Comparable estimates of the exchanges of other

Table 18-1. Symptoms of Indigestion, Based on a Survey in a Swedish Population

Symptoms	Age Groups (% with symptoms)		
	> 67	50–60	20–25
Abdominal distress	25–33	15–35	1–3
"Gas"	17–27	15–35	1
Constipation	15–30	10–30	1–5
Diarrhea	< 5	< 3	< 1
Fat intolerance	5–10	10	1

Source: Adapted from I. Werner and L. Hambraeus, The Digestive Capacity of Elderly People. In L. Carlson (Ed.), *Nutrition in Old Age.* Uppsala, Sweden: Swedish Nutrition Foundation, 1972.

nutrients across the intestine are generally lacking, but for nutrients such as zinc and copper, their flux may be expected to be large in relation to the daily intake or requirement for maintenance of nutrient balance.

CHANGES IN INTESTINAL FUNCTION WITH AGING

Information on age and intestinal enzyme activity, digestion, and absorption is not adequate. No reports have been published of nutrient utilization during old age as evaluated by the use of enzyme supplementation or of defined formula diets. Various dietary and metabolic factors and disease states may modify the changes brought about by aging and must be considered in assessing the significance of the available, but limited, data concerned with the digestion and absorption of foods and nutrients during human aging.

The pentose sugar, xylose, appears to be transported by an active transport mechanism, and the absorption of this sugar is considered to serve both as an index of the capacity of the small intestine to transport simple sugars (such as glucose and galactose) and of general mucosal function. Because of this, xylose absorption in aged individuals has been examined by a number of investigators. As seen in Table 18-2, peak blood levels of xylose are stable until age 80 and fall thereafter. While lower output of urinary xylose following a 25-g xylose load in the over 80 group implies reduced absorption from the intestinal lumen, part of the reduction in urinary xylose output is attributed to reduced renal clearance [6].

Data are also limited on lipid digestion and absorption. Werner and Hambraeus [4] observed a reduction in fat absorption in the elderly. This was assessed by an increased output of neutral fat in the feces in eight apparently healthy elderly subjects, 67 to 72 years old, when fat intake was raised from 85 to 90 g per day, as provided by a self-chosen diet, to 115 to 120 g per day. Although the nutritional and metabolic significance of their findings is

Table 18-2. D-Xylose Tolerance Test at Different Ages in Adult Subjects

Age Groups (yrs)	Urine Xylose (g/5 L)	Peak Concentration Blood Xylose (mg/dl)	"Relative" Renal Clearance (%)*
30–49	4.9	46	100
50–59	4.7	48	97
60–69	4.8	50	83
70–79	3.6	48	66
80+	2.7	36	63

Source: Summarized from P. H. Guth, Physiologic alteration in small bowel function with age. The absorption of D-xylose. *Am. J. Dig. Dis.* 13:565, 1968.
* Expressed as percent of value for the 30- to 49-year-old group.

unclear, a reduction in digestion and/or absorption of lipid at physiologic intake level may have significance in relation to fatty acid and bile levels in the large intestine and colon cancer. Hence, it should be established, if an actual impairment in fat digestion exists, whether the defect is at the intra-luminal phase of micellular formation or at the point of triglyceride entry into the mucosal epithelial cell and/or its subsequent incorporation into chylomicrons.

The digestion and absorption of dietary protein might be assessed crudely from measurement of the difference between dietary intake and fecal nitro-gen output. Studies have not detected any evidence to indicate that the over-all digestability of a high-quality dietary protein differs between healthy young adult and elderly subjects.

The absorption of many vitamins and minerals occurs by means of active and regulated processes. However, the influence of aging per se on vitamin absorption has received little attention. For example, studies of folic acid absorption from everted gut sacs from rats have not revealed major changes with advancing old age [7]. This finding agrees with a limited series of studies in human subjects [8]. However, because dietary folate exists in the polyglutamate form, it will be necessary to explore in more detail the effect of old age on folic acid absorption and metabolism.

Organ and Whole Body Metabolism
NUTRIENT LEVEL IN BODY FLUIDS

After absorption from the intestinal lumen, nutrients are transported across the mucosal epithelium and enter the circulation where the utilization and fate of nutrients depend on the metabolic status of body organs. Transport of nutrients between the various organs and into cells involves the partici-pation of a number of different mechanisms, ranging from the movement of molecules in free solution and simple diffusion across a semipermeable mem-brane to the binding of nutrients to specific carrier molecules in serum, as in the case of transferrin and iron or the transcobalamins and vitamin B_{12}, and their passage across cell membranes by active transport or carrier-medi-ated systems.

Information on blood and tissue levels of nutrients provides some clues concerning the utilization of essential dietary nutrients, but few reports have appeared in which these levels are considered critically as a function of adult age. For many constituents (e.g., sodium, potassium, bicarbonate, mag-nesium, total protein, albumin, inorganic phosphate) there may be little change with age, but for others such as urea, creatinine, calcium, alkaline phosphatase, and uric acid changes may occur. Accurate interpretation of the nutritional significance of levels of nutrients in blood, or their metabolites and compounds, that reflect the activities of metabolic pathways in which these nutrients function, awaits the development of adequate age-adjusted guidelines.

BODY COMPOSITION IN RELATION TO NUTRIENT UTILIZATION

Cross-sectional and longitudinal studies indicate a decline in lean body mass (or body cell mass) with advancing human age. Although the contribution made by each of the major body organs to this reduction is not precisely known, postmortem studies indicate that skeletal muscles account for a significant and perhaps the major proportion of the decline in body protein content [9]. Figure 18-1 shows that during early growth and development, the skeletal muscles account for an increasing contribution to total body weight, amounting to about 45 percent of body weight in the young adult. However, as the adult years progress, muscle mass continues to decline, decreasing to approximately 27 percent of total body weight by about age 70. Atrophy of skeletal muscles is a prominent clinical feature of advancing old age.

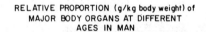

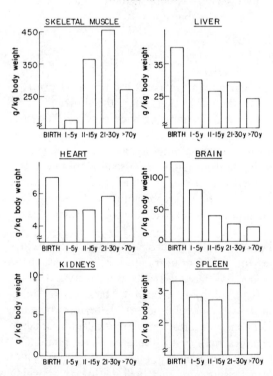

Figure 18-1. Relative proportion (g/kg of body weight) of major organs at various stages of life in humans. (Drawn from V. Korenchevsky, *Physiological and Pathological Ageing.* New York: Hafner, 1961.)

The decline in muscle mass with advancing adult age may be predicted to have an influence on nutrient utilization and perhaps overall nutritional health. The etiology of the loss of lean body and muscle mass is not known, but it has been suggested that the decline in physical activity may be of causal significance. Active middle-age men have a higher body cell mass than inactive men [10]. Also, a program of moderate physical activity in elderly persons has been shown to result in favorable effects on body nitrogen content [11].

The fall in body cell mass is accompanied by an increase in the amount and percentage of body fat, at least during the period of middle age. From this observation, it is to be concluded that there is a small, but perceptible, excess of energy intake over energy expenditure. The metabolic basis for changes in body composition during the passage of adult life remains unclear. The control of body energy content, including the fat-free cell mass, is still a matter of considerable speculation, but a resolution of this problem is of considerable great public health importance, in view of the prevalence of obesity and problems of overweight in our society.

Energy Metabolism and Utilization
BASAL ENERGY EXPENDITURE

Daily energy expenditure is the sum of basal energy metabolism, a small loss due to the heat increment after food ingestion and that associated with physical activity. Basal or resting energy metabolism represents the combustion of substrates required to meet the energy needs of the metabolic processes involved in maintaining cell function and integrity, and the mechanical processes necessary for survival. Synthetic processes (protein, nucleic acid, and lipid synthesis, urea synthesis, and gluconeogenesis), transport processes (including the pumping of ions to maintain ion gradients within cells and organelles), and mechanical processes (involving muscular activity) all require energy inputs. These are obtained from high-phosphate compounds such as adenosine triphosphate (ATP) and guanosine triphosphate (GTP) generated during the oxidation of energy-yielding substrates. Various nutritional, physiologic, and pathologic factors alter the activities of these processes and the types and sources of substrate used for supplying their energy needs.

Basal metabolic rate (BMR) falls with increasing adult age. This decline appears to be due to the loss of cell mass rather than to a reduction in the metabolic activity of body tissues, since there is little decline in basal metabolic rate when the latter is expressed per unit of body cell mass [12]. However, because of the importance of the brain, liver, and muscle in total body energy metabolism it is to be expected that alterations in the relative mass of these organs would lead to differences in the contribution made by each of them to total body energy expenditure during advancing adult age.

In support of this, Tzankoff and Norris [13,14] examined the relationships between basal oxygen consumption and creatinine excretion, the latter as an index of muscle mass, in adults of varying ages. They observed an age-dependent linear relation between basal oxygen and creatinine excretion, and calculated the contribution made by nonmuscle tissue to basal oxygen consumption. As shown in Figure 18-2, nonmuscle consumption showed no age-related changes, indicating that the loss of muscle mass may be responsible for the age-related decrease in BMR.

FUEL SOURCES

As discussed earlier, the major sources of energy in mammalian tissues are glucose, fatty acids, ketone bodies, amino acids, and lactate. The pattern of fuel sources changes markedly if food is withheld for longer than the usual overnight fast [15]. Hence, for a fast that lasts for two or three days or longer, glucose oxidation is decreased, together with a reduced rate of gluconeogenesis. In parallel with the diminished glucose metabolism, mobilization of triglyceride from adipose tissue and utilization of fatty acids in peripheral tissues, particularly muscle, are increased, and the brain utilizes ketone bodies as its principal fuel source with a continuation of the fast. This pattern of change in fuel utilization during short- and long-term fasts is accompanied by alterations in substrate availability and hormonal balance, and is achieved, in part, by the regulatory effects of ketone bodies on protein turnover and amino acid oxidation in peripheral tissues. Whether older individuals main-

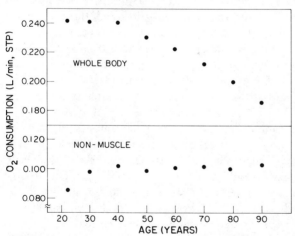

Figure 18-2. An estimate of the age-related changes in oxygen consumption by the skeletal muscles and nonmusculature tissues in men at various stages of adult life. STP, standard temperature and pressure. (From S. P. Tzankoff and A. H. Norris. Effect of muscle mass decrease on age-related BMR changes. *J. Appl. Physiol.* 43:1001–1006, 1977.)

tain a capacity similar to that in young adults to effectively bring out these changes in the pattern of fuel utilization when dietary energy intake is reduced is not clear.

Lipid Metabolism

Most available data on changes in lipid metabolism and utilization during aging are derived from studies in experimental animals. Investigations in humans are less extensive and most have been concerned with measurement of blood lipid levels. These studies are often cross-sectional, and since elevated levels of certain lipid moieties are risk factors for death from cardiovascular disease, the elderly groups may be viewed as "survivors" and thus represent a selected group. Even longitudinal studies may be difficult to interpret in view of the marked secular changes regarding diet and exercise over the past several decades. Nonetheless, the presently available data would indicate that the circulating level of low-density lipoproteins, which are associated with increased risk of atherosclerosis, increase with age whereas levels of high-density lipoproteins, which appear to offer protection against atherosclerosis, do not change with age. Alteration of lipid levels by diet, exercise, weight reduction, or administration of medications is of uncertain value in the elderly and would seem to be particularly out of place in the very elderly. Thus, the appropriate management of the patient with abnormal circulating lipoprotein levels must take into account the patient's age, capacity to comply with recommended regimens, and likelihood of benefit.

Since adipose-tissue lipids serve as an important source of fuel, the effects of aging on the capacity for mobilization of fatty acids from these depots is of interest. There is a reduction in hormone-stimulated fat mobilization with progressive aging in the rat, and this may be the case in humans [16]. Whether this implies a diminished capacity in the aged individual to adapt successfully to a deficient energy intake remains to be determined and is clinically relevant in view of the increased frequency of periods of short- and longer-term food restriction in the aged due to infectious episodes, physical trauma, and psychologic stress.

Protein Metabolism
WHOLE-BODY NITROGEN METABOLISM
Alterations in energy balance and in fuel metabolism have important consequences for body and tissue protein metabolism and vice versa. Changes in the rate of tissue and organ protein synthesis will lead to alterations in substrate need, particularly because whole protein synthesis is thought to account for a significant proportion of basal energy utilization. Skeletal muscles account for about 30 percent of whole-body protein breakdown in young adult men and for about 20 percent in elderly men.

INDIVIDUAL PROTEINS

Most studies of the metabolism of individual proteins in human subjects have focused on albumin metabolism. A low plasma albumin is a frequent finding (in the absence of nephrosis and liver disease) in nutritional surveys among the elderly. In a recent study it was reported that albumin synthesis in older subjects is regulated at a lower "set-point" than in healthy young adults [17]. This suggests that the response of albumin metabolism to nutritional repletion in older subjects may differ from that in young adults.

RESPONSE OF NITROGEN METABOLISM
TO ALTERED PROTEIN INTAKE

Body nitrogen losses, after adaptation to a brief period of very low or protein-free feeding (obligatory nitrogen losses) in elderly men, are essentially the same as those for young men. However, when expressed per unit of creatinine excretion or per unit of body cell mass, obligatory urinary nitrogen losses are apparently higher in the elderly [18]. These differences in nitrogen output parallel those found for changes in rates of whole-body protein breakdown (and synthesis) with aging, implying a relationship between whole-body protein turnover and obligatory nitrogen losses.

The effect of aging on nitrogen metabolism may also be examined from the comparative response of nitrogen metabolism in young adults and elderly subjects given differing protein intakes within the submaintenance range of nitrogen intake. Such studies indicate that the mean nitrogen intake necessary to maintain body nitrogen balance in the elderly is greater than 120 mg N/kg per day for women and 110 mg N/kg per day for men.

The nitrogen balance response pattern for elderly subjects is similar, in qualitative terms, to that observed for healthy young adults. Comparisons suggest that the efficiency of dietary nitrogen utilization for maintenance of nitrogen equilibrium might be less in quantitative terms for older subjects [19].

Carbohydrate Metabolism

The influence of age on carbohydrate metabolism is discussed in detail in Chapter 9. In brief, advancing age is associated with slight increases in fasting glucose levels and substantial increases in postprandial glucose levels. These decreases in glucose tolerance are so great as to require use of age-adjusted criteria for the diagnosis of chemical diabetes. Present data indicate that resistance to the effect of insulin on peripheral tissues is the primary physiologic abnormality underlying the age-related carbohydrate intolerance.

Vitamin and Mineral Metabolism

The effects of human aging per se on the utilization of vitamins and minerals remain largely unexplored. The major problems of osteoporosis and of calcium and vitamin D metabolism in relation to human aging are discussed in Chapter 15. Iron and potassium metabolism in the elderly have been explored only to a limited extent, and there are insufficient data to draw any definitive conclusions concerning the impact of aging on the utilization of these essential nutrients in the human. Some nutritional surveys have suggested that vitamin insufficiency may occur with considerable frequency in the elderly, but there are no comprehensive studies on the utilization and metabolism of individual vitamins [20]. Although adult age may influence the plasma levels of some vitamins, such as vitamin B_6 and vitamin C, interpretation of the biochemical, physiologic, and nutritional significance of such findings is difficult at present.

Nutrient Requirements in the Elderly

In the foregoing section we have considered some of the more basic aspects of nutrition and progressive human aging. The available knowledge is quite limited, and there is an obvious need for much greater inquiry into this aspect of human nutrition because it would help provide a better basis for assessing nutritional status and nutrient requirements in elderly persons. However, there is a pressing and continued need to supply estimations of the nutrient requirements of older people, and in the following section we will review briefly the current recommendations for dietary allowances for this age group.

FACTORS AFFECTING NUTRIENT REQUIREMENTS

In addition to the possible influence of adult age per se, humans are affected by various factors. These are listed in Table 18-3 according to host, environmental, and agent (dietary) factors [21]. The variable importance of these factors, interacting in complex ways, for different individuals makes a definition of the quantitative nutrient requirements of the elderly a difficult task.

Not everyone of the same age, body build, and sex has the same requirement; these differences may be due in part to variations in genetic background. In relation to practical human nutrition, it is generally thought that the effects of various environmental, physiologic, psychologic, and pathologic influences are of greater importance in determining the variability in nutrient needs among individuals. For example, the growing infant or child requires higher nutrient intakes per unit of body weight than does the young adult. Therefore, nutrient needs are relatively high during the early growth and developmental phase of life, declining as adulthood is approached. However, other than for energy, for which the daily requirement declines due to lowered physical activity, it is uncertain whether the requirement for essential nutrients changes in the healthy individual with the progression of the adult years. On the basis of quite limited knowledge, the nutrient needs in healthy aged subjects do not appear to differ significantly from those of young adults. Nevertheless, a characteristic of aging is increased disease incidence and morbidity, and these are conditions that appear to be far more

Table 18-3. Agent, Host, and Environmental Factors That Influence Nutrient and Nutritional Status in the Elderly

---

Agent (dietary) factors
  Chemical form of nutrient
  Energy intake
  Food processing and preparation (may increase or decrease dietary needs)
  Effect of other dietary constituents
Host factors
  Old age
  Sex
  Genetic makeup
  Pathologic states
    Drugs
    Infection
    Physical trauma
    Chronic disease, cancer
Environmental factors
  Physical (unsuitable housing, inadequate heating)
  Biologic (poor sanitary conditions)
  Socioeconomic (poverty, dietary habits and food choices, physical activity)

Source: From V. R. Young, Diet and Nutrient Needs in Old Age. In J. A. Behnke, C. E. Finch, and G. B. Moment (Eds.), *The Biology of Aging.* New York: Plenum Press, 1978.

important than age per se in determining practical differences between young adults and elderly people in their need for nutrients.

Numerous dietary factors determine the amounts of a particular nutrient sufficient to meet the body's needs. For example, all forms of dietary iron are not equally available and, in addition, the type of diet and composition of individual meals influence the availability of the iron consumed. Another factor of particular importance in our considerations of diet and nutrient needs during old age is the effect of stressful stimuli, such as those arising from infection or physical trauma or even those of psychologic origin. Thus, early in the infectious episode there is an increased rate of synthesis of immunoglobulins and other proteins. This is followed by a net catabolic response that results in increased losses of body nitrogen and of some vitamins and minerals and in decreases in blood levels of these nutrients. Furthermore, absorption of nutrients may be interfered with if the gastrointestinal tract is significantly involved by either acute or chronic infections. The net result is depletion of body nutrients followed by a physiologic increase in the need for nutrients during the recovery phase to promote recovery and to compensate for the earlier losses. However, while it is appreciated that acute and chronic infections and other stressful stimuli, including anxiety, pain, and physical trauma, generally increase the requirement for many essential nutrients, there are inadequate quantitative data to help determine how much nutrient intakes should be increased to meet the additional nutritional demands created by these conditions that may be frequent in elderly people.

Finally, various drugs may have profound effects on nutrient requirements by decreasing nutrient absorption or by altering the utilization of nutrients. The effects of drugs on nutrient requirements will depend on the dose and period of administration, and, furthermore, the multiple administration of drugs may have synergistic effects, thus increasing further nutrient needs. Reduced appetite is a frequent consequence of drug therapy, and this will exaggerate the effects of drug treatment on the individual's nutritional status, particularly if the diet is marginal in adequacy to begin with. Mention of alcohol (ethanol) might be made here because nutritional deficiency is often seen in alcoholics. Although this is due in part to an inadequate diet, ethanol interferes with the absorption and/or utilization of various nutrients, thereby effecting increasing nutrient needs above those required by healthy individuals.

RECOMMENDED DIETARY ALLOWANCES (RDAs)
Because the minimum requirement for a nutrient to maintain health varies among apparently similar individuals, the RDAs are designed so that they would be adequate to meet the nutritional needs of practically all healthy persons within a particular population. The question of the extent of the variation in nutrient needs among individuals is of particular importance, therefore, in the development of appropriate dietary standards. In healthy populations of adults, this variation is assumed to be normally distributed, and the mean requirement plus two standard deviations above the mean is now considered to be a reasonable objective for establishing an RDA. This should then be sufficient to cover the requirements of about 97.5 percent of the population.

The situation differs for energy requirements, and the RDA for energy is based on the *average* requirement for the population. Intakes of energy nutrients either well above or well below the individual's true requirement would result eventually in a deterioration of health, and it is assumed that most individuals select diets providing energy intakes that meet or approximate their actual needs. Thus, the average energy requirement is given as a guideline rather than recommending the intake level that would suit those few individuals in a population whose energy requirements are much higher than the mean.

Table 18-4 summarizes the most recent recommended dietary allowances for adults as proposed by the U.S. Food and Nutrition Board. It should be noted that insufficient information is available on human requirements on which to make a reliable recommendation for all of the known essential nutrients. Accordingly, the Food and Nutrition Board has proposed a range

Table 18-4. RDAs and Estimated Safe and Adequate Daily Dietary Intakes of Selected Vitamins for Adults of 51 Years and Older[a]

	Men	Women
Weight (lbs)	154	120
Height (in)	70	64
Recommended dietary allowances (RDAs)		
Energy (kcal)	2400	1800
Protein (g)	56	44
Fat-soluble vitamins		
Vitamin A (μgRE)[b]	1,000	800
Vitamin D (μg)[c]	5	5
Vitamin E activity		
(mg α-TE)[d]	10	10
Water-soluble vitamins		
Vitamin C (mg)	60	60
Folic acid (μg)	400	400
Niacin (mg NE)[e]	16	13
Riboflavin (mg)	1.4	1.2
Thiamin (mg)	1.2	1.0
Vitamin B_6 (mg)	2.2	2.0
Vitamin B_{12} (μg)	3.0	3.0
Minerals		
Calcium (mg)	800	800
Phosphorus (mg)	800	800
Iodine (μg)	150	150
Magnesium (mg)	350	300
Zinc (mg)	15	15
Safe and adequate intakes		
Vitamin K (μg)	70–140	
Biotin (μg)	100–200	
Pantothenic acid (mg)	4–7	
Copper (mg)	2.0–3.0	
Manganese (mg)	2.5–5.0	
Fluoride (mg)	1.5–4.0	
Chromium (mg)	0.05–0.2	
Selenium (mg)	0.05–0.2	
Molybdenum (mg)	0.15–0.5	
Sodium (mg)	1100–3300	
Potassium (mg)	1875–5625	
Chloride (mg)	1700–5100	

[a] These intakes are designed to be sufficient for the maintenance of good nutrition in practically all *healthy* persons. Diets should be based on a variety of common foods in order to provide other nutrients for which human requirements have been less well defined. Further details regarding these allowances are described in *Recommended Dietary Allowances* (9th ed., from the Food and Nutrition Board, National Research Council, National Academy of Sciences, Washington, D.C., 1980.
[b] Retinol equivalents; RE = 1 μg retinol or 6 μg carotene.
[c] As cholecalciferol; 10 μg = 400 IU vitamin D.
[d] α-tocopherol equivalent; 1 mg d-α-tocopherol = 1 α-TE.
[e] One niacin equivalent (NE) is equal to 1 mg niacin or 60 mg tryptophan.

of intake that is considered safe and sufficient to meet the physiologic needs for those nutrients for which RDAs have not been determined. These intake ranges are also given in Table 18-4.

It must be emphasized strongly that the recommended allowances are amounts considered sufficient for the maintenance of health in nearly all adults. Recommendations are concerned with health maintenance, and they are not intended to be sufficient for therapeutic purposes. Thus, they are not designed to cover the additional requirements that may occur during and after recovery from infection, or under conditions of malabsorption, trauma, metabolic disease, or other significant stress. The possible benefits that might occur with considerably higher intakes of individual nutrients in a variety of clinical situations are not relevant to RDAs, and proposals for very much higher intakes of nutrients relative to those intakes proposed in Table 18-4 as a normal dietary practice cannot be justified for healthy old people on the basis of current information.

SPECIFIC CONSIDERATIONS OF DIET AND NUTRIENT REQUIREMENTS IN THE AGED

A broad range of conditions that accompany old age may have important effects on the nutritional status of the elderly. A listing of such factors is given in Table 18-5 [22].

Physical and mental disabilities affect the mode of living and this may lead to changes in dietary pattern and a deterioration of nutritional status. Under-

Table 18-5. Factors That May Lead to Inadequate Nutrition in the Elderly

Depression
Loneliness, psychologic problems
Physical disability: immobility at home, poor vision, arthritis, etc.
Disease: infection, cancer, and other chronic illness
Malabsorptive and gastrointestinal disorders and discomfort
Poverty
Mental deterioration
Inadequate knowledge of dietetic principles: food fads, poor dietary habits
Alcoholism
Medications
Increased requirements (?)

Source: Adapted from A. N. Exton-Smith, Nutritional Problems of Elderly Populations. In W. W. Hawkins (Ed.), *Nutrition of the Aged*. Quebec: Nutrition Society of Canada, 1978.

lying medical problems, emotional disturbance, loneliness, and poverty are all factors that may reduce the desire or ability to consume an adequate, well-balanced diet. Thus, risk of nutritional deficiencies will increase under these circumstances, and these are common causes for inadequate nutrition in elderly people. Because the energy requirements are reduced with inactivity, an adequate intake of other essential nutrients may not be met without a change in the dietary pattern toward foods of increased nurient density. This problem may be compounded by the decrease in taste sensitivity that occurs with old age, and the poor health of the oral tissues that may restrict the selection of foods to those that are bland, soft, and readily masticated. The net result is a further worsening in the condition of the oral tissues and an increase in the intensity of the vicious cycle leading to nutrient depletion, one that produces a reduced capacity to respond favorably to infection and disease, which in turn produces a gradual deterioration in health.

The vulnerable groups of old people therefore must be identified and a means must be developed for improving nutrient intakes. Only a small percentage of the elderly population may be affected, and many elderly individuals will never experience nutritional deficiencies. However, with the increasing numbers of elderly persons in our society, a small percentage translates into many lives.

References

1. Shank, R. E. Nutritional Characteristics of the Elderly: An Overview. In M. Rockstein and M. L. Sussman (Eds.), *Nutrition, Longevity and Aging*. New York: Academic Press, 1976.
2. Finch, C. E., and Hayflick, L. (Eds.). *Handbook of the Biology of Aging*. New York: Van Nostrand Reinhold, 1977.
3. Nordin, B. E. C., et al. Calcium and Bone Metabolism in Old Age. In L. A. Carlson (Ed.), *Nutrition in Old Age*. Uppsala, Sweden: Swedish Nutrition Foundation, 1972.
4. Werner, I., and Hambraeus, L. The Digestive Capacity of Elderly People. In L. A. Carlson (Ed.), *Nutrition in Old Age*. Uppsala, Sweden: Swedish Nutrition Foundation, 1972.
5. Fauconneau, G., and Michel, M. C. The Role of the Gastrointestinal Tract in the Regulation of Protein Metabolism. In H. N. Munro (Ed.), *Mammalian Protein Metabolism*. New York: Academic Press, 1970. Vol. IV.
6. Guth, P. H. Physiologic alteration in small bowel function with age. The absorption of D-xylose. *Am. J. Dig. Dis.* 13:565, 1968.
7. Bhanthumnavin, K., Wright, J. R., and Halsted, C. H. Intestinal transport of tritiated folic acid (^{3}H-PGA) in the everted gut sac of the rat at different ages. *Johns Hopkins Med. J.* 135:152, 1974.
8. Hurdle, A. D. F., Picton, T. C., and Williams, T. C. Folic acid deficiency in elderly patients admitted to hospital. *Br. Med. J.* 2:202, 1966.
9. Korenchevsky, V. *Physiological and Pathological Ageing*. New York: Hafner, 1961.

10. Brozek, J. Changes in body composition in man during maturity and their nutritional implications. *Fed. Proc.* 11:784, 1952.
11. Sidney, K. H., Shephard, R. J., and Harrison, J. E. Endurance training and body composition of the elderly. *Am. J. Clin. Nutr.* 30:326, 1977.
12. Shock, N. W. Energy Metabolism, Caloric Intake and Physical Activity of the Aging. In L. A. Carlson (Ed.), *Nutrition in Old Age.* Uppsala, Sweden: Swedish Nutrition Foundation, 1972.
13. Tzankoff, S. P., and Norris, A. H. Effect of muscle mass decrease on age-related BMR changes. *J. Appl. Physiol.* 43:1001, 1977.
14. Tzankoff, S. P., and Norris, A. H. Longitudinal changes in basal metabolism in man. *J. Appl. Physiol.* 45:536, 1978.
15. Cahill, G. J., Jr. Starvation in man. *Clin. Endocrinol. Metab.* 5:397, 1976.
16. Masoro, E. J., et al. Nutritional probe of the aging process. *Fed. Proc.* 39:3178, 1980.
17. Gersovitz, M., et al. Albumin synthesis in young and elderly subjects using a new stable isotope methodology: response to level of protein intake. *Metabolism* 29:1075, 1980.
18. Bricker, M. L., and Smith, J. M. A study of endogenous nitrogen output of college women, with particular reference to use of the creatinine output in the calculation of the biological values of the protein of egg and sunflower seed. *J. Nutr.* 44:553, 1951.
19. Uany, R., Scrimshaw, N. S., and Young, V. R. Human protein requirements: nitrogen balance response to graded levels of egg protein in elderly men and women. *Am. J. Clin. Nutr.* 31:771, 1978.
20. Brin, M., and Bauernfield, J. C. Vitamin needs of the elderly. *Postgrad. Med.* 63:155, 1978.
21. Young, V. R. Diet and Nutrient Needs in Old Age. In J. A. Behnke, C. E. Finch, and G. B. Moment (Eds.), *The Biology of Aging.* New York: Plenum Press, 1978.
22. Exton-Smith, A. N. Nutritional Problems of Elderly Populations. In W. W. Hawkins (Ed.), *Nutrition of the Aged.* Quebec: Nutrition Society of Canada, 1978.

Suggested Reading

Albanese, A. A. *Nutrition for the Elderly.* New York: Alan R. Liss, 1980.
Exton-Smith, A. N., and Caird, F. I. *Metabolic and Nutritional Disorders in the Elderly.* Bristol, England: John Wright and Sons, 1980.
Munro, H. N. Nutrition and Ageing. *Br. Med. Bull.* 37:83, 1981.
Watkin, D. M. Nutrition for the Aging and Aged. In R. S. Goodhart and M. E. Shils (Eds.), *Modern Nutrition in Health and Disease.* Philadelphia: Lea & Febiger, 1978.
Young, V. R., Gersovitz, M., and Munro, H. N. Human Aging: Protein and Amino Acid Metabolism and Implications for Protein and Amino Acid Requirements. In G. B. Moment (Ed.), *Nutritional Approaches to Aging Research.* Boca Raton, Florida: CRC Press (in press).

19. *Immune System*

Richard M. Rose
Richard W. Besdine

The study of the immune system and aging has, more than any other aspect of the biology of aging, fostered hope for a fountain of youth. An extensive investigative effort, begun in the 1960s to define specific alterations in immune function with age, is based on the premise that these alterations are at least in part responsible for the aging process and age-related disease. Were this assumption valid, reconstitution of normal immune function might then lead to increased life span.

The notion that immunity is impaired in the elderly has historic precedent based on clinical experience. Sir William Osler [1] recognized the exceptional susceptibility of the elderly to fatal bacterial pneumonia. "The old are likely to die, the young to recover. . . . At about sixty the death rate is very high, amounting to 60 to 80 percent. From the reports of its fatality in some places, one may say that to die of pneumonia is almost the natural end of old people."

Osler attributed this excess mortality to "generalized debility of the organs" in the aged. Although Osler's observations on impaired resistance to infection in the elderly are shared by many contemporary physicians, it is surprising to find that a paucity of information still exists on the specific alterations in host defenses responsible for this apparent age-related phenomenon.

Perhaps greater impetus for the study of the role of the immune system in the aging process has come from observations based on a variety of naturally occurring and experimentally induced immunodeficiency states [2]. In humans, as well as in laboratory animals, immunodeficiency is strongly associated with increased frequency of autoantibodies [3] and certain malignancies [4]. Furthermore, in laboratory animals such as the NZB mouse, a primary alteration in immune regulation is causally related to the development of an autoimmune disease resembling human lupus erythematosus, increased risk of amyloidosis, and premature death [3].

On a human population level, these processes—autoantibodies, amyloidosis, and neoplasia—all appear to have an increased prevalence with age [5]. As such, they can be considered biologic markers for the aging process. It seems logical then to ask if aging or age-related diseases in man have an immunologic basis. If so, alterations in immune function might be similarly age-related and perhaps amenable to correction.

Immunologic Theory of Aging

Stated simply, the immunologic theory of aging views senescence as the consequence of an age-related decline in the immune system (Fig. 19-1). Mammalian lymphocytes occur as either thymus-derived T cells or, by analogy

335

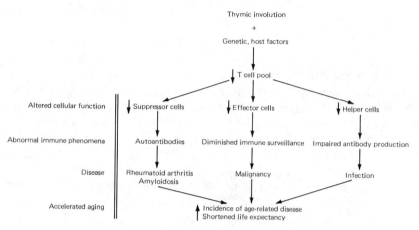

Figure 19-1. Schematic view of the immunologic theory of aging.

to the avian bursa of Fabricius, bursa-derived or bone marrow–derived B cells. T cells mediate the array of cellular immune functions, including delayed hypersensitivity, histocompatibility recognition, the helping function, the killing function, antigen-induced blastogenesis, and the suppression function. B cells are the precursors of plasma cells that synthesize antibody. Altered T cells function allegedly produces diminished self-tolerance [6] and immune surveillance [7], thereby accounting for the age-related increase in autoimmune phenomena and malignancy. A decline in B cell function may be partly responsible for increased severity of infection in older individuals.

A decline in immune function in old laboratory animals is evident at a cellular level. Immunocompetent murine lymphocytes exhibit an age-related diminution in ability to proliferate and differentiate in response to a variety of antigens, including those involved in rejection of tumors and heterologous grafts [8]. Although the precise mechanism is unclear, several explanations have been offered: enhanced suppressor cell activity in aged animals [9], alterations in the extracellular milieu [10], accumulated damage to genetic material [11], or running down of an intrinsic biologic clock in the nucleus of immunocompetent cells [12].

Further support for the immunologic theory of aging comes from immunodeficient strains of animals, such as the neonatally thymectomized or congenitally athymic nude mouse that lacks functional T lymphocytes but is otherwise normal. These short-lived animals are prone to a variety of autoimmune diseases, severe infection, malignant tumors, and a wasting syndrome that bears some pathologic similarities to degenerative vascular changes in aged humans. When these animals are immunologically reconstituted with thymic transplants or syngeneic lymphocytes, premature death and the aforementioned diseases are averted [13].

In humans congenital thymic hypoplasia associated with hypoparathyroidism (the DiGeorge syndrome) results in profoundly diminished cell-mediated immunity, which may be partially reconstituted by injections of calf thymus extract [14]. Although children with this disorder are particularly prone to infection, they do not appear to undergo the accelerated aging of their murine counterparts. The dissimilarities between animal and human models is further suggested by the postthymectomy state in adult humans, in which no immunologically mediated reduced life expectancy is apparent [15]; and by progeria, a disease of premature aging that begins in childhood, in which no immune deficit has consistently been found [16].

Some support for the immunologic theory of aging comes from human population studies. In a prospective, longitudinal study of residents in Busselton, Australia, the presence of an autoantibody was associated with excess cancer and vascular disease mortality over the ensuing five years and is statistically significant, even when age-adjusted mortality is considered [17]. In another study, impaired cutaneous delayed hypersensitivity in individuals over 80 years old predicted excess mortality over a two-year period [18]. Although these studies attempt to relate a specific immune parameter to life expectancy, they are limited by small numbers and an inability to clearly exclude underlying or age-related disease as the primary cause of altered immune function and mortality.

Additionally, while a number of human population studies allegedly show an age-related decline in various parameters of immune function, many of these studies are cross-sectional in design and consequently are often ambiguous. Is an age-related decline in immune function a true risk factor for aging or could it be a marker for longevity [19]?

The immunologic theory of aging is far from proved. Nevertheless, it provides an important historic perspective for the study of the immune system in aged humans and raises provocative questions about the role of immune function in senescence and the pathogenesis of aging.

Morphologic Alterations in Lymphoid Tissue With Age

The thymus is the first lymphoid organ to develop during fetal life, and the first to show involution, beginning shortly after puberty. By the fifth decade of life, the thymus is markedly atrophied. Histologic changes consist of cortical thinning, diminished numbers of lymphocytes and secretory granules, and widespread replacement with connective tissue [20].

These changes suggest that thymic ability to modulate the differentiation of bone marrow–derived prothymocytes into mature T cells would be impaired substantially. However, quantitative assessment of circulating T lymphocytes in healthy aged humans is normal [2], or only mildly diminished when hospitalized individuals are included in the analysis [21]. Nevertheless, serum levels of thymic hormone activity generally decline around age 50 [20], perhaps accounting for the loss in weight of secondary lymphoid organs, the lymph nodes and spleen, at about the sixth decade [22]. These changes result in part from depletion of lymphocytes from thymus-dependent regions in the deep cortical areas and interfollicular regions of superficial cortex. The functional significance of these morphologic alterations in secondary lymphoid tissue is thus far unclear.

Humoral Immunity

Analysis of humoral immunity in elderly humans has several potential benefits. Quantitative assessment of naturally occurring antibodies in an aged population permits an estimation of normal reference levels. Significant deviation from these norms may then be used as one variable in the study of the aging process and age-related disease. Furthermore, study of the humoral response to immunization in the elderly has important implications for preventive therapy in clinical practice.

With advancing age the absolute number of circulating B lymphocytes, the precursors of antibody-forming cells, is unchanged [21]. Cross-sectional analysis of serum immunoglobulin levels demonstrates a peak in the third decade, followed by a statistically significant fall in IgG and IgM levels [23] (Fig. 19-2). In longitudinal studies of patients beyond the seventh decade of life a small upward trend in serum IgG and IgA levels has been found [24,25]. These changes may result in part from the inclusion of individuals in the study population with underlying systemic disease. When criteria for health are rigorously defined, serum IgM levels are found to be diminished with age, while IgG and IgA are unchanged [2]. Alterations in IgE levels have shown no consistent age-related trend [2,26]. A pattern of midlife

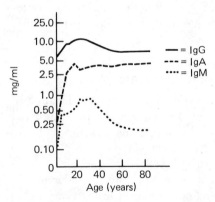

Figure 19-2. Relation of serum immunoglobulin subclass concentration to age. Mean value plotted on log scale. (From C. E. Buckley and F. C. Dorsey, The effect of aging on human serum immunoglobulin concentrations. *J. Immunol.* 105:964, 1970. By permission of The Williams & Wilkins Co., Baltimore.)

decline has been found for other naturally occurring antibodies, such as iso-hemagglutinins [27] and *Salmonella* flagellar antigen [28]. Quantitative decline of these antibodies could reflect a general decrease of IgM subclass with age or increasing time from antigenic exposure usually occurring early in life.

The importance of these changes in naturally occurring antibody is unclear. Although certain trends are apparent, there is greater variability in the concentration of most immunoglobulins in healthy old people than in their younger counterparts. This variability could reflect the impact of age-related disease and nutritional status rather than the aging process per se. Longitudinal study of a large cohort over several decades would be helpful in distinguishing these possibilities.

In vitro studies of human humoral immune responses have been extended by investigation of the mechanisms of the diminution in antigen-specific and polyclonal responses in B lymphocytes from aged humans. It was shown that age-related deficits in B lymphocyte function were usually associated with abnormalities of regulatory T lymphocytes and rarely seemed secondary to intrinsic B cell aberrations [29].

The humoral response to exogenous antigen in the elderly has been best studied using vaccines directed against respiratory pathogens. In 1976, nationwide studies on bivalent influenza vaccine A/New Jersey–A/Victoria were carried out in the elderly [30–32]. In all instances the rate of local and systemic reactions was low and comparable to that of individuals receiving placebo. Antibody response was excellent for A/New Jersey: nearly 100 percent developed hemagglutination inhibition titers of greater than 1 : 40, a level normally considered protective [30,31]. Response to A/Victoria, although protective in the majority of individuals, was not as high. This differential response may be a reflection of augmented antibody synthesis to a previously infecting virus sharing antigenic determinants with the strain causing primary influenza infection of an individual. For persons over 50 years of age, primary exposure to an Hsw/N1 influenza virus similar to A/New Jersey occurred in the epidemic years 1918 to 1930, perhaps thereby accounting for the "booster" effect in the 1976 trials [32].

This immunologic phenomenon has been termed original antigenic sin and was initially described by T. Francis and his colleagues [33] and Fazekas de St. Groth and R. G. Webster [34,35] in studies of the humoral response to influenza virus. They showed that humans or animals immune to one influenza strain who were primarily immunized with another antigenically related strain did not show the expected slow primary antibody response to the second strain. Furthermore, antibody did not appear as rapidly as in a classic anamnestic response. Instead, accelerated production of antibody more reactive with the original immunizing strain, but also with the new strain, was observed. The antibody produced was IgG with no early IgM detectable. Thus, each time influenza vaccine is given or infection occurs in a person immune to an antigenically related strain of virus, original antigenic sin may modify the antibody response. This is likely to be a more important consideration in old than young individuals since the elderly have necessarily had experience with a greater variety of influenza viruses.

Immune response to polyvalent pneumococcal polysaccharide vaccine has also been examined in the elderly. Over 95 percent of healthy older individuals given pneumococcal vaccine develop a twofold or greater antibody rise to the majority of serotypes [36].

Although peak antibody titers after vaccination may be lower in elderly persons than in younger individuals, protection appears to be equivalent with influenza vaccine [37]. Efficacy studies also are now accumulating that suggest similar protection with pneumococcal vaccine.

Cell-Mediated Immunity

Quantitative analysis of the circulating T lymphocyte pool shows no difference between healthy old and young individuals [2,38,39]. Cutaneous delayed hypersensitivity to a variety of viral and bacterial antigens is also similar in these groups; however, the number of positive tests per person tends to decline with age [40]. Although tuberculin reactivity has been reported to wane with age [41], it is unclear from the population studied whether this reflects generalized anergy consequent to intercurrent illness or debilitation, or a primary immune impairment.

In vitro assessment of cellular immune function has consistently demonstrated diminished lymphocyte blastogenic response to plant lectins as well as to allogeneic lymphocytes in mixed culture in the elderly [2,24,38,39]. The deficit is moderate in degree: reactivity to phytohemagglutinin of lymphocytes from aged donors ranges from 50 to 75 percent of young control subjects. Kinetically, lymphocyte blastogenesis in the elderly is characterized by decreased numbers of mitogen-responsive cells and diminished proliferative capacity of those cells that respond [42].

Other components of the cellular immune response, such as generation of lymphokines and cell-mediated cytotoxicity, have not been studied in aged humans. However, cell-mediated killing of allogenic tumor cells has been found to be reduced in older mice in spite of prior sensitization with tumor-specific antigens [43].

The mechanism and significance of diminished lymphocyte blastogenesis in elderly humans are unknown but are consistent with the Hayflick theory of cellular aging [12] at the level of the T lymphocyte. This theory postulates that the age-related proliferative capacity of cells in vitro is dependent on factors within the cell nucleus. The idea of a nuclear clock is one way to account for age-related changes in cellular immunity. It may be that as this intranuclear clock runs out, the T lymphocyte becomes less able to respond to mitogens, a process that entails cell division and differentiation.

The Hayflick theory is not only speculative, but the observation it attempts to explain—the age-related decline in cellular immunity—is itself a non-specific observation, since it has not been clearly associated with suscepti-bility to infection or malignancy and has not been related epidemiologically to rate of aging, age-related disease, or mortality.

Maximal immune responses to strongly antigenic substances require the interaction of competent B cells and T cells, and in the case of particulate antigen, local macrophages. These responses are regulated at the cellular level by subclasses of T cells that can suppress or augment the host response [44].

Outbred aged mice exhibit diminished antibody and cell-mediated immune responses compared to younger mice of the same strain. The decline is greater for antigens that require T cell participation than for antigens that do not [8,45]. The mechanism of this age-related decline appears to be associated with an abnormality in cellular immune regulation, showing changes in both the helper and suppressor T cell function [46]. Since these changes are temporally related to thymic involution and are reversible using thymic extract [47], abnormal regulation of immune response in old mice may result from altered T cell differentiation into suppressor and effector subclasses as a consequence of thymic aging [48].

In has been shown that stimulated lymphocyte cultures from elderly donors produce less T cell growth factor (TCGF) and incorporate less triti-ated thymidine than do cultures from young donors. The aged lymphocytes also respond less to exogenous TCGF. These data suggest that defects in response to and production of TCGF may be important in decreased im-mune function of aging [49].

Inflammatory Response and Aging

Nonspecific factors in host defense have received limited attention in elderly humans. In vitro neutrophil killing of *Staphylococcus aureus* is comparable in old and young individuals [2]. Moreover, in vivo clearance of labeled albumin by the reticuloendothelial system apparently exhibits no age-related changes [50]. In the murine system, circulating monocytes show no age-related alteration in phagocytic capacity, lysosomal content, or ability to process antigen [51].

The complement system similarly shows no functional decline with age; in fact, levels of C_3 and properidin are increased in elderly humans [2].

Conclusions

When age-related immune function is measured, only subtle differences are found between healthy elderly and young individuals. In the presence of age-related disease, these differences are likely to be exaggerated. The im-portance of altered immune function in the human aging process is uncer-tain, although there is a large body of indirect evidence suggesting a causal relationship in animals. Unless causality is established in humans, attempts at increasing life span via the reconstitution of normal immune function are unwarranted.

References

1. Osler, W.   The Principles and Practice of Medicine. In A. M. Harvey and V. A. McKusick (Eds.), *Osler's Textbook Revisited*. New York: Appleton-Century-Crofts, 1967.
2. Phair, J. P., et al.   Host defenses in the aged: evaluation of components of the inflammatory and immune responses. *J. Infect. Dis.* 138:67, 1978.
3. Good, R. A., and Yunis, E.   Association of autoimmunity, immunodeficiency, and aging in man, rabbits, and mice. *Fed. Proc.* 33:2040, 1974.
4. Cerilli, J., and Hatten, D.   Immunosuppression and oncogenesis. *Am. J. Clin. Pathol.* 62:218, 1974.
5. Mackay, I. R., Whittingham, S. F., and Mathews, J. D.   The Immuno-epidemiology of Aging. In T. Makinodan and E. Yunis (Eds.), *Immunology and Aging*. New York: Plenum Press, 1977.
6. Walford, R. L.   Immunologic theory of aging: current status. *Fed. Proc.* 33: 2020, 1974.
7. Burnet, F. M.   An immunological approach to aging. *Lancet* 1:35, 1970.
8. Makinodan, T., and Adler, W. H.   Effects of aging on the differentiation and proliferation potentials of cells of the immune system. *Fed. Proc.* 34:153, 1975.
9. Singhal, S. K., Roder, J. C., and Duwe, A. K.   Suppressor cells in immunosenescence. *Fed. Proc.* 37:1245, 1978.
10. Price, G. B., and Makinodan, T.   Immunologic deficiencies in senescence. II. Characterization of extrinsic deficiencies. *J. Immunol.* 180:413, 1972.
11. Walford, R. L.   *The Immunologic Theory of Aging*. Copenhagen: Munksgaard, 1969.
12. Hayflick, L.   The cell biology of human aging. *N. Engl. J. Med.* 295:1302, 1976.
13. Fernandes, G., Good, R. A., and Yunis, E. J.   Attempts to correct age-related immunodeficiency and autoimmunity by cellular and dietary manipulation in inbred mice. In T. Makinodan and E. Yunis (Eds.), *Immunology and Aging*. New York: Plenum Press, 1977.
14. Wara, D. W., et al.   Thymosin activity in patients with cellular immunodeficiency. *N. Engl. J. Med.* 292:70, 1975.
15. Vessey, D.   Thymectomy and cancer—a follow-up study. *Br. J. Cancer* 26:53, 1972.
16. Debush, F. L.   The Hutchinson-Gilford progeria syndrome. Report of 4 cases and review of the literature. *J. Pediatr.* 80:697, 1972.
17. Mathews, J. D., et al. Association of autoantibodies with smoking, cardiovascular morbidity, and death in the Busselton population. *Lancet* 2:754, 1973.
18. Roberts-Thomson, I. C., et al.   Aging, immune response and mortality. *Lancet* 2:368, 1974.
19. Rowe, J. W.   Clinical research on aging: strategies and directions. *N. Engl. J. Med.* 297:1332, 1977.

20. Lewis, M., et al. Age-thymic involution, and circulating thymic hormone activity. *J. Clin. Endocrinol. Metab.* 47:145, 1978.
21. Diaz-Jouanen, E., Strickland, R. G., and Williams, R. C. Studies of human lymphocytes in the newborn and the aged. *Am. J. Med.* 58:620, 1975.
22. Fernandez, G., and Schwartz, J. M. Immune responsiveness and hematologic malignancy in the elderly. *Med. Clin. North Am.* 60:1253, 1976.
23. Buckley, C. E., and Dorsey, F. C. The effect of aging on human serum immunoglobulin concentrations. *J. Immunol.* 105:964, 1970.
24. Hallgren, H. M., et al. Lymphocyte phytohemagglutinin responsiveness, immunoglobulins, and autoantibodies in aging humans. *J. Immunol.* 111:1101, 1973.
25. Buckley, C. E., Buckley, E. G., and Dorsey, F. C. Longitudinal changes in serum immunoglobulin levels in older humans. *Fed. Proc.* 33:2036, 1974.
26. Delespesse, G., et al. IgE mediated hypersensitivity in aging. *Clin. Allergy* 7:155, 1977.
27. Somers, H., and Kuhns, W. J. Blood group antibodies in old age. *Proc. Soc. Exp. Biol. Med.* 141:1104, 1972.
28. Rowley, M. J. "Natural" antibody in man to flagellar antigens of *Salmonella adelaide. Aust. J. Exp. Biol. Med. Sci.* 48:249, 1970.
29. Pahwa, S. G., Pahwa, R. N., and Good, R. A. Decreased in vitro humoral immune responses in aged humans. *J. Clin. Invest.* 67:1094, 1981.
30. Douglas, R. G., Bentley, D. W., and Brandriss, M. W. Responses of elderly and chronically ill subjects to bivalent influenza A/New Jersey/8/76 (Hsw/ N1)–A/Victoria/3/75 (H3N2) vaccines. *J. Infect. Dis.* 136:S526, 1977.
31. Cate, T. R., et al. Clinical trials of bivalent influenza A/New Jersey/76– A/Victoria/75 vaccines in the elderly. *J. Infect. Dis.* 136:S518, 1977.
32. Noble, G. R., et al. Age-related heterologous antibody responses to influenza virus vaccination. *J. Infect. Dis.* 136:S686, 1977.
33. Francis, T., Davenport, F. M., and Hennessy, A. V. Epidemiological re-capitulation of human infection with different strains of influenza virus. *Trans. Assoc. Am. Physicians* 66:231, 1953.
34. de St. Groth, F., and Webster, R. G. Disquisitions on original antigenic sin. I. Evidence in man. *J. Exp. Med.* 124:331, 1966.
35. de St. Groth, F., and Webster, R. G. Disquisitions on original antigenic sin. II. Proof in lower creatures. *J. Exp. Med.* 124:347, 1966.
36. Bentley, D. W., et al. Responses to Pneumococcal Vaccines in Healthy Elderly Volunteers. Abstract presented at Fourteenth Interscience Conference of Antimicrobial Agents and Chemotherapy, San Francisco, 1974. P. 187.
37. Howells, C. H. L., Vesselinova-Jenkins, C. K., and Evans, A. D. Influenza vaccination and mortality from bronchopneumonia in the elderly. *Lancet* 2:381, 1975.
38. Hallgren, H. M., et al. Lymphocyte subsets and integrated immune function in aging humans. *Clin. Immunol. Immunopathol.* 10:65, 1978.
39. Weksler, M. E., and Hutteroth, T. H. Impaired lymphocyte function in aged humans. *J. Clin. Invest.* 53:99, 1974.
40. Grossman, J., et al. The effect of aging and acute illness on delayed hyper-sensitivity. *J. Allergy Clin. Immunol.* 55:268, 1975.
41. Gianni, D., and Sloan, R. S. A tuberculin survey of 1285 adults with special reference to the elderly. *Lancet* 1:525, 1957.

42. Innes, J. B., et al.   Immunological studies of aging. III. Cytokinetic basis for the impaired response of lymphocytes from aged humans to plant lectins. *J. Exp. Med.* 145:1176, 1977.
43. Shigemoto, S., Kishimoto, S., and Yamamura, Y.   Change of cell-mediated cytotoxicity with aging. *J. Immunol.* 115:307, 1975.
44. Hallgren, H. M., and Yunis, E. J.   Suppressor lymphocytes in young and aged humans. *J. Immunol.* 118:2004, 1977.
45. Nordin, A. A., and Makinodan, T.   Humoral immunity in aging. *Fed. Proc.* 33:2033, 1974.
46. Goidl, E. A., Innes, J. B., and Weksler, M. E.   Immunological studies of aging: loss of IgG and high avidity plaque-forming cells and increased suppressor cell activity in aging mice. *J. Exp. Med.* 144:1037, 1976.
47. Weksler, M. E., Innes, J. B., and Goldstein, G.   Immunological studies of aging. IV. The contribution of thymic involution to the immune deficiencies of aging mice and reversal with thymopoietin. *J. Exp. Med.* 148:996, 1978.
48. Kay, M. M. B.   Effect of age on T cell differentiation. *Fed. Proc.* 37:1241, 1978.
49. Gillis, S., et al.   Immunological studies of aging. Decreased production of and response to T cell growth factor by lymphocytes from aged humans. *J. Clin. Invest.* 67:937, 1981.
50. Palmer, D. L., Rifkind, D., and Brown, D. W.   ^{131}I-labelled colloidal human serum albumin in the study of reticuloendothelial system function. II. Phagocytosis and catabolism of a test colloid in normal subjects. *J. Infect. Dis.* 123:457, 1971.
51. Teller, M. N.   Age changes and immune resistance to cancer. *Adv. Gerontol. Res.* 4:25, 1972.

20. *Infectious Disease*

Richard M. Rose
Richard W. Besdine

Infectious diseases characteristically have the greatest impact on survival at the extremes of life. Fatal respiratory infection, for instance, occurs three times more frequently in infants in the first year of life than in the general population. By the second decade of life, the risk of dying from pneumonia approximately doubles for each succeeding decade, and by the seventh decade the risk of succumbing to pneumonia is nearly 20 times that of the overall population [1]. Bacteremia is another infectious disease in which both the age-specific attack rate and mortality rate increase with age [2].

The continued importance of infection in the elderly is paradoxical in the antibiotic era. Of the common causes of mortality in individuals over age 65 (Table 20-1), respiratory infection is the only one that is both potentially preventable with vaccines and curable with appropriate antimicrobial therapy. Moreover, the accumulated immunologic experience of an elderly individual with a lifetime of infectious agents might be expected to provide enhanced resistance to infection based on acquired immunity. Yet, elderly individuals appear to be more likely than younger people to develop and die from certain infections. What is the basis of this susceptibility? Is it an intrinsic aspect of aging, or are some elderly individuals more prone to infection than others?

Antimicrobial Defenses in the Elderly
GENERAL DEFENSES

As discussed in Chapter 19, aging is associated with alterations in the immune system. There is an age-related decline in the number of circulating T lymphocytes and their response to mitogens. The humoral response to some exogenous antigens is also diminished in the elderly. The relationship of these findings to susceptibility to and severity of infection in the elderly is unclear, since the immune response to naturally occurring infection has not been rigorously evaluated in aging humans. In one study, no correlation could be found between in vitro tests to evaluate host defenses against infection and risk of pneumonia in older persons [3]. It is clear, however, that the magnitude of age-related abnormalities in humoral and cell-mediated immunity is greater in aged individuals with underlying systemic disease, such as malignancy or rheumatoid arthritis, than in apparently healthy older people.

Other general aspects of host defense against infection, such as granulocyte function and complement level, appear to be normal in the healthy elderly [4]. On the other hand, the febrile response to infection may be impaired in some elderly individuals [5]. It is not known whether this is due to deficiency in release of leucocyte pyrogen or altered sensitivity of the hypothalamus to mediators of the febrile response. The consequence of the abnormal febrile

Table 20-1.   Comparison of the Leading Causes of Mortality in the General Population and the Aged (1976)

All Ages			Age Group 75+		
Causes of Death	Rate per 100,000	Percent	Causes of Death	Rate per 100,000	Percent
Diseases of heart	337.2	37.9	Diseases of heart	3,289.0	41.4
Malignant neoplasms	175.8	19.8	Cerebrovascular diseases	1,243.0	15.6
Cerebrovascular diseases	87.9	9.9	Malignant neoplasms	1,204.0	15.2
Influenza and pneumonia	28.8	3.2	Influenza and pneumonia	322.8	4.1
All other accidents	25.0	2.8	Diabetes	205.5	2.6
Motor vehicle accidents	21.9	2.5	Arteriosclerosis	190.2	2.4
			All other accidents	115.1	1.4
All causes	889.6	100.0	All causes	7,941.9	100.0

Source: Adapted from U.S. DHEW, *Leading Causes of Death and Probabilities of Dying, United States 1975–1976.* Washington, D.C.: U.S. Government Printing Office, 1979.

response to infection is obscured by the lack of a clear-cut role for the elevation of body temperature per se in host defense. The major importance of the relative hypothermia exhibited by some elderly individuals in response to infection seems to be that it may retard recognition of infection and delay institution of therapy.

LOCAL DEFENSES
Age-related changes in local defenses may also predispose to infection. The aging respiratory system is characterized by diminished compliance because of increased stiffness of the chest wall that results, in part, from configurational changes associated with loss of lung elastic recoil (Chapter 21). One consequence of these alterations in pulmonary function is diminished effectiveness of cough as a means of clearing central airways of particulate matter and mucus. Although the cough mechanism has not been studied directly in older humans, it can be extrapolated from investigations of cough in individuals with chronic airflow obstruction that the less compliant chest wall of the elderly person will diminish the capacity to generate the high airflow rates necessary to effectively propel mucus upward during cough. Moreover, the loss of lung elastic recoil with age means that the greatest shearing forces

during cough will be on peripheral airways. This could limit the ability of the cough mechanism to clear central airways and predispose to mucus plugging and infection.

Other pulmonary reflexes such as the aspiration reflex have not been systematically evaluated in healthy aged individuals. It is clear, though, that pulmonary aspiration of oropharyngeal contents is a common occurrence in elderly individuals with alterations in consciousness, swallowing disorders, and abnormalities of the upper airway [6]. Whether lesser degrees of aspiration occur in apparently normal old people during sleep or after receiving sedative-hypnotic drugs is not known, but given the importance of pulmonary aspiration in the pathogenesis of pneumonia, and the exceptional impact of pneumonia upon the health of the aged, further study of aspiration in this setting seems warranted.

Antimicrobial defenses of the lower respiratory tract, which include pulmonary macrophages and the mucociliary clearance mechanism, have not been well characterized in old age. In one study tracheal mucus velocity was diminished in nonsmoking elderly individuals compared to young nonsmoking controls [7]. This could be a reflection of age-related changes in the viscoelastic properties of mucus or the functional properties of cilia.

Defects in local defenses against infection occurring in a variety of aging organ systems are summarized in Table 20-2 and are discussed in other chapters.

Table 20-2. Local Defects in Host Antimicrobial Defense in the Elderly

Organ System	Physiologic Change	Alteration in Host Defense
Respiratory system	↓Compliance and ↓lung elastic recoil	Diminished effectiveness of cough
	Unknown	Decreased mucociliary clearance
	Alteration in consciousness or defect in upper airway	Diminished aspiration reflex
Skin	↓Vasculature	↓Healing
	↓Release of mediators of inflammatory response	↓Inflammation
	↓In thickness of stratum corneum	↓Barrier against bacterial penetration
Gastrointestinal tract	↓Gastric acid production	Loss of gastric acid barrier ↓Motility
Genitourinary tract	Prostatic hypertrophy ↓Bladder tone	Urinary stasis

*INTERACTION OF DISEASE AND AGE-RELATED LOSS
OF ANTIMICROBIAL DEFENSES*

Age-related alterations in systemic and local antimicrobial defenses play a major role in the enhanced susceptibility of certain elderly individuals to infection. In the normal old person, the magnitude of these abnormalities may be insufficient to increase the risk of serious infection. However, as the severity and complexity of underlying disease increase in an older individual, one can expect a proportionate decline in the ability of host defenses to resist infection. In the elderly population, as in any group, debilitated, bedridden, and malnourished individuals are at greatest risk from infection. Under these circumstances alterations in host defense not only enhance susceptibility to infection, but also make infections more difficult to treat and prevent. In the chronically ill elderly person with pneumococcal pneumonia, ineffective cough, altered mucociliary clearance, and diminished humoral immune response all conspire to cause severe or even lethal disease in spite of the extreme sensitivity of the *Pneumococcus* to penicillin. Furthermore, because of age-related defects in immune response accentuated by chronic underlying disease, the same individual may not develop a protective antibody level after pneumococcal vaccination [8]. Thus, the elderly individual at highest risk from lethal pneumococcal infection still may be at risk despite the availability of modalities that are highly efficacious in treating and preventing disease in healthier individuals.

Epidemiology of Infection in Old Age
REACTIVATION OF LATENT INFECTION

Different infectious agents are most likely to cause disease at various stages of the life cycle. Prevalance of chicken pox declines with advancing age as a greater proportion of people in each successive age group have developed primary infection and lifelong immunity to reexposure. Since the virus that causes chicken pox also has the potential for remaining latent in dorsal root ganglia, it can be predicted that an increasing number of individuals will harbor latent virus as they grow older. Reactivation of this latent focus of infection occurs in association with many conditions that depress host immune function, such as malignancy and steroid therapy. Not surprisingly, the incidence of shingles (the localized cutaneous manifestation of reactivation) increases with age [9].

An analogous situation exists for tuberculosis. There has been a steady decline in new cases of pulmonary tuberculosis in the United States in the past three decades. This means that individuals who were born in the early part of this century were more likely to contract infection than those born later when exposure to active cases of tuberculosis was less likely. This hypothesis is substantiated by comparing the prevalence of positive tuberculin reactors in various age groups. For every socioeconomic group studied, the prevalence of positive reactors increases with age [10]. Thus the greatest reservoir of latent foci of tuberculosis is the elderly population. Because both the prevalence of latent tuberculosis and the conditions that predispose to reactivation of tuberculosis (e.g., altered host immunity) increase with age, the incidence of active infection also increases with age [11] (Fig. 20-1).

CHANGE IN ATTACK RATE OF INFECTION WITH AGE

For some infectious agents age still has its benefits. If childhood infection results in long-term immunity against a pathogen that has no potential for developing latency, it could be predicted that the likelihood of infection with the organism would decline with age. This is true for measles, for instance, and probably also explains the well-documented decline of *Mycoplasma pneumoniae* infection with age [12]. Another possible explanation for the rarity of *Mycoplasma* infection in the elderly is the limited contact many older individuals have with the reservoir of infection, young children and teenagers.

Conversely, some infectious agents introduced into a population of susceptible individuals will characteristically have higher attack rates in the elderly than in the young. A striking example was the introduction of a new vector-borne viral encephalitis into St. Louis in 1933. Although the entire population was potentially susceptible to infection, the majority of clinically apparent and almost all of the fatal cases occurred in elderly individuals [13]. This epidemic pattern has not been explained adequately, even though it is frequently found during endemic outbreaks of viral encephalitis each summer.

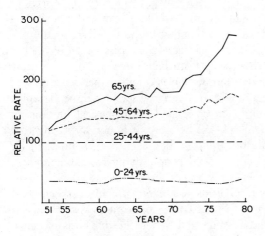

Figure 20-1. Relative rates of tuberculosis by age group in the United States, 1953–1979. (Reprinted from K. E. Powell and L. S. Farer, The rising age of the tuberculosis patient: a sign of success and failure. *J. Infect. Dis.* 142:946, 1980. By permission of The University of Chicago Press. Copyright © 1980, by The University of Chicago Press.)

Special Infections

In the following sections the discussion is not meant to be comprehensive in the scope of infections covered or in the detail of each disease. Rather, several infections with special features in the elderly are discussed in light of their particular problems for aged patients. Pneumonia, tuberculosis, bacterial endocarditis, and urinary tract infection are chosen as infections especially likely to present different features and special problems in patients who are old, and it is these features and problems that are discussed.

PNEUMONIA
Diagnosis
The importance of infections of the lower respiratory tract in the elderly cannot be overemphasized. Pneumonia is the most common infection to require hospitalization of adults, the second most common infection to complicate hospitalization, and the infection accounting for most fatalities in the elderly. The impact of pneumonia may be attributed, in part, to defects in host antimicrobial defenses related to coincident disease states and advancing age, as mentioned earlier. Clinical features of pneumonia in older individuals also contribute to poor outcome. For instance, delay in recognition or misdiagnosis of pneumonia in the elderly can lead to late or inappropriate therapy. Although the spectrum of signs and symptoms has not adequately been defined for an older population, it is axiomatic that some older individuals fail to exhibit the typical findings of pneumonia seen in other old people or healthy young people. Symptoms that may be absent include fever, dyspnea, cough, and chest pain. Instead, pneumonia may present with the effects of infection and hypoxia on other organ systems. An old person with pneumonia may develop behavioral abnormalities or congestive heart failure as the primary manifestation of infection. Indolent infectious processes may have even more subtle manifestations, such as sleep disturbance, weight loss, or simply "failure to thrive." Unfortunately, examination is often neither sensitive nor specific for the diagnosis of pneumonia. In one large series roentgenographic evidence of parenchymal consolidation correlated with physical findings in only 41.5 percent of adult patients [14]. Therefore, it is not surprising that the presence of severe lung infection may go unrecognized in some elderly individuals. In a retrospective series of old people dying from pneumonia, nearly 20 percent had been either undiagnosed or misdiagnosed [15]. This situation could be prevented by recognition of the varied clinical presentation of pneumonia in the elderly and the need for simple noninvasive tests of high sensitivity, such as the chest radiograph, when the diagnosis of pneumonia is suspected.

Determination of Etiology: Obtaining Cultures of the Lower Respiratory Tract
Another aspect of pneumonia in the elderly that contributes to morbidity and mortality is difficulty in establishing a specific etiologic diagnosis. In

recent series of community-acquired [16] and nosocomial pneumonia [17] in adults, a specific pathogen was identified in only 50 to 60 percent of cases. This suggests that a substantial number of patients with pneumonia are treated empirically. Potential hazards of empiric antibiotics in an older individual are great: unnecessary exposure to toxic drugs, increased risk of super-infection, ineffective therapy, and prolonged hospitalization. Unfortunately, empiric therapy is often instituted in an elderly person with pneumonia who is either too weak, too uncooperative, or too dehydrated to produce sputum. Even when sputum can be obtained, the diagnostic usefulness of routine culture is limited by contamination with oropharyngeal flora and lack of sensitivity for common pathogens such as *S. pneumoniae* [18]. Similar limitations apply to bronchoscopically obtained specimens, which may also be mixed with upper airway flora [19].

These limitations can be minimized by a careful examination of the sputum Gram's stain. An adequate specimen should have inflammatory cells and fewer than 10 epithelial cells per high-power field [20]. The presence of pulmonary macrophages confirms the origin of the sample as the lower respiratory tract. The greatest diagnostic value will be derived from evaluating the microbial flora in an area of the specimen in which inflammatory cells are most abundant. A single predominant organism inside or around phagocytes is very likely to be the causative agent.

In some individuals with pneumonia, a diagnostic procedure may be considered to clarify the microbiology of infection. Transtracheal aspiration has been shown to be a safe and effective procedure for obtaining secretions from the lower respiratory tract, even among elderly persons [21]. Although occasional complications occur, they can be minimized by careful selection of patients. Transtracheal aspiration should not be performed on patients with chronic bronchitis, uncorrectable bleeding disorder or hypoxia, and in patients who are uncooperative or cannot control coughing. An alternative method of establishing an etiologic diagnosis of pneumonia is percutaneous needle aspiration. Like transtracheal aspiration, this is a safe and highly sensitive means of identifying the causative agent [22]. However, direct lung aspiration requires the patient to hold his or her breath while the needle is inserted, in order to avoid laceration of the underlying parenchyma. This restriction makes needle aspiration impractical for many older persons who cannot voluntarily control respiration because of pain, cough, or hypoxia.

The decision to undertake one of these diagnostic procedures in an elderly individual with pneumonia may be influenced by a variety of factors, including local expertise in performing the procedure, the presence of patient factors that affect procedural morbidity, and the risk of empiric therapy in an individual patient. The last is often the most difficult to assess. In an elderly person with preexisting renal disease, the empiric use of aminoglycosides may have enough potential morbidity to outweigh the small risk of a complication from transtracheal aspiration. Another situation in which the value of a diagnostic procedure may outweigh its risks is the moderately or severely ill person in whom the bacteriology cannot be predicted adequately because of prior antibiotic therapy or prolonged hospitalization.

Importance of Local Epidemiology

In many patients the therapeutic approach to lung infection can be accurately guided by an appreciation of local epidemiology, tempo of illness, and host factors affecting oropharyngeal colonization (Table 20-3).

In outpatient-acquired pneumonia, an important initial consideration is the prevalence of respiratory disease in the community. In some cases this simply means recognizing that influenza-related respiratory illness is most common in the winter months, or in other situations, noting that the patient's roommate has active tuberculosis or that pneumonia secondary to *Neisseria meningitidis* has been endemic in the nursing home recently.

Tempo of Illness

The tempo of illness also provides an important clue to the nature of community-acquired pneumonia. Because of the adverse effect of many respiratory viruses on antimicrobial defenses of the lung [23], bacterial pneumonia is frequently preceded by a viral upper respiratory infection. This usually results in a diphasic illness in which the early phase consists of mild "cold" symptoms, followed by an abrupt worsening and shift in symptomatology to the lower respiratory tract. In a previously healthy elderly person with this pattern of respiratory illness, the most common etiologic agent is *Streptococcus pneumoniae,* followed by *Staphylococcus aureus* and aerobic gram-negative bacilli. In one adult series, the pneumococcus was associated with 53 percent of all community-acquired lung infections requiring hospitalization, while gram-negative organisms accounted for 9.5 percent and staphylococci for 7 percent [16].

Since the pathophysiology of bacterial pneumonia following viral infection involves microaspiration of oropharyngeal secretions, colonization of the oropharynx with potential pathogens, such as aerobic gram-negative bacilli, is a forerunner of pneumonia with these organisms. In a carefully performed cross-sectional study of the prevalence of oropharyngeal colonization with gram-negative bacilli in the elderly [24], carriage rates were found to increase as older individuals required increasing levels of care (Table 20-4). Even ambulatory, elderly persons who were living independently had a higher colonization rate than young control subjects. The local factors that normally inhibit attachment of gram-negative rods to epithelial cells of the oropharynx appear to be altered by age and underlying systemic disease. The precise nature of defects that predispose to colonization need to be better defined, but could include poor oral hygiene, altered salivary gland flow or composition, and altered binding sites on the epithelial cell membrane.

Progressive outpatient-acquired pneumonia of acute onset without prodromal symptoms should lead to consideration of necrotizing infection with

Table 20-3. Clinical Approach to Pneumonia in the Elderly

Tempo of Illness	Radiologic Appearance	Causative Organisms	Therapy First Choice	Second Choice
Community-acquired				
Acute with prodrome	Acinar or lobar consolidation	*S. pneumoniae*	Penicillin	Erythromycin
	Patchy or homogeneous segmental consolidation	*S. aureus*	Semisynthetic penicillin	Cephalosporin
		H. influenzae	Ampicillin	Trimethoprim-sulfamethoxazole
Acute without prodrome	Necrotizing pattern (cavities, pneumatoceles, abscesses, nodules)	*S. aureus*	Semisynthetic penicillin	Cephalosporin
		Aerobic gram-negative rods	Aminoglycoside	Cephalosporin
	Interstitial pattern with or without air space consolidation	Influenza Adenovirus	Amantadine None	
		Legionella pneumophila	Erythromycin	Tetracycline
Subacute	Necrotizing pattern in dependent segments	Anaerobes	Penicillin	Clindamycin
	Acinar infiltrate with or without cavitation in apical-posterior segment of upper lobe	*M. tuberculosis*	Isoniazid Rifampin	Ethambutol Streptomycin
Hospital-acquired				
Acute without prodrome	Air space consolidation or necrotizing pattern	*S. aureus*	Semisynthetic penicillin	Cephalosporin
		Aerobic gram-negative rods	Aminoglycoside	Cephalosporin

Table 20-4. Prevalance of Gram-Negative Bacilli in the Oropharynx of Elderly Subjects According to Level of Care

Location	Percent with Gram-Negative Bacilli
Acute hospital ward	60
Skilled nursing facility	37
Health-related facility	42
Private proprietary nursing home	23
Independent apartments	19
Employees	8

Source: Reprinted by permission of the *New England Journal of Medicine* from W. M. Valenti, R. G. Trudell, and D. W. Bentley, Factors predisposing to oropharyngeal colonization with gram negative bacilli in the aged. *N. Engl. J. Med.* 298:1108, 1978.

staphylococci, aerobic gram-negative rods, influenza, and Legionnaire's disease. Sporadic cases of infection with *Legionella pneumophila* are being recognized with increasing frequency as the clinical characteristics of the disease are defined and diagnostic methods are improved. Compared to pneumococcal pneumonia, Legionnaire's disease is distinguished by a higher mean age, lack of prodrome, presence of encephalopathy, and abnormalities in urine sediment and serum transaminases [25]. Diagnosis may be established by a fourfold rise in antibody titer, culture of respiratory secretions on special media, and direct immunofluorescence of transtracheal aspirate [26].

Respiratory viruses such as influenza generally occur in epidemics and are characterized by high attack rates among susceptible hosts and an incubation period of several days. Influenza is a lower respiratory tract infection, with symptoms of tracheobronchitis common early in the illness. In a few percent of individuals with influenza infection, signs and symptoms of parenchymal pulmonary involvement develop. The mildest form of lung infection is associated with dry cough, focal findings on chest examination such as rales or wheezes, but no radiologic abnormality. This form of infection probably corresponds to bronchiolitis pathologically. A more common presentation of influenza is bacterial superinfection with *S. aureus, S. pneumoniae,* group A streptococci, or *Hemophilus influenzae.* In this situation, cough produces frankly purulent sputum and there are focal roentgenographic abnormalities. The most severe form of influenza lung infection is fulminant diffuse pneumonitis, which develops over one to two days and rapidly produces respiratory failure. Many of these patients have underlying cardiopulmonary disease, and some have early superinfection with *S. aureus.*

Chronic Pneumonia
In elderly individuals with a subacute or chronic pneumonic process of infectious origin, consideration should be given to anaerobic infection or tuber-

culosis. Clues to the presence of anaerobic lung infection include putrid sputum, periodontal disease, predisposition to aspiration, and infiltrate in a dependent lung segment [27]. The majority of patients with documented anaerobic lung infection also have systemic manifestations of infection, such as anemia and weight loss, and approximately one-third have associated empyema. Definitive diagnosis can be made by isolating anaerobes in pure or mixed culture from lung abscess or pleural fluid or by transtracheal aspiration [28].

Nosocomial Pneumonia

Nosocomial, or hospital-acquired, pneumonia differs from community-acquired lung infection in terms of predisposing conditions, spectrum of causative agents, and prognosis. Data from the National Nosocomial Infections Study suggest that lower respiratory tract infection complicates 0.6 percent of all medical/surgical hospital admissions, and comprises 10 to 20 percent of all nosocomially acquired infections [33]. Major risk factors for the development of nosocomial pneumonia are severe underlying disease, surgical procedures requiring general anesthesia, administration of antimicrobial or immunosuppressive drugs, and ventilatory assistance [17]. Because there is an age-related increase in the prevalence of the underlying systemic diseases associated with nosocomial pneumonia, such as diabetes and malignancy, it is reasonable to assume that age-specific attack rates for nosocomial pneumonia will be higher in an elderly than in a younger population.

The microbiology of nosocomial pneumonia is characterized by a greater incidence of infection with aerobic gram-negative rods and coagulase-positive staphylococci than is found in community-acquired infections. In the National Nosocomial Infections Study, these organisms produced approximately 50 percent of all lung infections, while *S. pneumoniae* caused only 9 percent [33]. This bacteriology reflects a change in the microbial flora of the oropharynx of hospitalized patients. Colonization of the oropharynx with aerobic gram-negative bacilli in this setting correlates best with clinical severity of illness [34] and increasing age [35].

The prognosis for nosocomial pneumonia is expectedly worse than for community-acquired infection. Fatal outcome occurs in over one-third of cases of nosocomial pneumonia; and in gram-negative infection, nearly half the patients succumb [17]. The high mortality reflects the virulence of the infecting organisms and the severity of underlying defects in host defense that lead to infection. Moreover, late sequelae like empyema, cavitation, or slow radiologic resolution of pneumonia occur more frequently in nosocomial pneumonia and may complicate infection in nearly one-quarter of cases [17]. Delayed resolution of pneumonia as seen radiologically may also be associated with increasing age per se. In one study, resolution of pneumococcal pneumonia occurred in half of normal individuals under age 50 by two weeks, while it took almost eight weeks for half the individuals over 50 years of age to show complete radiologic clearing of their infiltrates [36].

Management

Optimal treatment of pneumonia, regardless of the patient's age, requires accurate identification of the infecting organism and administration of an effective antibiotic in proper dose. Principles of antibiotic use in elderly patients are discussed later in this chapter. In addition to antibiotic administration, pneumonia patients are helped by other management strategies that require special consideration in aged individuals. Altered presentation, unusual complications, and delayed resolution must be anticipated and have already been discussed. Adequate nutrition and hydration are essential for the elderly pneumonia patient. Chest physical therapy is universally prescribed for pneumonia victims, but elderly patients are usually more exhausted by the vigorous thumping and twisting of pulmonary hygiene than they are benefited. Humidified air and encouragement to cough and breathe deeply are most useful. Suctioning of tracheal secretions is done for those patients who cannot raise sputum any other way. Antipyretic drugs should be avoided unless fever is very disturbing to the patient, since the temperature chart can give valuable information concerning antibiotic efficacy and development of complications. Nasal oxygen is certainly useful in relieving the hypoxemia commonly associated with pneumonia (especially in view of the diminishing oxygen saturation noted with normal aging [Chapter 2]). Since chronic lung disease and hypercapnia are more common in the elderly, special attention must be given to the danger of hypoventilation and even apnea in the chronically hypercapnic patient whose hypoxemic respiratory drive is turned off by oxygen at more than 1 to 2 liters per minute. Although not particularly more common in elderly patients, pleuritic chest pain, by producing alveolar hypoventilation and increasing the work of breathing, causes trouble more quickly for the frail, elderly pneumonia patient. Relief of pleurisy, either by topical heat or cold or treatment with codeine or even meperidine, is preferable to the impact of pleurisy on respiration.

TUBERCULOSIS

Tuberculous infection presents clinical features similar to those of chronic pneumonia. The illness is generally subacute or chronic and associated with nonspecific systemic symptoms. The characteristic apical-posterior location of reactivation tuberculosis is also seen in anaerobic infection. Distinction of tuberculosis (TB) from anaerobic pneumonia is made definitively by demonstrating acid-fast bacilli in respiratory secretions, or strongly suggested by the presence of cutaneous reactivity to tuberculin. Although it is often thought that the waning reactivity to tuberculin with advancing age limits the diagnostic value of the skin test in an elderly person with suspected tuberculosis [29], it should be pointed out that a majority of older persons with active disease will be reactors. In one series, the frequency of a positive skin test in individuals greater than 50 years of age with active tuberculosis was 70.4 percent compared to 90.2 percent for individuals less than 50 years of age [30]. Retesting nonreactive individuals with active disease may elicit a positive reaction.

The spectrum of extrapulmonary tuberculosis in the elderly is similar to that in younger persons, although the manifestations of disease are characteristically more subtle in the elderly person. Low-grade fever and mild peripheral blood and liver function abnormalities may be the only clues to disseminated infection. These cases often present as fever of unknown origin. Of the myriad causes of this syndrome in the elderly [31], tuberculosis is common; it may be differentiated from other causes of fever of unknown origin by tuberculin testing and examination of liver or bone marrow biopsy specimens [32].

ENDOCARDITIS IN THE ELDERLY
Incidence
Recent series of infective endocarditis (IE) in adults suggest that the incidence of IE in individuals over 60 years of age has increased from that found by studies done in the preantibiotic era. In a review of IE published in 1955, nearly 18 percent of all cases occurred in those over 60 years of age [37], while in reports published in the past 10 years, the incidence of IE in this age group ranged from 30 to 50 percent [38–40]. It is doubtful that this reflects a true change in the nature of IE; it is more likely a reflection of increased life expectancy, which places more older people at risk for developing IE than in years past. Additionally, older people may be at greater risk of IE as a consequence of having more episodes of bacteremia than younger people. Although age-specific attack rates for bacteremia increase in hospitalized patients [2], it is unclear if this is true for outpatient bacteremia, in which the majority of IE develops.

Prognosis
Endocarditis, like pneumonia, has a greater case fatality rate in the elderly than in a younger age group [41,42]. There are several potential reasons for this. As mentioned earlier, defects in antimicrobial defenses that occur with age and concomitant systemic disease may alter host response to infection and to therapy of infection. Two other factors that may adversely affect outcome are the nature of underlying heart disease in the elderly and difficulty in establishing a diagnosis.

Underlying Pathology
In pathologic studies of the valvular lesions predisposing to IE in the elderly, approximately half had no detectable abnormality while the majority of the remaining cases had rheumatic fibrosis or bicuspid or calcified aortic valves [43]. Both congenital bicuspid aortic valves and calcific degeneration of normal aortic valves are more commonly associated with aortic valve stenosis and endocarditis in the elderly than is rheumatic deformity. Although this

different valvular pathology in the elderly may not directly influence the course or prognosis of IE [42], other aspects of underlying heart disease, particularly atherosclerosis, may have a profound effect on outcome. Pre-existing coronary disease or myocardial infarction can severely limit the capacity to adapt to hemodynamic alterations resulting from valvular incompetence, coronary emboli, or conduction system disturbance occurring in the course of IE. Even though the cardiac complications of IE in the elderly appear to be similar in nature and frequency to those occurring in younger individuals with IE [41], the impact of these complications is likely to be far greater on the older cardiovascular system.

Diagnosis
Difficulty in detecting IE in the elderly also contributes to poor prognosis. In one retrospective series, the premortem diagnosis of IE was made in only 40 percent of elderly individuals [43]. Although the absence of fever, leuko-cytosis, and heart murmur in the elderly with IE has been stressed in the past, in recent series fever has been reported in 93 percent of cases [43], leukocytosis and anemia in 60 percent [41], and murmur in 68 percent [43]. In patients with murmur, the diagnosis is often neglected because the auscultatory findings are considered insignificant. It should be emphasized that systolic murmurs are common in the elderly and often do not change during IE, particularly early in the course. In patients without murmur, the diagnosis of IE should be suggested by nonspecific systemic complaints (e.g., weight loss or myalgias), in conjunction with focal or generalized neuro-logic disturbance, abnormalities in urine sediment and renal function, splenomegaly, and cutaneous manifestations of IE, such as petechiae, Osler's nodes, and Janeway lesions. The diagnosis of IE may be confirmed in greater than 95 percent of patients without recent antibiotic exposure by demonstrat-ing continuous bacteremia of varying magnitude [44].

The microbiology of IE in the elderly is similar to that in younger indi-viduals without prosthetic valves or intravenous drug usage [42]. Approxi-mately two-thirds of cases are caused by streptococci, and the remainder by coagulase-positive and coagulase-negative staphylococci. Unusual pathogens such as gram-negative rods, fungi, and anaerobes are equally uncommon in the elderly and the young [41,43].

Management
Therapy of IE in the elderly, as with any age group, should be guided by careful assessment of the antimicrobial sensitivities of the causative organism. Since preexisting renal or auditory disease may predispose the elderly indi-vidual to antibiotic toxicity, particularly from aminoglycosides, the serum concentration of these drugs should be monitored carefully. In one study, low doses and short courses of antibiotics in older persons with IE were a major risk factor for fatal outcome [45]. Ineffective therapy and inadequate

clinical recognition of IE are potentially remedial aspects of this disease in the elderly that, if corrected, could improve outcome substantially.

URINARY TRACT INFECTION

Asymptomatic Bacteriuria

The urinary tract is the most common site for bacterial infection in elderly individuals, but classic concepts of infection and pathology must be set aside when considering bacteriuria. Asymptomatic bacteriuria (ASB) is defined as greater than 10^5 of the same bacterial species per milliliter of urine on two consecutive, aseptically collected urine cultures in an individual without symptoms, fever, or other signs referable to the urinary tract. Asymptomatic bacteriuria is epidemic in the elderly, rising in prevalence from 3 percent in middle age to over 20 percent after age 70 years, and approaches 30 percent among residents of long-term care facilities [46,47]. Women are at greater risk than men. Among community-dwelling elders, diabetes, dementia, cerebrovascular disease, and decreased physical activity are important risk factors. Asymptomatic bacteriuria alone is not an indication for anatomic evaluation of the urinary tract.

Age-related factors of possible importance in the establishment of ASB include poor hygiene, decreased immune competence, and the presence of bladder outlet obstruction or neuropathic changes leading to residual urine. Absence of long-term studies on the natural history of ASB in the elderly makes management uncertain. Present evidence suggests that ASB rarely leads to serious acute illness or loss of renal function. In view of the increased risk of adverse drug reactions in the elderly, withholding antibiotics seems best.

Cystitis

Management of acute symptomatic lower urinary tract infection is less influenced by age than by the level of renal function, a prior history of infection, or the presence of renal stones, anatomic abnormalities, or an indwelling catheter. In addition to the usual symptoms of cystitis in young adults, incontinence assumes increasing importance as an indicator of cystitis with advancing age. In uncomplicated cases, a 10- to 14-day course of an oral organism-specific antibiotic will suffice. Recurrence of infection after an initial antibiotic course is not unusual and more frequently represents reinfection (a new infection) rather than relapse (failure to eradicate original infection). Reinfection, when identified by the presence of a new organism, is best managed with a second 10- to 14-day course of antibiotics, while relapse requires a six-week course. When infection recurs after the second course of antibiotics, the patient should be evaluated for the presence of underlying pathology. In resistant cases, chronic suppressive therapy is indicated. If renal function is normal and the organism is sensitive, a single nightly dose of trimethoprim-sulfamethoxazole or nitrofurantoin is often an effective suppressant.

Management of bacteriuria and infection in the presence of permanent transurethral bladder catheterization requires special guidelines [48]. Virtually all these patients have bacteriuria and pyuria, and neither should provoke antibiotic treatment. When pyuria makes urine sediment so thick as to impede catheter drainage, several daily dilute (⅛ % to ¼ %) acetic acid irrigations may reduce the sludge. Periodic (at least monthly) culture of the catheter drainage can provide useful information for antibiotic choice in the likely future development of invasive infection. When the catheterized patient develops signs of invasive infection, catheter patency must first be verified. Antibiotic treatment, directed by surveillance urine culture data, should be aimed at eradicating any bacteremia and reducing the bacterial load in the urine. Relapse or reinfection after antibiotics are stopped is certain, and treatment should continue only long enough to eradicate signs and symptoms of infection, unless blood cultures were positive, in which instance antibiotics should be continued for 7 to 10 days.

Renal function is an important guide in choosing an antibiotic regimen for urinary infection. Nitrofurantoin is not excreted into the urine in patients with azotemia and tends to induce peripheral neuropathy as it accumulates in blood. Tetracyclines, with the exception of doxycycline, should not be given to azotemic patients both because of nephrotoxicity and because anti-anabolic effects increase BUN levels dramatically in patients with impaired renal function. Trimethoprim-sulfamethoxazole should be given in reduced dosage (two regular strength tablets daily) in moderate renal insufficiency (creatinine 2.0–5.0 mg/dl), and should be avoided in cases of severe renal impairment (creatinine greater than 5.0 mg/dl). Gentamicin and other aminoglycosides are effective in urinary infection but dose must be adjusted carefully for renal function (Chapter 11).

Pyelonephritis

Acute pyelonephritis with bacteriuria, pyuria, fever, and flank pain or renal tenderness is a life-threatening disorder in the elderly. Diagnosis is more difficult than in younger patients since bacteriuria is nonspecific, being seen in many elderly patients without acute pyelonephritis, and since fever and localizing findings may be less prominent than in young adults. Initial therapy should consist of parenteral organism-specific antibiotics and repletion of any deficits in extracellular fluid. In choosing antibiotics, the possibility of enterococcal infection in patients previously receiving chronic trimethoprim-sulfamethoxazole must be kept in mind. The urine Gram's stain should not be overlooked in any bacteriuric patient, since it can identify the gram-positive cocci that indicate possible enterococcal infection. Conversely, when gram-negative rods are the only morphology seen, treatment need not be directed against the enterococcus.

When appropriate antibiotics are given in adequate doses, the urine is generally sterile within 24 hours. Nevertheless, fever, abdominal discomfort, weakness, and poor intake may persist for several days; they should not necessarily be considered indications for intravenous pyelography, a procedure performed far too frequently in view of its increased risk to elderly patients with acute pyelonephritis. Treatment failure is more frequently secondary to incorrect antibiotic therapy than to obstruction.

Chronic renal infection is an important and often overlooked cause of the "failure-to-thrive" syndrome in the elderly. Perinephric abscess may develop, especially in the presence of renal stones, and leads to insidious weight loss, weakness, altered mental state, and sometimes fever. Antibiotics may be ineffective and the treatment of choice is often surgery.

Immunization

The statistically significant age-related decline in antibody response to foreign antigens is only quantitative and small, and it should not impede enthusiasm for vaccination of elderly individuals at risk for preventable infection. Given the sharply increased prevalence of infection in the elderly, and the tendency to late presentation for treatment of established disease, any efforts likely to prevent infection should be vigorously encouraged. Although certain disease states (hematologic malignancy, immune disorders, and so on) that are more prevalent in the elderly do interfere with humoral immunity, the great majority of older individuals, including frail elders with chronic diseases, can be expected to produce adequately protective but lower levels of antibody when appropriate vaccines are administered [49]. Influenza and pneumococcal vaccines are discussed in detail in view of the especial virulence and prevalence of these infections in the elderly.

INFLUENZA

The United States Public Health Service (USPHS) advises annual immunization of elderly individuals with the current vaccine containing the influenzal agent (usually one or several type As and sometimes a type B) prevalent in the southern hemisphere in the spring preceding the fall of the vaccination year. Although recommendations for vaccination are more urgent for the oldest and sickest individuals, wholesale immunization of fit community-dwelling elderly is also advised and takes place in many American neighborhoods annually. Generally vaccine provokes protective antibody to hemagglutinin and neuraminidase surface antigens of the inactivated virus, but individuals who are most at risk for severe influenzal diseases and complications are most likely to produce inadequate antibody. Although a lifetime of exposure would be expected to confer cumulative immunity on aged persons, most annual influenza outbreaks do not spare the elderly, and annual revaccination should be encouraged. From the first availability of vaccine throughout the winter, any contact with a health provider or facility should provide an opportunity for immunization, in addition to the wide advertising of public vaccination sessions. Protective antibody begins to appear in seven days and peaks in two to four weeks. Protection is short-lived, a year or less, and type-specific immunization protects no more than 70 percent of vaccinated persons. Adverse reactions are generally limited to local inflammation and a day or two of fever, but the 1976 "swine flu" vaccination campaign appears to have produced a statistically significant increase in vaccine-related Guillain-Barré syndrome.

PNEUMOCOCCUS

In the early twentieth century, experimental immunity to type-specific pneumococcal polysaccharides was produced in laboratory animals, and antibody was detected in humans recovering from infection. In the 1940s, a commercial vaccine was marketed and thought to be effective in preventing pneumonia in elderly nursing home residents. However, immunization was never widespread, and with the dramatic appearance of cheap, effective penicillin to treat pneumococcal infections (largely pneumonia), vaccine use became less and less frequent; by the early 1950s it had been withdrawn from the market. During the subsequent two decades, persuasive evidence was collected, largely by Robert Austrian's perseverance [50,51], documenting age-related increases in death and complications from pneumococcal pneumonia as well as an apparently irreducible early mortality in spite of prompt initiation of antibiotic treatment, again largely in elderly patients. Additional theoretical impetus for vaccine development came from multiple reports of relatively penicillin-resistant pneumococci in worldwide settings, although certainly clinical problems due to resistant pneumococci are still case report rarities in the western hemisphere.

Pneumococcal vaccine, containing the 14 most common serotypes producing bacteremic infection in North America, is commercially available and produces a protective antibody response in young and old recipients with a variety of chronic diseases. Illnesses affecting humoral immunity and advanced debility interfere with antibody production and thus negate vaccine efficacy. Additionally, infants under two years of age do not make adequate protective antibody after vaccination. Ironically, since humoral immunity is a major natural defense against pneumococcal infection, some of the very individuals most in need of vaccine protection will not respond to immunization. One well-documented such situation is the postsplenectomy patient with hematologic malignancy who is doubly vulnerable to pneumococcal infection by virtue of splenectomy and disease.

With clear understanding of efficacy limitations, pneumococcal vaccination is being suggested (there are no formal USPHS Advisory Committee on Immunization Practices recommendations, only guidelines for vaccine use) for closed populations of elderly individuals such as those in nursing homes for frail chronically ill elderly, for splenectomized individuals, and in circumstances of epidemic spread [52]. Vaccination confers protective immunity for three to five years, and adverse reactions are generally limited to local inflammation and soreness. Although several studies show that aged individuals produce adequate levels of protective type-specific antibody, most studies of the immune response and virtually all current studies of clinical efficacy have been done in young subjects. There has to date been no documentation of the concern that vaccine use would merely result in substitution of another group of infecting serotypes for the ones in the vaccine. As vaccine use becomes more widespread, documentation of prior immunization becomes important in the acutely ill pneumonia patients, since pneumococcal infection, the most common bacterial pneumonia, is much less likely in vaccinatees.

Antimicrobials

Numerous good reviews and textbooks discuss principles and specifics of antibiotic usage in patients of all ages, and efforts will be made to avoid duplication here. General principles of antibiotic use specifically relevant to elderly individuals will be identified, and a few agents with special problems or characteristics in old patients will be discussed.

GENERAL PRINCIPLES

The impact of physiologic change on pharmacokinetics and pharmacodynamics has been discussed generally in Chapter 4, but several principles are especially relevant to antibiotic use and deserve mention. Because of diminished gastric acid secretion, acid-labile penicillins that are usually not given by mouth may be used if achlorhydria is documented. Slowed gastrointestinal transit time may elevate levels of penicillins and tetracyclines that are usually incompletely absorbed. Highly protein-bound drugs such as methicillin and cefazolin will have a higher percentage of a dose in the unbound form and available because of diminished albumin levels. However, the most important change is the predictable physiologic decline in creatinine clearance and glomerular filtration rate, which slow the excretion of all drugs but especially those cleared unchanged by the kidney. The physiologic decline in renal function occurs without elevation of BUN or creatinine (Chapter 11) and must be anticipated in all elderly patients. When BUN or creatinine is elevated, renal function is compromised even further and drug dose must be reduced even more. Specific guidelines for each antibiotic are available and should be consulted [53,54]. For drugs filtered but not secreted, such as the aminoglycosides or amantadine, doses should be reduced by roughly 10 percent per decade in patients over 40 years of age if BUN and creatinine are normal. Alternatively, creatinine clearance can be measured directly and doses adjusted. Antibiotics that are filtered and secreted, primarily the penicillins and cephalosporins, require only slight dose reduction until urine flow diminishes or creatinine clearance falls to very low levels (less than 20 ml per minute) as a result of renal disease superimposed on renal aging.

When using antibiotics, the same guidelines for choice of an agent apply regardless of the patient's age. After all available materials are cultured, treatment for serious infection is initiated based on the epidemiology, site, and clinical behavior of the illness and on the Gram's stain appearance of relevant specimens. Agents should be changed according to sensitivity data from cultures, and the least toxic drug should always be used. The special vulnerability of the elderly to antibiotic toxicity, pseudomembranous colitis, and superinfection demands narrow spectrum agents and prompt termination following cure.

SPECIFIC DRUGS
Penicillins
Penicillins have already been mentioned. One special note of caution in elderly individuals concerns use of the disodium penicillins such as carbenicillin. These agents contain nearly 5 mEq of sodium per gram, and their rapid clearance requires dozens of grams for effective daily treatment; this results in administering the equivalent of up to one liter of physiologic saline per day just in antibiotics. The precipitation or exacerbation of congestive heart failure is a genuine concern when such agents are used in elderly patients with heart disease.

Aminoglycosides
Aminoglycosides are drugs broadly effective against gram-negative infections, which are increasingly prevalent and dangerous in the elderly, often producing bacteremia originating from the gut or urinary tract and pneumonia. These agents are also especially hazardous in the elderly, poisoning and further damaging the same renal tubules whose diminished physiologic function engenders drug accumulation in the first place. It has been suggested that tobramycin is less nephrotoxic than other agents, but the differences are small. Aminoglycosides are ototoxic as well as nephrotoxic when serum levels rise. There is differential toxicity among different agents for the auditory and vestibular portions of the eighth cranial nerve. Streptomycin, gentamicin, and tobramycin are more toxic to the vestibule, whereas kanamycin and amikacin are likely to produce deafness before balance difficulties. Depending upon existing problems in the hearing, mobility, and balance, and upon an individual's life-style, choice of an agent from one group or the other, given equal efficacy, may be wiser. Whatever aminoglycoside is used, serum levels should be monitored carefully, keeping peak levels below the toxic range but high enough to be therapeutic.

Isoniazid
Isoniazid (INH) chemoprophylaxis has been recommended for several situations indicating prior untreated, currently inactive tuberculosis to prevent

subsequent reactivation [55,56]. As the major reservoir of TB in developed nations, elderly individuals are most often considered for one year of prophylactic INH; however, the incidence of INH hepatitis appears to rise with age, as does the severity of illness. Thus, great caution should be exercised in using INH prophylaxis in an asymptomatic elderly person with inactive TB. The greater the life expectancy, the stronger the indication for INH, since most reactivation risks do not change from year to year. Accordingly, in an extremely elderly person with only a few years of life expectancy but a 10 percent or greater risk of INH hepatitis, careful monitoring of tuberculosis status by chest x-ray and clinical examination may be wiser than INH chemoprophylaxis.

Amantadine

Amantadine, an agent useful in treating parkinsonism, was found experimentally to prevent penetration of host cells by type A influenza viruses. Clinical studies have shown that amantadine prevents acquisition of epidemic influenza A disease in roughly 70 percent of susceptible individuals, approximately the same protection rate as vaccination. The drug must be taken before and throughout exposure to be effective. Although reputed to have exaggerated toxicity in the elderly, amantadine at 200 mg a day produces a less than 10 percent adverse reaction rate in aged subjects. Toxicity is either anticholinergic or central nervous system, characterized by lethargy, dizziness, or confusion. Although certainly disturbing, such toxicity is readily apparent and quickly reversible when the drug is stopped. In influenza A outbreaks in unvaccinated or inappropriately vaccinated populations of high-risk frail elderly, mass administration of prophylactic amantadine would likely prevent numerous cases and complications of influenzal disease. Additionally, when begun shortly after onset of illness, amantadine ameliorates influenza and hastens overall improvement and recovery of pulmonary functional impairment. When the onset of influenza A is especially severe in especially vulnerable elderly persons, therapeutic amantadine can help and probably should be used.

References

1. U.S. DHEW. *Leading Causes of Death and Probabilities of Dying, United States 1975–1976.* Washington, D.C.: U.S. Government Printing Office, 1979.
2. Myerowitz, R. L., Medeiros, A. A., and O'Brien, T. F. Recent experience with bacillemia due to gram negative organisms. *J. Infect. Dis.* 124:239, 1971.
3. Phair, J. P., Kauffman, C. A., and Bjornson, A. Investigation of host defense mechanisms in the aged as determinants of nosocomial colonization and pneumonia. *J. Reticuloendothel. Soc.* 23:397, 1978.
4. Phair, J. P., et al. Host defenses in the aged: evaluation of components of the inflammatory and immune response. *J. Infect. Dis.* 138:67, 1978.

5. Gardner, I. D. The effect of age on susceptibility to infection. *Rev. Infect. Dis.* 2:801, 1980.
6. Zavala, D. C. The threat of aspiration pneumonia in the aged. *Geriatrics* 32:46, 1977.
7. Goodman, R. M., et al. Relationship of smoking history and pulmonary function tests to tracheal mucous velocity in non-smokers, young smokers, ex-smokers, and patients with chronic bronchitis. *Am. Rev. Respir. Dis.* 117:205, 1978.
8. Broome, C. V., Facklam, R. R., and Fraser, D. W. Pneumococcal disease after pneumococcal vaccination: an alternative method to estimate the efficacy of pneumococcal vaccine. *N. Engl. J. Med.* 303:549, 1980.
9. Meyers, M. G. Varicella and herpes zoster: comparisons in the old and young. *Geriatrics* 32:77, 1977.
10. Reichman, C. B., and O'Day, R. Tuberculosis infection in a large urban population. *Am. Rev. Respir. Dis.* 117:705, 1978.
11. Powell, K. E., and Farer, L. S. The rising age of the tuberculosis patient: a sign of success and failure. *J. Infect. Dis.* 142:946, 1980.
12. Foy, H. M., et al. Long term epidemiology of infections with *Mycoplasma pneumoniae*. *J. Infect. Dis.* 139:681, 1979.
13. Burnet, M., and White, D. O. *Natural History of Infectious Disease* (4th ed.). Cambridge, England: Cambridge University Press, 1972. P. 99.
14. Osmer, J. C., and Cole, B. K. The stethoscope and roentgenogram in acute pneumonia. *South. Med. J.* 59:75, 1966.
15. Rossman, I., Rodstein, M., and Bornstein, A. Undiagnosed diseases in an aging population. *Arch. Intern. Med.* 133:366, 1974.
16. Sullivan, R. J., et al. Adult pneumonia in a general hospital: etiology and host risk factors. *Arch. Intern. Med.* 129:935, 1972.
17. Graybell, J. R., et al. Nosocomial pneumonia: a continuing major problem. *Am. Rev. Respir. Dis.* 108:1130, 1973.
18. Connor, E. B. The nonvalue of sputum culture in the diagnosis of pneumoccocal pneumonia. *Am. Rev. Respir. Dis.* 103:845, 1971.
19. Bartlett, J. G., et al. Should fiberoptic bronchoscopy aspirates be cultured? *Am. Rev. Respir. Dis.* 114:73, 1976.
20. Murray, P. R., and Washington, J. A. Microscopic and bacteriologic analysis of expectorated sputum. *Mayo Clin. Proc.* 50:339, 1975.
21. Valenti, W. M., Jenzer, M., and Bentley, D. W. Type specific pneumococcal respiratory disease in the elderly and chronically ill. *Am. Rev. Respir. Dis.* 117:233, 1978.
22. Davidson, M., Tempest, B., and Palmer, D. L. Bacteriologic diagnosis of acute pneumonia: comparison of sputum, transtracheal aspirates, and lung aspirates. *J.A.M.A.* 235:158, 1976.
23. Loosli, C. G. Influenza and the interaction of viruses and bacteria in respiratory infections. *Medicine* 52:369, 1973.
24. Valenti, W. M., Trudell, R. G., and Bentley, D. W. Factors predisposing to oropharyngeal colonization with gram negative bacilli in the aged. *N. Engl. J. Med.* 298:1108, 1978.
25. Helms, C. M., et al. Comparative features of pneumococcal, mycoplasmal and Legionnaire's disease pneumonias. *Ann. Intern. Med.* 90:543, 1979.

26. Edelstein, P. H., Meyer, R. D., and Finegold, S. M. Laboratory diagnosis of Legionnaire's disease. *Am. Rev. Respir. Dis.* 121:317–327, 1980.
27. Bartlett, J. G., and Finegold, S. M. Anaerobic infections of the lung and pleural space. *Am. Rev. Respir. Dis.* 110:56, 1974.
28. Bartlett, J. G., Rosenblatt, J. E., and Finegold, S. M. Percutaneous transtracheal aspiration in the diagnosis of anaerobic pulmonary infection. *Ann. Intern. Med.* 79:535, 1973.
29. Johnson, R. N., Ritchie, R. T., and Murray, I. H. F. Declining tuberculin sensitivity with advancing age. *Br. Med. J.* 2:720, 1963.
30. Holden, M., Dubin, M. R., and Diamond, P. H. Frequency of negative intermediate strength tuberculin sensitivity in patients with active tuberculosis. *N. Engl. J. Med.* 285:1506, 1971.
31. Esposito, A. L., and Gleckman, R. A. Fever of unknown origin in the elderly. *J. Am. Geriatr. Soc.* 26:498, 1978.
32. Heinle, E. W., Jensen, W. N., and Westerman, M. P. Diagnostic usefulness of marrow biopsy in disseminated tuberculosis. *Am. Rev. Respir. Dis.* 91:701, 1965.
33. Sanford, J. P., and Pierce, A. K. Lower Respiratory Tract Infections. In J. V. Bennett and P. S. Brachman (Eds.), *Hospital Infections.* Boston: Little, Brown, 1979.
34. Johanson, W. G., et al. Nosocomial respiratory infections with gram negative bacilli: the significance of colonization of the respiratory tract. *Ann. Intern. Med.* 77:701, 1972.
35. Tillotson, J. R., and Finland, M. Bacterial colonization and clinical superinfection of the respiratory tract complicating antibiotic treatment of pneumonia. *J. Infect. Dis.* 119:597, 1969.
36. Jay, S. J., Johanson, W. G., and Pierce, A. K. The radiologic resolution of *Streptococcus pneumoniae* pneumonia. *N. Engl. J. Med.* 293:798, 1975.
37. Anderson, H. J., and Staffurth, J. S. Subacute bacterial endocarditis in the elderly. *Lancet* 2:1055, 1955.
38. Lerner, P. I., and Weinstein, L. Infective endocarditis in the antibiotic era. *N. Engl. J. Med.* 274:199, 259, 323, 388, 1966.
39. Weinstein, L., and Rubin, R. H. Infective endocarditis—1973. *Prog. Cardiol. Dis.* 16:239, 1973.
40. Tan, J. S., Watanakunakorn, C., and Terhune, C. A. *Streptococcus viridans* endocarditis: favorable prognosis in geriatric patients. *Geriatrics* 28:68, 1973.
41. Applefeld, M. M., and Hornick, R. B. Infective endocarditis in patients over age 60. *Am. Heart J.* 88:90, 1974.
42. Ries, K. Endocarditis in the Elderly. In D. Kaye (Ed.), *Infective Endocarditis.* Baltimore: University Park Press, 1976.
43. Thell, R., Martin, F. H., and Edwards, J. E. Bacterial endocarditis in subjects 60 years of age and older. *Circulation* 51:174, 1975.
44. Werner, A. S., Cobbs, C. G., and Kaye, D. Studies on the bacteremia of endocarditis. *J.A.M.A.* 202:127, 1967.
45. Habetz-Gabr, E., January, L. E., and Smith, I. M. Bacterial endocarditis: the need for early diagnosis. *Geriatrics* 28:164, 1973.
46. Akhtar, A. J., et al. Urinary tract infection in the elderly: a population study. *Age Ageing* 1:48, 1972.

47. Brocklehurst, J. C., et al. Bacteriuria in geriatric hospital patients. *Age Ageing* 6:240, 1977.
48. Stamm, W. E. Guidelines for prevention of catheter-associated urinary tract infections. *Ann. Intern. Med.* 82:386, 1975.
49. Gladstone, J. L., and Recco, R. Host factors and infectious diseases in the elderly. *Med. Clin. North Am.* 60:1225, 1976.
50. Austrian, R., and Gold, J. Pneumococcal bacteremia with special reference to bacteremic pneumococcal pneumonia. *Ann. Intern. Med.* 60:759, 1964.
51. Austrian, R. Random gleanings from a life with the pneumococcus. *J. Infect. Dis.* 131:474, 1975.
52. Center for Disease Control. *Morbidity Mortality Weekly Rep.* 27:25, 1978.
53. Appell, G. B., and Neu, H. C. The nephrotoxicity of antimicrobial agents. *N. Engl. J. Med.* 296:663, 722, 784, 1977.
54. Bennett, W. M., et al. Guidelines for drug therapy in renal failure. *Ann. Intern. Med.* 86:754, 1977.
55. Ferebee, S. H. Controlled chemoprophylaxis trials in tuberculosis: a general review. *Adv. Tuberc. Res.* 17:28, 1969.
56. Comstock, G. W., and Edwards, P. O. The competing risks of tuberculosis and hepatitis for adult tuberculin reactors. *Am. Rev. Respir. Dis.* 111:573, 1975.

21. Pulmonary System

Scott T. Weiss

A comprehensive approach to aging and pulmonary function involves consideration of the interaction of normal physiologic changes with environmental factors to produce pulmonary symptoms and disease in the elderly. The substantial interindividual variability in the effect of normal aging on pulmonary function is evident in the wide range of lung volumes or flow rates considered to be within the normal range. After correction for age, sex, and body size, considerable variability in level of pulmonary function remains unexplained. Although subject effort and the inability of commonly used tests of pulmonary function to detect small changes may account for part of this variability, epidemiologic and environmental factors, notably cigarette smoking, are important modifiers of normal age changes.

This chapter will cover the normal physiology of aging in the areas of (1) pulmonary mechanics, (2) gas exchange in the lung, (3) control of respiration, and (4) pulmonary defense mechanisms, and will integrate these physiologic data with epidemiologic risk factors such as cigarette smoking, atopy, and respiratory illness history. The interaction of physiologic and epidemiologic changes with age will be discussed in the context of chronic airflow obstruction and pneumonia in the elderly. Pneumonia is discussed in detail in Chapter 20.

Normal Physiology of Aging
COMPLIANCE

The mechanical properties of the respiratory system depend primarily on the compliance (e.g., change in volume for a given change in pressure applied, $\Delta V/\Delta P$) of the lung and chest wall. The lungs and chest wall are bound together by the potential pleural space and function as a bellows, with the lung having a natural tendency to collapse inward and the chest wall a natural tendency to expand outward.

Because respiratory system compliance changes at different lung volumes, individual compliance measurements are not comparable unless the lung volume at which they were made is known. Cross-sectional studies have shown that the lung becomes more compliant, that is, has less tendency to collapse, with age [1]. There is a linear increase in lung compliance after ages 20 to 25 that results in a greater change in volume for a given change in pressure. This loss of elastic forces cannot be accounted for by loss of connective tissue (collagen and elastin) in pulmonary parenchyma [2,3].

The compliance of the chest wall changes with age as well. After age 20, as a result of ossification of the costochondral cartilage forming a more rigid thorax, the chest wall becomes less compliant (i.e., stiffer) with a greater tendency to expand. The result of these age-related changes in compliance—the lung having less tendency to collapse and the chest wall having a greater tendency to expand—explains the changes in static lung volumes with age.

VOLUMES

The influence of age on lung volumes is depicted in Figure 21-1. Total lung capacity, or the total amount of air in the lungs following a maximum inspiration, does not change with age after adulthood is attained. However, functional residual capacity (FRC), or the amount of air in the lungs at the end of a normal expiration, increases with age. FRC is the resting point of the lung, i.e., that point at which the tendency of the lung to collapse inward is exactly balanced by the tendency of the chest wall to expand outward. Because compliance changes with age, FRC increases as individuals age. This increase in FRC is accompanied by a decrease in vital capacity (the amount of air exhaled following a maximal inhalation) and an increase in residual volume or the amount of air in the lungs at the end of a maximum expiration.

FLOW

Airflow in the lungs is dependent on airway size and airway resistance, muscle strength, and elastic recoil [4,5]. None of these factors have received careful attention with respect to the impact of age. Muscular strength, most important for flow at large lung volumes, and elastic recoil, the major determinant of flow at low lung volumes, both decline as a person ages. The loss of elastic recoil (increased compliance) leads to the dynamic collapse of airways on expiration, with trapping of gas in the lung and a decrease in flow rates as a result of the increased resistance.

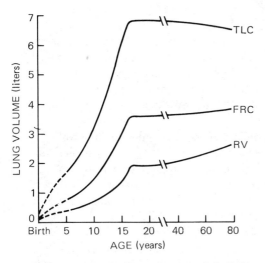

Figure 21-1. Total lung capacity (TLC), functional residual capacity (FRC), and residual volume (RV) as a function of age from birth to 80 years for an "average" body build. (From J. F. Murray, *The Normal Lung.* Philadelphia: Saunders, 1976.)

All indices of airflow, the forced vital capacity (FVC), the forced expiratory volume in one second (FEV_1), and the forced expiratory flow$_{25-75}$, or the flow between 25 and 75 percent of the vital capacity (FEF_{25-75}), decline with age, although not at equal rates. The greatest decline is seen in FEF_{25-75}, reflecting abnormal flow at low lung volumes and the primacy of a decrease in elastic recoil. FEV_1 and FVC reflect flows at high lung volumes and thus depend more on muscular strength than elastic recoil. Both tests decrease with increased age, with FEV_1 declining at a somewhat greater rate.

Since the most important clinical variables that determine flow rates and lung volumes are age, height, and sex, normal values for pulmonary function tests are routinely corrected for these characteristics. Pulmonary function is one of the few clinical parameters that normally corrects for age. The predictive value of any single determination is low because of the high variability associated with the tests. For example, normal FEV_1 is considered to range from 80 percent predicted to 120 percent predicted. However, repeated values in the same individual are helpful in plotting intraindividual trends in disease.

GAS EXCHANGE

Gas exchange is primarily determined by the distribution of ventilation and blood flow. The relationship of ventilation to blood flow is very close to unity for the lung as a whole, despite important regional variations. The most notable departures from this one-to-one relationship are seen at the top and the bottom of the upright lung. Since ventilation and, to a greater extent, blood flow increase as one goes from top to bottom in the upright lung, the ratio of ventilation to perfusion (V_A/Q) is greater than one at the apex and less than one at the base. Although alveoli are smaller at the base than at the apex, there are a greater number of alveoli at this point, offsetting the decrease in alveolar size. This mild ventilation-perfusion mismatch in the normal lung yields an overall V_A/Q ratio of 0.8 for the whole lung and results from venous admixture (blood not in contact with gas-exchanging alveoli) and physiologic dead space (air spaces not in contact with blood vessels). Normally, mild regional differences in V_A/Q do not lead to clinically significant hypoxemia, but they are responsible for the age-related decline in arterial oxygen tension (PaO_2).

As summarized in Figure 21-2, there is a steady linear decline in PaO_2 with increasing age, going from 90 at age 30 to 75 at age 80. This decline is related primarily to changes in the mechanical characteristics of the lung noted earlier and their effect on ventilation and perfusion. Loss of elastic recoil causes some airways, particularly in dependent regions, to be closed during all or part of the normal respiratory cycle. The net result of this airway closure is resorption of gas and alveolar collapse and atelectasis. This results in blood flowing to alveoli that are only partly oxygenated or not oxygenated at all, creating venous admixture. In addition, loss of elastic

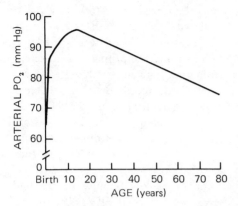

Figure 21-2. Arterial PO_2 as a function of age from birth to 80 years. (From J. F. Murray, *The Normal Lung*. Philadelphia: Saunders, 1976.)

recoil leads to dilation of air spaces and larger gas-containing areas without access to blood flow, or physiologic dead space. Primarily as a result of these mechanical lung changes, V_A/Q imbalance in the form of venous admixture contributes to age-related hypoxemia.

CONTROL OF RESPIRATION
The control of respiration is complex, involving central and peripheral mechanisms and a number of reflexes. The medullary respiratory control center is responsive to changes in carbon dioxide tension mediated by the cerebrospinal fluid concentration of hydrogen ion and bicarbonate. Peripheral chemoreceptors located in the carotid and aortic bodies in the neck respond to changes in arterial PaO_2. Normal ventilatory drive depends on these chemical responses to low PaO_2 and to neural output to the respiratory muscles. Ventilatory drive can be measured as the change in ventilation that occurs when the respiratory system is challenged.

Presently available data suggest that both central and peripheral drives are blunted with increasing age [6]. It is unclear whether this decrease results from decreased responsiveness to normal respiratory stimuli (i.e., PaO_2, $PaCO_2$) or whether decreased output (neural or muscular) from the central respiratory center is responsible.

DEFENSE MECHANISMS
The lung is open to the atmosphere to a much greater extent than are most other organ systems. Normal protection of the lung involves the epiglottis and upper airway, which prevent aspiration, and the cough reflex, which expels mucus or unwanted material from the lung. In addition to these local

mechanisms, cellular and humoral immunity play an important role in defending the lung from infectious agents.

There is no evidence at present for a decrease in humoral immunity with increasing age, and, although cellular immune function as measured by skin test declines with age, the relationship of this to pulmonary disease in the elderly is unclear. However, local airway protection does change with age. Both cough and laryngeal reflexes decrease with age. There is a marked age-related reduction in sensitivity to inhaled ammonia as a cough stimulus [7]. Older subjects have much less of a cough response than do younger individuals. This response is heterogeneous, however, and a few elderly subjects have a response similar to that of younger individuals. The linkage of this decrease in cough and laryngeal reflexes to increased aspiration is as yet unclear. Employing radioactive-tagged albumin and lung-scanning techniques, the occurrence of aspiration has been found to increase in subjects with diseases that depress consciousness, such as coma, stroke, and so on [8]. While the mean age of these patients was greater than that of normal control subjects, no normal elderly subjects were studied, leaving unanswered the question of whether depressed consciousness or age was the major determinant of the breakdown in local defenses.

Other factors besides attenuation of reflexes may be important. It has been observed (using radiopaque disks) that mean tracheal mucus velocity is slower in nonsmoking elderly subjects [9], although, as can be seen in Figure 21-3, there is considerable overlap of the young and old subjects.

These changes in local defenses need further definition and investigation because of the major problem presented by pneumonia in elderly populations. A summary of the effects of normal aging on respiratory physiology is presented in Table 21-1.

Development of Pulmonary Disease in an Aging Population

The development of pulmonary disease in adult life is determined by (1) maximal level achieved and (2) rate of decline of pulmonary function. Maximal level of pulmonary function, as measured by many different parameters, is attained in the early twenties. As shown in Figure 21-3, loss of pulmonary function is relatively linear, but it does accelerate with increase in age. Early life events could conceivably influence the development of adult symptoms by preventing the lung from attaining its maximum growth potential. Thus, an individual who started at age 25 with low normal (80 percent of predicted) pulmonary function (Fig. 21-4, curve B) might develop dyspnea late in life without acceleration of the normal age-related decline or without overt disease in adult life [10].

In general, patients do not develop dyspnea until their pulmonary function

Table 21-1. Effect of Age on Respiratory Function

Respiratory Function	Anatomic Site	Comment	Effect of Aging
Regulation of ventilation	Central: medulla, pons; peripheral: carotid and aortic bodies	Adjust rate and depth of breathing to achieve appropriate PO_2 and PCO_2 with minimal work	Decreased central responsiveness to hypoxia and hypercarbia
Bellows function and muscular strength	Diaphragm: accessory muscles, ribs, and chest wall	Influenced by conditioning	Decreased strength of respiratory muscles; increased stiffness of chest wall
Gas transport to and from periphery	Conducting airways	All airways to the respiratory bronchioles	Expiratory flow decreases due to parenchymal (elastic recoil) changes
Gas exchange	Lung parenchyma	V/Q close to 1 represents maximal efficiency	Loss of recoil; ventilation-perfusion mismatch produces hypoxemia

Source: Adapted from E. J. Campbell and S. S. Lefrak, How aging affects the structure and function of the respiratory system. *Geriatrics* 1:68, 1978.

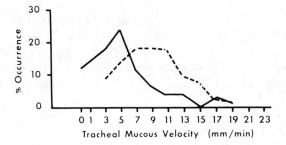

Figure 21-3. Frequency histogram of tracheal mucous velocity (percent of total number of analyzed disks) of individual disk velocities in young (broken line) and elderly (solid line) nonsmokers. (From R. M. Goodman et al., Relationship of smoking history and pulmonary function tests to tracheal mucous velocity in nonsmokers, young smokers, ex-smokers, and patients with chronic bronchitis. *Am. Rev. Respir. Dis.* 117:205, 1978.)

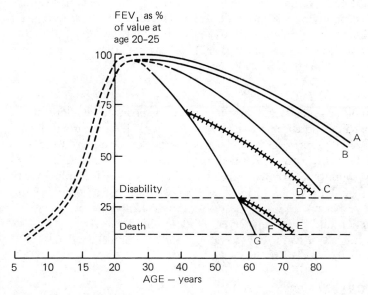

Figure 21-4. Theoretical curves representing varying rates of change in FEV$_1$ by age. Curve A depicts normal decline in FEV$_1$, curve B normal, and curve C the accelerated decline in FEV$_1$ with cigarette smoking. Curve D depicts the effect of smoking cessation also seen in disabled individuals (curve E). However, often the disability-related decline continues (curve G). (From F. E. Speizer and I. B. Tager, Epidemiology of mucus hypersecretion and obstructive airways disease. *Epidemiol. Rev.* 1:124, 1979.)

is roughly half of the normal value for age 20, which, for an average-sized man, corresponds to an FEV_1 of approximately two liters. The higher the initial level (Fig. 21-4, curve A) and the slower the decline in adult life, the longer the time to develop symptoms. Although loss of pulmonary function is progressive, the patient will often ascribe the new onset of dyspnea to recent life events that may have only a trivial influence on the development of the symptoms.

Chronic Obstructive Airways Disease

Chronic bronchitis is defined as cough and phlegm production on most days for three consecutive months for two consecutive years. The prevalence of chronic bronchitis increases with increasing age. *Emphysema* is a pathologic term referring to dilatation and destruction of air spaces distal to the terminal bronchiole. The clinical term reflecting the pathologic entity of emphysema is *chronic airflow obstruction*. Chronic airflow obstruction generally refers to decreased flow rates (an FEV_1 usually less than 65 percent of predicted for age, sex, and height and often less than 50 percent of predicted) and increased lung volumes (total lung capacity [TLC], residual volume [RV], FRC), signifying loss of elastic recoil. The important risk factors for the development of chronic bronchitis and chronic airflow obstruction are: (1) cigarette smoke ("active" or "passive"), (2) air pollution, (3) respiratory illness, (4) familial factors, and (5) atopy.

CIGARETTE SMOKING
Cigarette smoking is the single most important factor in the development of chronic bronchitis and chronic airflow obstruction [11]. The normal decline in FEV_1 of 20–30 ml per year is doubled in the smoker (see Fig. 21-4, curves C and G). This markedly accelerated loss in pulmonary function will lead to clinically significant airflow obstruction early in life in individuals with low initial (age 25) levels or in those who smoke a greater amount (assuming a dose response). Smoking leads to cough symptoms by increasing mucus secretion and irritating nerves. Airflow obstruction is produced by actual plugging of airways with secretions and by parenchymal tissue destruction, leading to loss of elastic recoil.

RESPIRATORY ILLNESS
Respiratory illness in adult life has no significant impact on rate of decline of FEV_1 or vital capacity [11]. However, in the patient with chronic airflow obstruction, any respiratory illness, bacterial or viral, can lead to the worsening of both symptoms and function.

ATOPY, AIR POLLUTION, AND FAMILIAL FACTORS
When Burrows and coworkers [12] compared old and young patients with obstructive airways disease, older patients were less likely to have positive

allergy skin tests and eosinophils in their sputum. However, Barter and Campbell [13] have reported that those patients with an allergic diathesis are more susceptible to the adverse effects of cigarette smoke. Atopy declines with increasing age and at present its relationship to lower levels of pulmonary function is unclear.

Except for severe changes in air quality, air pollution has not been shown to be a significant risk factor. The major known familial factor, α_1-antitrypsin deficiency, is important for selected individuals but, because of its relative rarity, has little significance in large populations.

Therapy for Chronic Airflow Obstruction

The basic principles of therapy for airflow obstruction do not change simply because the patient is elderly. However, recognition of age-related physiologic changes leads to some important modifications. For example, hypoxemia caused by inadequate pulmonary function is important because it could worsen congestive heart failure, arrhythmias, or delirium, all common problems in the elderly.

For the patient with chronic symptoms of dyspnea secondary to bronchospasm, bronchodilators (sympathomimetics, methylxanthines) are the mainstay of a therapeutic regimen. However, since loss of elastic recoil may play a major role in a decrease in airflow and because this is not amenable to bronchodilator therapy, recognition of the limits of bronchodilators is necessary [14].

In addition, the frequent association of occult heart failure in the elderly with airflow obstruction may be important, although difficult to detect. Home oxygen therapy is necessary relatively infrequently at sea level and a consistent PaO_2 of less than 60 mm Hg and polycythemia (hematocrit greater than 50) in the presence of cor pulmonale should be present prior to the institution of therapy. Oxygen must be used for a minimum of 12 to 15 hours a day to effectively decrease pulmonary artery pressure [15]. Finally, for the stable outpatient, it is sometimes noted that cessation of smoking will revert the rate of loss of pulmonary function to normal in two to three years.

Acute exacerbations of chronic airflow obstruction are common and are the most frequent cause of hospitalization for patients with chronic airflow obstruction. The common causes of acute exacerbations of chronic airflow obstruction are (1) respiratory infection, (2) myocardial infarction, (3) sedative drugs (narcotics, sleep medications), (4) air pollution, and (5) systemic illness (sepsis or other organ failure).

Although respiratory infection is the most common cause for acute exacerbations in any age group, in the elderly, "silent" myocardial infarction presenting as respiratory failure and respiratory failure second to sepsis or other organ system failure are of increased importance. Because of the decrease in respiratory drive noted with increased age, the prescription of hypnotic, psychotropic, and sedative drugs can precipitate respiratory failure in the elderly. The coexistence of other diseases such as heart failure can increase work of breathing or predispose to infection, and use of drugs such as diuretics may exacerbate respiratory failure by inducing chloride depletion and metabolic alkalosis, with further respiratory depression. Finally, although respiratory infections will not permanently decrease pulmonary function, the transient effect in a patient with severe airflow obstruction can be life-threatening. The elderly patient is more susceptible for two reasons. First, a decrease in respiratory drive implies less pulmonary reserve to cope with the increased stress. Second, the mechanical work of moving the chest is greater in an older person. For example, Turner and coworkers [1] estimate that the work of breathing is 20 percent greater in a 60-year-old than in a 20-year-old.

Treatment for the acute exacerbation involves the use of oxygen, bronchodilators, and antibiotics, if appropriate. Bronchodilator dosage must be adjusted carefully in the elderly. Lower doses of sympathomimetics, 0.2–0.3 cc of 1 : 1,000 epinephrine and 0.25 mg subcutaneously or 2.5 mg by mouth should be used in the elderly patient because of the risk of cardiac arrhythmias. Similarly, the effect of aminophylline is directly dependent on liver function and hepatic blood flow. Silent loss of hepatic function in many elderly patients makes a downward adjustment in dose mandatory. Therapeutic levels (10–20 μg/ml) of aminophylline can be achieved with a standard loading dose (5 mg/kg), given only if the patient has not had the drug before. A maintenance infusion of from 0.2–0.4 mg/kg per hour should be used, as opposed to the rate of 0.8–1.2 mg/kg per hour used in young adults.

References

1. Turner, J. M., Mead, J., and Wohl, M. E. Elasticity of human lungs in relation to age. *J. Appl. Physiol.* 25:644, 1968.
2. Pierce, J. A., and Ebert, R. V. Fibrous network of the lungs and its change with age. *Thorax* 20:469, 1965.
3. John, R., and Thomas, J. Chemical composition of elastins isolated from aortas and pulmonary tissues of humans of different ages. *Biochem. J.* 127:261, 1972.
4. Murray, J. F. *The Normal Lung.* Philadelphia: Saunders, 1976.
5. Rahn, H., et al. The pressure-volume diagram of the thorax and lung. *Am. J. Physiol.* 146:161, 1946.
6. Kronenberg, R. C., and Drage, C. W. Attenuation of the ventilatory and heart rate responses to hypoxia and hypercapnea with aging in normal men. *J. Clin. Invest.* 52:1812, 1973.
7. Pontoppidan, H., and Blecker, H. K. Progressive loss of protective reflexes in the airway with the advance of age. *J.A.M.A.* 174:2209, 1960.
8. Huxley, E. J., et al. Pharyngeal aspiration in normal adults and patients with depressed consciousness. *Am. J. Med.* 64:564, 1978.

9. Goodman, R. M., et al. Relationship of smoking history and pulmonary function tests to tracheal mucous velocity in nonsmokers, young smokers, ex-smokers, and patients with chronic bronchitis. *Am. Rev. Respir. Dis.* 117:205, 1978.
10. Campbell, E. J., and Lefrak, S. S. How aging affects the structure and function of the respiratory system. *Geriatrics* 1:68, 1978.
11. Fletcher, C., et al. *The Natural History of Chronic Bronchitis and Emphysema.* New York: Oxford University Press, 1976.
12. Burrows, B., et al. Chronic obstructive lung disease. Clinical and physiological findings in 175 patients and their relationship to age and sex. *Am. Rev. Respir. Dis.* 91:521, 1965.
13. Barter, C. E., and Campbell, A. H. Relationship of constitutional factors and cigarette smoking to decrease in 1 second forced expiratory volume. *Am. Rev. Respir. Dis.* 113:305, 1976.
14. Lertzman, M. M., and Cherniack, R. M. Rehabilitation of patients with chronic obstructive pulmonary disease. *Am. Rev. Respir. Dis.* 114:1145, 1976.

22. Skin

Barbara A. Gilchrest

Skin is the interface between humans and their environment that protects the other organs of the body against excessive temperature changes, mechanical injury, ultraviolet irradiation, toxic chemicals, and microbial pathogens. It is also a tactile organ through which individuals receive pleasurable stimuli and assess their physical surroundings. With age, the skin performs each of these vital functions less well. Skin is also readily visible and hence of great psychologic and social, as well as physiologic, importance. For this reason the morphologic changes that accompany aging in the skin often affect an individual as greatly as do the functional changes.

Consideration of age-induced changes in the skin is complicated by the fact that the skin is subjected to repeated and often cumulative environmental damage that is difficult to distinguish from true aging. In the minds of the public and many physicians actinically altered skin is synonymous with old skin. In addition, portions of the skin and some of its appendages are very sensitive to hormonal stimulation, so that age-related hormonal shifts (e.g., puberty and menopause) may produce skin changes not directly attributable to aging itself.

The following sections review the physiologic, morphologic, biochemical, and biophysical changes that occur in aging skin and discuss the skin lesions that frequently or disproportionately affect the elderly. Figure 22-1 illustrates in schematic form the anatomic compartments, specialized structures, and specific cell types of normal human skin.

Normal Changes Associated with Aging
MORPHOLOGIC CHANGES

The major aging changes in gross morphology of the skin include "dryness" (by which is meant roughness), wrinkling, laxity, uneven pigmentation, and a variety of proliferative lesions, discussed below. The morphologic features that have been associated with aging in human skin are listed in Table 22-1.

The most striking and consistent change in biopsies of old skin is flattening of the dermoepidermal junction with effacement of both the dermal papillae and epidermal rete pegs, shown schematically in Figure 22-2. This results in a tremendously smaller contiguous surface between the two compartments and presumably less "communication" and nutrient transfer. A decrease of approximately 10 to 20 percent per decade in the density of enzymatically active melanocytes has been repeatedly documented. It is not known whether the cells truly disappear or simply become undetectable by ceasing to produce pigment [1], but in either case the body's protective barrier against ultraviolet light is reduced. The number of melanocytic nevi also progressively decreases with age beginning in the third or fourth decade.

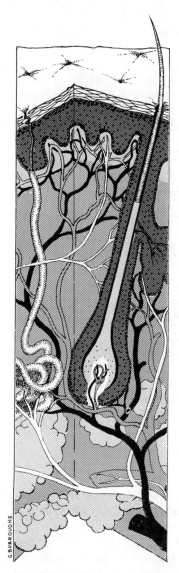

Figure 22-1. Schematic three-dimensional drawing of normal human skin. Epidermis is typically 0.1 to 0.2 mm thick; dermal thickness varies from 1 to 4 mm depending on body site. (From T. B. Fitzpatrick et al., *Dermatology in General Medicine.* New York: McGraw-Hill, 1971. P. 226. Copyright © 1971 by McGraw-Hill Book Co. Used with the permission of McGraw-Hill Book Company.)

Table 22-1. Morphologic Features of Aging Human Skin

Epidermis	Dermis	Appendages
Flat dermoepidermal junction	Atrophy	Greying of hair
Variable thickness	Fewer fibroblasts	Loss of hair
Variable cell size and shape	Fewer blood vessels	Conversion of terminal to vellus hair
Occasional nuclear atypia	Shortened capillary loops	Abnormal nail plates
Loss of melanocytes	Abnormal nerve endings	Fewer glands

Loss of dermal thickness is pronounced in elderly individuals and accounts for the paper-thin, sometimes nearly transparent, quality of their skin. The remaining dermis is relatively acellular and avascular. The marked reduction of vascular bed and especially of the vertical capillary loops that occupy dermal papillae in young skin is felt to underlie many of the physiologic alterations in old skin discussed in the following section. The marked reduction in the vascular network surrounding hair bulbs and eccrine, apocrine, and sebaceous glands may be responsible for their gradual atrophy and fibrosis with age.

Pacinian and Meisner's corpuscles, cutaneous end organs responsible for pressure perception and light touch, display progressive disorganization and histologic degeneration with age. Free nerve endings appear not to change substantially.

Age-related changes in hair color, density, and distribution are widely recognized. Greying, which is pronounced in about half the population by age 50, is due to progressive and eventually total loss of melanocytes from

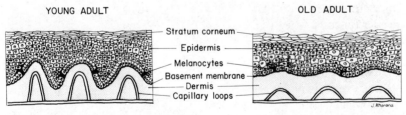

Figure 22-2. Histologic changes associated with aging in normal human skin. Note flattening of the dermoepidermal junction and shortening of capillary loops in older skin. Variability in size and shape of epidermal cells, irregular stratum corneum, and loss of melanocytes are also apparent. Age-associated loss of dermal thickness and subcutaneous fat are not shown, since the diagram includes only the epidermis and superficial or papillary dermis.

the hair bulb. This process is believed to occur more rapidly in hair than in skin because melanocytes are called upon to proliferate and manufacture melanin at maximal rates during the anagen or growth phase of the hair cycle, while epidermal melanocytes are relatively inactive throughout their life span. Scalp hair is believed to grey more rapidly than other body hair because its anagen (growth phase) : telogen (resting phase) ratio is considerably greater than that of other body hair. Advancing age is also accompanied by a gradual decrease in number of hair follicles over the entire body, with atrophy and fibrosis of many follicles. Appreciable hair loss on the scalp, commonly called balding, results primarily from the androgen-dependent conversion of the relatively dark, thick scalp hairs to lightly pigmented, short, fine hairs similar to those on the ventral forearm. By age 50, the process is at least moderately advanced in approximately 60 percent of men and noticeable in perhaps 20 percent of women. Since hair density must decrease by at least 50 percent to be clinically detectable, it is apparent that this loss of hair is substantial. Axillary hair is virtually absent in 30 percent of women and in 7 percent of men by age 60, and pubic hair also thins markedly. Remaining scalp and body hairs grow more slowly and may be smaller in diameter.

Eccrine, apocrine, and sebaceous glands become smaller, less numerous, and fibrotic throughout the skin, coincident with their reduced activity. With age, fingernails and toenails develop longitudinal ridges (onychorrhexis), an expression of alternating hyperplasia and hypoplasia of the nail matrix, as well as generalized thinning. Frequently traumatized or relatively ischemic nails, usually on the feet, may thicken, as apparent overcompensation for the injury.

PHYSIOLOGIC CHANGES
The major functions of the skin that decline with age include:

1. Growth rate
2. Injury response
3. Barrier function
4. Chemical clearance rates
5. Sensory perception
6. Resistance to infection
7. Vascular responsiveness
8. Thermoregulation
9. Sweat production
10. Sebum production

An age-related decrease in epidermal turnover rate of approximately 50 percent between the third and seventh decades has been documented by a study of desquamation rates for cells of the stratum corneum at selected body sites [2]. Forty-five minutes after intradermal injection of ^{3}H-thymidine, the percent of cells of the basal layer of the epidermis (site of production for all the cells destined to form the stratum corneum) that are labeled averages 5.5 percent in adults aged 18 to 25 years, but only 3 percent in adults aged 71 to 86 years. Growth rates for hair and nails also slow considerably with age. Fingernail linear growth rates decrease approximately 0.5 percent annually from an average of 0.9 mm per week in the third decade to 0.5 mm per week in the tenth [3]. Repair rate likewise declines with age, whether measured in terms of wound closure, regeneration of blister roofs (epidermal cell migration and mitosis), or excision of thymine dimers in UV-irradiated DNA of dermal fibroblasts [4].

Comparison between adults below age 35 years and those above age 65 years reveals an approximately 50 percent prolongation in the average time required to reepithelialize a blistered skin site—from 3.5 to 5.5 weeks. The time required for blister formation following topical application of irritant chemicals doubles between young and old adulthood, while the intensity of erythema (sunburn) following a standardized ultraviolet light exposure decreases, illustrating two other forms of compromised tissue response to injury (transudation and vasodilation).

An age-related decrease in the barrier function of intact stratum corneum has been documented by measuring percutaneous absorption of various substances [5]. This increased permeability is accompanied by a decreased clearance of the absorbed materials from the dermis, probably due to alterations in the vascular bed and in the extracellular matrix. These combined changes render old skin quite susceptible to irritant and allergic reactions, both of which require local accumulation of the offending substance.

In vitro, an age-related decline in cell-mediated immunity has been well documented. This may reflect itself in the skin of the elderly as a high prevalence of certain chronic infections such as tinea pedis. The tendency in many older patients toward bacterial superinfection of cuts and abrasions, especially on the legs, probably results from compromised tissue perfusion and inherently slow healing in those areas.

Decreased vascular responsiveness in the skin of older individuals has been documented by observing vasodilation after application of standardized irritants to young and old subjects. Compromised thermoregulation, which predisposes the elderly both to heat stroke and hypothermia, may be due in part to reduced vasodilation or vasoconstriction of dermal arterioles, in part to decreased eccrine sweat production, and in part to loss of subcutaneous fat, all of which occur with advancing age.

The decrease in sebum production that accompanies advancing age in both men and women results in part from the concomitant decrease in production of gonadal androgen, to which sebaceous glands are exquisitely sensitive. The clinical effects of decreased sebum production, if any, are unknown. There is no direct relationship to xerosis.

Finally, both nerve conduction velocity and stimulation thresholds for cutaneous fibers and end organs increase with age, undoubtedly contributing to the risk of mechanical or chemical injury to the skin.

BIOCHEMICAL CHANGES

The numerous investigations in the area of biochemical changes in the skin have been restricted to consideration of the dermis. Changes occurring during fetal development and early childhood are much greater than those occurring after maturity but reflect growth and development rather than aging and will not be reviewed.

Collagen constitutes 70 to 80 percent of dermal dry weight. With advancing age, collagen fibers become progressively cross-linked, less soluble, and less hydrated. These biochemical changes are accompanied by a decrease in extensibility and an increase in isometric tension. Elastin, which constitutes approximately two percent of dermal dry weight, increases nearly threefold in amount with age, and elastin fibers become progressively cross-linked and may calcify. These combined changes in collagen and elastin are responsible for the laxity and inelasticity of old skin.

The nonfibrous matrix of the dermis, the ground substance, is a hydrated gel composed of mucopolysaccharides and proteins. Numerous, sometimes contradictory studies have revealed little if any change in its composition [3]. Only hexosamine content has been documented to decrease slightly during adulthood; the proportions of hyaluronic acid, dermatan, and heparin sulfates appear constant. However, the ratio of ground substance to collagen definitely decreases with age, undoubtedly affecting tissue turgor.

Skin Diseases Associated with Aging
PREVALENCE

Inflammatory disorders, infections, and neoplasms of the skin increase in prevalence throughout life among otherwise healthy individuals. The best documentation of this fact derives from a 1971–1974 survey of over 20,000 representative noninstitutionalized Americans aged 1 to 74 years in which each person underwent a physical examination and laboratory testing [6]. In the first decade, approximately 15 percent of those surveyed had a dermatologic disorder at the time of examination sufficiently severe to warrant at least one physician visit; and in almost all of these cases, a single problem was present. In contrast, nearly 40 percent of the population at age 70 years had at least one skin disease of similar severity, and affected individuals averaged more than 1.5 disorders each. Not all dermatologic disorders disproportionately affect the elderly, however. Many common conditions, such as psoriasis and seborrheic dermatitis, affect young and old adults equally, whereas warts and acne are virtually restricted to children and young adults. The disorders discussed here are those that occur most commonly, although certainly not exclusively, in the elderly.

XEROSIS

Xerosis—the "dry" or rough quality of skin mentioned earlier—may be generalized but is especially prominent on the lower legs and is exacerbated by a low-humidity environment. This condition may reflect minor abnormalities in the epidermal maturation process; to date it has not been investigated experimentally. Affected skin is often pruritic and may show evidence of inflammation, probably as a result of breaks in the stratum corneum with secondary entry of irritating substances into the dermis. The resulting condition, called erythema craquele or winter eczema, responds promptly to topical corticosteroids and emollients.

TUMORS

The numerous proliferative growths manifested in old skin (Table 22-2) are so nearly universal [7] that they might be considered part of the normal aging process. These lesions suggest that loss of modulation or control of growth in the skin may be more characteristic of aging than is the simple decrease in proliferative capacity.

Malignant neoplasms of the skin increase in incidence throughout adulthood and account for nearly 50 percent of all malignancies reported annually in the United States. By far the most common are basal cell epitheliomas (BCE). These are slow-growing, encapsulated, locally invasive, and destructive proliferations of basilar cells that extend down from the epidermis and characteristically form multiple, nearly spherical masses in the dermis. Clinically, BCE begin as painless "pearly" or opalescent telangiectatic papules; 90 percent arise on the head or neck and virtually always on a background of markedly sun-damaged skin. The appearance is so distinctive that an experienced examiner can readily diagnose BCE less than 2 mm in diameter. As lesions enlarge, central ulceration and crusting may occur ("rodent ulcers"), but the epidermis remains intact over many lesions exceeding a centimeter in diameter. Cure rates for small lesions approach 100 percent, utilizing any of several therapeutic modalities (excision, cryotherapy, currettage, or x-irradiation). Large, neglected BCE may be virtually impossible to eradi-

Table 22-2. Proliferative Growths Associated with Aging in Human Skin

Lesion	Participating Cells or Tissues
Acrochordon (skin tag)	Dermis, keratinocytes, melanocytes
Cherry angioma	Capillaries
Seborrheic keratosis	Dermis, keratinocytes, melanocytes
Lentigo	Melanocytes
Sebaceous hyperplasia	Sebaceous glands

cate and may result in major disfigurement, loss of an eye, or death from debility and sepsis. Even the largest BCE rarely metastasize.

Squamous cell carcinomas are overwhelmingly lesions of sun-exposed skin with an increasing incidence throughout adulthood. In addition to ultraviolet light, other environmental carcinogens established as causes of cutaneous squamous cell carcinomas include x-irradiation, arsenic, soot, coal tar, and numerous industrial oils. Because such environmental carcinogens are often present in small amounts over long time periods and because induction time following adequate exposure is usually many years, most squamous cell carcinomas arise in older individuals. In addition, there is evidence in rodents that older animals are more prone to develop skin cancers following a standard challenge than are younger animals. Probably as a result of combined environmental and host factors, individuals with a history of cutaneous squamous cell carcinoma or BCE are at much higher risk of developing a new lesion than are those without a prior history.

Squamous cell carcinomas usually present as firm, painless, slightly erythematous nodules or plaques. The surface may be scaly or ulcerated. Most often, lesions are found on severely sun-damaged skin, although areas of radiation dermatitis, chronic inflammation (such as a nonhealing burn scar), or even normal skin may give rise to this malignancy. The rate of local growth and tendency to metastasize vary with the location and clinical setting of the lesion. The prognosis for squamous cell carcinomas involving a mucous membrane is poor, as it is for those unrelated to chronic sun exposure. Actinic keratoses, extremely common, minimally raised "sandpaper-like" patches in sun-exposed areas are acknowledged precursor lesions of squamous cell carcinomas, but rarely evolve into true malignancies. Even those lesions that meet all the histologic criteria for invasive carcinoma metastasize in fewer than 3 percent of cases. This is in contrast to a nearly 50 percent rate of metastases for squamous cell carcinoma of the skin in other settings. Treatment is based on the size and location of the tumor, as well as the setting in which it arises. Electrosurgery, excision, or x-irradiation is appropriate for most lesions.

Lentigo maligna melanomas, which account for approximately 10 percent of all melanomas, and keratoacanthomas, self-healing lesions that closely resemble squamous cell carcinomas histologically, also occur almost exclusively in the sun-exposed skin of the elderly. Other cutaneous malignancies not clearly related to environmental damage are rare in all age groups.

HERPES ZOSTER

Herpes zoster ("shingles") is a familiar vesicular dermatomal eruption caused by reactivation of latent varicella virus in the dorsal ganglia of a partially immune host. The disorder has a peak incidence between 50 and 70 years of age and usually affects otherwise healthy individuals, although immunosuppressed patients are at higher risk. The major difference between herpes zoster in the elderly versus the young adult is the incidence of postherpetic neuralgia, which increases sharply with age to approximately 40 percent beyond the age of 60 years. Moreover, the duration and severity of the discomfort increase even more markedly with age than does the incidence. Acyclovis, an antiviral agent, has been found to be beneficial in reducing discomfort during the acute phase of the illness, but does not influence the incidence or severity of postherpetic neuralgia [8]. Levodopa, in combination with peripheral decarboxylase inhibitor, has been shown to be effective in speeding healing and reducing pain during the acute phase and lessening late sequelae in elderly patients with herpes zoster [9]. Prednisone, 40–60 mg a day, or its equivalent given during the active eruption also appears to reduce the risk of postherpetic neuralgia in elderly patients.

PEMPHIGUS VULGARIS AND BULLOUS PEMPHIGOID
Two dermatoses for which immunologic alterations may be responsible occur with much greater frequency in older patients: pemphigus vulgaris and bullous pemphigoid. These blistering diseases may be differentiated by their characteristic clinical presentations and by immunofluorescent stains of biopsied skin. In pemphigus vulgaris, a rare disorder, autoantibodies directed against the intercellular substance of the epidermis cause the keratinocytes literally to fall apart from each other, forming intraepidermal bullae. Increasingly large areas of skin are denuded, especially in the mouth and frequently traumatized sites. Apparently normal skin may erode (slough its epidermis) after firm lateral pressure (Nikolsky's sign). Intact blisters are transient and rarely seen because the roofs consist only of the stratum corneum. Untreated patients uniformly succumb to sepsis. High-dose systemic steroids (equivalent to prednisone, 200–300 mg/day) can halt the blistering process but are themselves associated with a high morbidity and mortality.

Bullous pemphigoid is a much more common affliction of the elderly. Complement and in most cases immunoglobulins are fixed at the dermoepidermal junction of perilesional skin, and circulating anti–basement-membrane antibodies are usually detectable. These abnormalities result histologically in subepidermal bullae and clinically in mixed erosions and intact bullae, arising either from normal-appearing skin or from erythematous macules. The process is usually generalized but may be localized to small areas of the body. Untreated patients may remain in good general health for prolonged periods, although infection of denuded skin is a constant threat. Systemic steroids in doses equivalent to prednisone, 40 to 60 mg a day, are the mainstay of therapy and can be successfully tapered or discontinued after weeks to months in many patients.

MISCELLANEOUS DISORDERS
Some common skin lesions of the elderly, such as venous lakes and giant comedones, result from ectasia of the component structures. So-called senile purpura is the consequence of increased vascular fragility, itself the result of loss of connective tissue support and protective subcutaneous fat, as well

as slow resorption of extravasated blood in the dermis. The frequency of systemic diseases, circulatory insufficiency, and neurologic deficits in elderly individuals predisposes them to a variety of skin lesions, such as decubitus ulcers, stasis dermatitis, moniliasis, and drug eruptions.

Decubitus Ulcers

The decubitus ulcer or pressure sore is one of the most difficult management problems encountered in geriatric patients and is common among those confined to bed or wheelchair. The lesion is better classified as a systemic rather than a cutaneous disorder, as major illness involving at least one and usually several organ systems is invariably present. Indeed, decubitus ulcers are a major problem in clinical medicine precisely because the predisposing factors are of paramount importance and rarely correctable.

The ulcers occur over bony prominences: statistically, 65 percent in the pelvic area and 30 percent on the lower extremities [10]. Prolonged direct pressure, in excess of the 32 mm Hg average capillary perfusion pressure in the skin, produces tissue anoxia with necrosis of epidermis and superficial dermis. Since pressures up to 70 mm Hg may be generated at the sacrum and 45 mm Hg at the heels when the body is supine, it is not surprising that decubitus ulcers may arise after as little as an hour of total immobility. Additional contributing factors in the elderly often include: (1) folding of loose lax skin, with compromised blood flow in larger dermal vessels as well as increased compression of superficial capillaries; (2) reduced subcutaneous fat, which results in greater local pressure on the skin over bony prominences such as the ischial tuberosities and sacrum; and (3) reduction in baseline cutaneous blood flow by congestive heart failure, atherosclerosis, loss of intravascular volume, or other disorder common in advanced age. Perhaps more importantly, once an ulcer occurs, healing may be retarded by general inanition, by incontinence with secondary chemical irritation and bacterial contamination of the ulcer base, or by inadequate vascular supply of the involved area. These same factors are indeed responsible for the inexorable progression of many decubitus ulcers into the underlying fat, muscle, and ultimately, bone.

Prevention, although difficult in high-risk patients, is much easier than cure. All effective measures redistribute pressure from bony prominences. The simplest is frequent turning of the bedridden patient, at least every two hours. Air- or fluid-filled mattresses tend to equalize pressure over the entire area of contact and are thus a big improvement over conventional mattresses. Strategically placed pillows are theoretically helpful, but in practice rarely remain in place for long periods. Undoubtedly the best of the currently available support surfaces is the ripple mattress, a series of contiguous, 12 cm-diameter horizontally aligned inflatable tubes. A machine pump repeatedly inflates and deflates the tubes every 5 to 10 minutes in an alternating pattern, so that the patient is supported first by the even-numbered tubes, then by the odd-numbered tubes; no area is continuously weight-bearing for more than the 5- to 10-minute pump cycle time.

Once a decubitus ulcer is present, in addition to the previously mentioned measures, it is necessary to maintain the ulcer base in as optimal condition for healing as possible. Surgical debridement of necrotic tissue may be necessary initially. If an eschar is present, it should be removed in order to permit reepithelialization. Healing is always slowed by heavy colonization of the ulcer with bacteria, the species depending on body site, patient continence, and recent antibiotic administration. Frequent changes of wet-to-dry saline dressings, at least four times daily, provide gentle debridement and substantially reduce bacterial counts. Routine use of systemic antibiotics is ill-advised, since tissue levels are often subtherapeutic in the ulcer bed when sufficient elsewhere to dangerously alter bowel and skin flora. Topical antibiotics also penetrate granulation tissue poorly, may have a direct adverse effect on wound healing, and occasionally induce marked allergic sensitization with its attendant discomfort and risk of cross-reaction to subsequently administered systemic drugs. Antibiotic usage may be justified for two to three days preceding definitive surgical treatment of a decubitus ulcer, however, as the probability of a successful closure falls from greater than 90 percent to less than 20 percent when bacterial counts exceed 10^5 per gram of tissue. The choice of antibiotics should ideally be based on a recent culture of granulation tissue excised from the ulcer crater. Acetic acid, 0.25 to 1.0% solution, applied as a wet-to-dry dressing is especially helpful for *Pseudomonas* organisms; other agents are usually best given by the intramuscular or intravenous route.

Mixtures of trypsin, streptokinase, vitamin E, dextran polymers, estrogens, and androgens are among the other agents intended to speed healing of decubitus ulcers, but the experience with them is almost entirely anecdotal and uncontrolled. Maintaining a positive nitrogen balance with a normal serum protein level is undeniably beneficial and may require supplementary feedings via nasogastric tube or intravenous hyperalimentation line. Deficiencies of ascorbic acid and zinc, both implicated in wound healing, should be corrected if present. Finally, surgical closure of decubitus ulcers is often preferable to the extremely slow process of natural healing. Primary closure, grafting, or rotation of a skin flap are excellent procedures in appropriate patients.

References

1. Gilchrest, B. A., Blog, F. B., and Szabo, G. Effects of aging and chronic sun exposure on melanocytes in human skin. *J. Invest. Dermatol.* 73:219, 1979.
2. Leyden, J. J., McGinley, K. J., and Grove, G. L. Age-Related Differences in the Rate of Desquamation of Skin Surface Cells. In R. D. Adelman, J. Roberts, and V. J. Cristofalo (Eds.), *Pharmacological Intervention in the Aging Process*. New York: Plenum Press, 1978.

3. Selmanowitz, V. J., Rizer, R. L., and Orentreich, N. Aging of the Skin and Its Appendages. In C. E. Finch and L. Hayflick (Eds.), *Handbook of the Biology of Aging*. New York: Van Nostrand Reinhold, 1977.

4. Gilchrest, B. A. Some gerontologic considerations in the practice of dermatology. *Arch. Dermatol.* 115:1343, 1979.

5. Christophers, E., and Kligman, A. M. Percutaneous Absorption in Aged Skin. In W. Montagma (Ed.), *Advances in Biology of Skin*. Vol. 4, *Aging*. Oxford, England: Pergamon Press, 1965.

6. Johnson, M. L. T., and Roberts, J. Prevalence of dermatological disease among persons 1–74 years of age: United States. Advance Data No. 4. Washington, D.C.: U.S. DHEW, 1977.

7. Tindell, J. P. Skin changes and lesions in our senior citizens: incidence. *Cutis* 18:359, 1976.

8. Peterslund, N. A., et al. Acyclovis in herpes zoster. *Lancet* 2:827, 1981.

9. Kernbaum, S., and Hauchecorne, J. Administration of levodopa for relief of herpes zoster pain. *J.A.M.A.* 246:132, 1981.

10. Agris, J., and Spira, M. Pressure ulcers: prevention and treatment. *Clin. Symp.* Vol. 31, 1979.

23. Falls

John W. Rowe

Physicians dealing with the elderly frequently encounter individuals whose chief complaint is falling. In adult medicine, falling about is a geriatric syndrome with multiple causes and represents an important source of morbidity and mortality. Increasing age and debility are associated with a marked increase in the risk of and damage from falls. All geriatricians should be familiar with the mechanisms responsible for falls in the elderly and the management of this common problem.

Epidemiology of Falls in the Elderly

Surveys of community-dwelling elderly individuals in Great Britain and the United States have repeatedly shown that 35 to 40 percent of individuals over 65 will suffer at least one fall per year and that the risk of falling increases dramatically with advancing age [1–3]. Most of these falls are not associated with significant morbidity. Only 16 percent of patients referred to geriatric hospitals have a chief complaint of having fallen [4]. An important study in a long-term care facility by Gryfe and his colleagues [5] chronicled the experience of over 400 individuals for a period of five years. The overall incidence of falls in this study population was 45 percent. While this is somewhat higher than the incidence found in community-based studies, it is more likely to be accurate since individuals were in a supervised environment in which the staff was particularly interested in documenting episodes of falling. As shown in Table 23-1, and confirmed by other studies [1,2], Gryfe and colleagues found elderly women to be especially vulnerable to falls, and particularly prone to falling down stairs [6]. Falls are likely to be recurrent. In Gryfe's study, over the course of the five years the average man who had fallen was noted to have 2.7 episodes of falling and the average woman, 3.5.

Morbidity and Mortality of Falls in the Elderly

Most falls are of no clinical consequence [5]. Gryfe and colleagues [5] have shown that 54 percent result in no injury whatsoever, and an additional 28 percent were considered to be trivial; 18 percent were noted to be severe, with 6 percent resulting in fracture. In view of the high prevalence of falls in the elderly, this rather small percentage of severe injuries accounts for the major portion of traumatic illness in the elderly. The likelihood of significant fracture or death from a fall corresponds with the presence of severe osteopenia and is thus greater in whites than in nonwhites, greater in women than men, and increases progressively after age 65. The annual incidence of femur fracture increases from less than 100 per 100,000 population at age

Table 23-1. Falls in Elderly Residents of a Long-Term Care Facility

	Men		Women	
	Number	%	Number	%
At risk	138	31	303	69
"Fallers"	58	29	140	71
Falls	158	24	493	76
Falls/person yr at risk	0.55		0.72	
Serious injury	25	22	89	78

Source: Adapted from C. I. Gryfe, A. Amies, and M. J. Ashley, A longitudinal study of falls in an elderly population: I. Incidence and morbidity. *Age Ageing* 6:201, 1977.

40, to greater than 500 episodes per 100,000 population after age 60 [7]. With regard to mortality, death rates from falls are less than 50 per 100,000 at age 65 and increase progressively to 150 per 100,000 at age 75 and 525 per 100,000 over age 85.

Age-Related Changes in Maintenance of Postural Stability

Postural stability is maintained via a variety of proprioceptive reflexes that rely upon afferent input from visual cortex, inner ear, and mechanoreceptors in peripheral joints. The integration of this information in the central nervous system enables the individual to be aware of the orientation of the head and body in space and to maintain upright posture. Recent studies have demonstrated an important change with age in the cervical articular mechanoreceptors—the afferents of which produce phasic reflexes in the muscles of the neck, jaw, eye, and extremities—that play an important role in the maintenance of upright posture [8,9]. It has been shown that normal aging is associated with decreased sensitivity of the mechanoreceptors to changes in orientation of the head on the neck and that this age-related decline is particularly prominent in women. This provides a physiologic explanation for the decreased mechanical efficiency of movement and the increased vulnerability of apparently healthy individuals, especially women, to falling. In addition to these changes in proprioception, there are well-described alterations in peripheral vision that place the elderly at special risk.

The unsteadiness of the elderly was initially identified in the simple but elegant studies of Sheldon [10] on body sway during quiet standing. Recent studies have confirmed Sheldon's initial observations and quantified the effects of age on postural sway, showing that elderly individuals demonstrate between 50 and 125 percent greater postural instability than younger adults [11,12].

Predisposing Factors in Frail Elderly

It is clear from clinical experience that because of a number of specific conditions that are increasingly common in the elderly these individuals carry with them a special vulnerability for falling. Perhaps the most important is the use of medications associated with orthostatic hypotension, confusion, vertigo, lethargy, or slowness to respond. An important and commonly overlooked factor in this regard is alcohol use, which, whether admitted by the patient or surreptitious, is not only an important cause of falls in the elderly but also a frequent marker of underlying depression.

The general debility and frailty associated with weight loss, prolonged bed rest, and decreased mobility; nutritional deficits; and disorders of several specific systems, including the central nervous system, cardiovascular system, and musculoskeletal system, all markedly predispose to the likelihood of falling. In the elderly patient with a specific disease predisposing to postural instability, the risk of falling has been found to be further enhanced by increased numbers of medications prescribed for or coincident to the presence of heart disease [13].

Specific Causes

As seen in Table 23-2, there is remarkable constancy in studies evaluating the causes of falls in the elderly.

ACCIDENTAL (ENVIRONMENTAL) FALLS

Approximately 40 percent of falls in the elderly are accidental and are related to some factor in the environment such as a crack in the sidewalk, a loose scatter rug at the top of the stairs, poor lighting at a stairwell (especially the bottom and top steps), or ice or other slippery conditions on a

Table 23-2. Etiology of Falls in the Elderly

| Etiology | Percent of Patients | | |
	Sheldon [14]	Clark [15]	Lucht [16]
Extrinsic (accidental)	44	46	39
Intrinsic	41	40	45
Drop attacks	25	16	
Postural hypotension	4	4	
CNS lesions	5	16	
Vertigo	7	4	
Unknown or miscellaneous	15	14	16

walkway. The increased vulnerability of the elderly to fall under conditions in which many young healthy adults would be able to maintain their balance is related in part to the normal changes in postural control outlined previously and in part to the special risk attributed to the presence of medications or specific diseases. Accidental falls are particularly important since many injuries are preventable. Elderly patients who are falling at home should have a home visit by a health professional to evaluate the home for the presence of remediable predispositions to falling such as poor lighting, scatter rugs, low-lying tables, and so on. In addition, inappropriate footwear, failing to leave lighting on at night for trips to the bathroom, and poorly advised trips out in winter all represent preventable components of the increased risk of the elderly.

Studies of falls in institutions have shown that most falls occur in the bathroom or in the area near the bed. The process of transferring from bed or bathtub to chair and/or upright position involves cardiovascular readjustments, coordinated muscular movements, and reorientation of the balance-controlling systems. Multiple age-related and disease-related factors thus make transfers a crisis for maintaining balance, and when these are added to the urge to void in a hurry and incomplete arousal from sleep, it is understandable that falls are prominent at these times. Straining at stool can exert large intrathoracic pressure transients that can adversely influence the cardiovascular adjustment to upright posture. Counseling the elderly to use better judgment in performing transfers and performing them at optimal times, using appropriate aids, and having knowledge of and access to alarms should decrease the incidence and morbidity of falls. Falling causes physical insecurity in elderly patients, thus promoting immobility and further increasing the risk of falls. Prompt education and specific teaching are important to restore appropriate confidence to these patients.

DROP ATTACKS

Drop attacks are a particularly interesting and uniquely geriatric syndrome accounting for approximately 25 percent of falls in community-dwelling elderly (see Table 23-2). The typical drop attack is a sudden interruption of an individual's walking about or performing routine activities in the home. The patient finds himself on the ground, somewhat befuddled as to his whereabouts and the cause of his fall, and often paralyzed or at least very clumsy and unable to position himself upright. The period of confusion and incoordination is of variable length but may last several minutes. The attack occurs without premonition, pain, vertigo, or any feeling of instability. Attacks may occur repeatedly in the same individuals but are often separated by long periods of time.

A drop attack appears to be related to the sudden unexpected loss of postural tone. Since some drop attacks are clearly associated with turning of the head or trunk or looking upward, and since they may be particularly common in elderly individuals with marked cervical arthritis, it has been hypothesized that compression of the spinal cord or vessels supplying the spinal cord or medulla oblongata is responsible for many drop attacks. Some clinicians report a satisfactory response to treatment of cervical arthritis in an elderly individual suffering from drop attacks. At the very least it would appear that careful examination and x-rays of the neck to search for cervical arthritis is indicated if the history suggests drop attacks and, in questionable cases of recurrent attacks, trial of a cervical collar seems reasonable. Most drop attacks do not result in injury unless they occur in particularly dangerous circumstances, such as on stairways.

POSTURAL HYPOTENSION
Postural hypotension is generally overrated as a cause of falling in the elderly and accounts for only about 4 percent of falls in studies of community-dwelling elders. While as many as 20 percent of elderly individuals will show reductions of 20 mm Hg or more in systolic and 10 mm Hg or more in diastolic blood pressure on standing, this is generally not associated with orthostatic symptoms or falls. It is likely that the absolute blood pressure after standing is a more important determinant of the capacity to maintain posture than the difference between supine and upright pressure.

MISCELLANEOUS CAUSES
Whenever a fall is associated with loss of consciousness, central nervous system events (such as transient ischemic attacks or seizures) or cardiovascular events (such as arrhythmia) must be high on the list of suspected diagnoses. Syncope or "near-syncope" is a common admitting diagnosis for elderly individuals to general hospitals and often results in an expensive, time-consuming, high-technology evaluation, including 24-hour cardiac monitoring, CT scan, EEG, and other studies. It is important to distinguish the loss of consciousness from a more simple fall and to limit these special investigations to individuals with a reasonable likelihood of benefit from the studies. The most commonly overlooked causes of falls in the elderly include medications or drugs, particularly alcohol, local factors in the home, and drop attacks.

References

1. Droller, H. Falls and Accidents in a Random Sample of Elderly People Living at Home. In Proceedings of the Third Congress of the International Association of Gerontologists (London, 1954), *Old Age in the Modern World*. Edinburgh: Churchill Livingstone, 1955.
2. Sheldon, J. H. *The Social Medicine of Old Age*. London: Oxford Printing Press, 1948. Pp. 96–105.
3. Blumenthal, M. D., and Davie, J. W. Dizziness and falling in elderly psychiatric outpatients. *Am. J. Psychiatry* 137:203, 1968.

4. Cape, R. D. T. A Geriatric Service. Report to Birmingham, England, Regional Hospital Board, August 1968.
5. Gryfe, C. I., Amies, A., and Ashley, M. J. A longitudinal study of falls in an elderly population: I. Incidence and morbidity. *Age Ageing* 6:201, 1977.
6. vanZonneveld, R. J. The Health of the Aged. Organization for Health Research T.N.O. Hassen, Netherlands, 1961.
7. Saville, P. D., and Heaney, R. P. Osteoporosis. In H. P. van Hahn (Ed.), *Practical Geriatrics*. Basel: S. Karger, 1975.
8. Albansese, A. A., et al. Quantitative radiographic survey technique for detection of bone loss. *J. Am. Geriatr. Soc.* 17:142, 1969.
9. Wyke, B. Cervicular articular contributions to posture and gait: their relation to senile disequilibrium. *Age Ageing* 8:251, 1979.
10. Sheldon, J. H. The effect of age on the control of sway. *Gerontol. Clin.* 5:129, 1963.
11. Hasselkus, B. L. R., and Shambes, G. M. Aging postural sway in women. *J. Gerontol.* 30:661, 1975.
12. Exton-Smith, A. N. Lecture to Conference on Geriatric Medicine. University of Western Ontario, London, Ontario, Canada, May 1976.
13. Cape, R. D. T. *Aging, Its Complex Management*. New York: Harper & Row, 1978. Pp. 113–136.
14. Sheldon, J. H. On the natural history of falls in old age. *Br. Med. J.* 2:1685, 1960.
15. Clark, A. N. G. Factors and fractures of the female femur; clinical study of the environmental, physical, medical and preventive aspects of this injury. *Gerontol. Clin.* 10:257, 1968.
16. Lucht, U. A prospective study of accidental falls and resulting injuries in the home among elderly people. *Acta Socio-Med. Scand.* 2:105, 1971.

24. Urinary Incontinence in the Elderly

Neil M. Resnick
John W. Rowe

Urinary incontinence, the uncontrollable, frequently unexpected wetting of oneself with urine, is a malodorous social stigma ordinarily hastily dismissed with an uninformative urine culture. In community-dwelling elderly, incontinence is found in 5 to 15 percent of individuals and is often concealed by its embarrassed victims with a mountain of absorbent pads [1]. The prevalence rises to 50 percent of elderly patients in acute-care hospitals [2] and may be even higher in chronic-care institutions. Risk factors include immobility, female sex, and neurologic disease, but in some series up to 75 percent of patients with incontinence have significant cognitive impairment. Surprisingly, advanced age and bacteriuria are not by themselves powerful predictors of incontinence [3]. As much as 25 percent of nursing time in geriatric hospitals is consumed in dealing with incontinent patients, who require twice as much nursing care as their continent peers [4].

Anatomy and Control of Urination

The lower urinary tract can be divided into two portions: (1) the muscular storage component known as the detrusor, and (2) the outlet, which is controlled by both internal and external sphincters. The internal sphincter is part of the base of the bladder, is smooth muscle, and is autonomically innervated and under involuntary control. The external sphincter is distal to this and, as part of the pelvic musculature, consists of striated muscle; it is somatically innervated and under voluntary control.

Control of bladder emptying is attained by a series of increasingly complex neurologic pathways (Fig. 24-1). In the infant a local reflex is operative in the stretching of the bladder wall; increasing urine volume activates a center in the lower sacral cord and results in prompt detrusor contraction and voiding. Complete voiding requires coordination of bladder contraction with outlet opening and is accomplished by a micturition center located in the pons [5]. The next highest level of organization involves development of a connection between the sacral bladder center and the parietal cortex, which detects bladder fullness. An additional center in the anterior frontal cortex permits control of micturition by inhibition of the sacral reflex.

Classification of Causes of Incontinence

As a preliminary step it is helpful to classify causes of incontinence as either temporary or fixed.

CAUSES OF TEMPORARY INCONTINENCE
Common causes of temporary incontinence include the following:

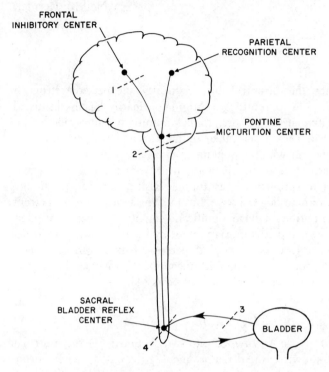

Figure 24-1. Simplified neuroanatomy of micturition, with classic lesions. Lesions correspond to types of neurogenic bladder: (1) uninhibited, (2) reflex, (3) atonic, (4) autonomous (see text).

1. Acute confusional states interfering with awareness of the need to void
2. Psychologic regression to forced dependency during hospitalization
3. Bed rest or immobility interfering with normal urination habits
4. Fecal impaction, producing acute urinary retention with overflow
5. Acute symptomatic bladder inflammation from infection, radiation, stones, or other causes that result in local irritation
6. Atrophic vaginitis/urethritis
7. Medications, especially anticholinergics and potent diuretics
8. Metabolic abnormalities that increase urinary flow such as hypokalemia, hypercalcemia, and hyperglycemia

PATHOPHYSIOLOGIC CLASSIFICATION
OF FIXED INCONTINENCE

Because clinical presentations of chronic incontinence often do not correlate with pathologic causes documented by sophisticated urodynamic testing, there is still no universally accepted classification. We prefer to separate the clinical categories of chronic incontinence, as recently proposed by the International Continence Committee [6], from the pathologic causes. The clinical entities are as follows:

1. Urge incontinence: the involuntary loss of urine accompanied by a strong urge to void
2. Reflex incontinence: the periodic involuntary voiding unassociated with a desire to micturate
3. Stress incontinence: the involuntary loss of urine only when intraabdominal pressure is transiently increased
4. Overflow incontinence: the involuntary loss of urine in the setting of a grossly distended bladder

The pathophysiologic causes of incontinence can be conceptualized as problems with bladder (detrusor) contraction or with outlet resistance. The muscular detrusor can either contract when it should not (detrusor instability) or fail to contract vigorously enough when it should (detrusor insufficiency). The outlet resistance can either be high when it should be low or vice versa. Thus there are four primary ways the lower urinary tract can malfunction. The correlation of clinical with pathophysiologic and disease entities is shown in Table 24-1.

Uninhibited Bladder (Detrusor Instability)
Detrusor instability occurs when the bladder escapes from central nervous system inhibition and contracts spontaneously at periodic intervals. This condition is also known as bladder instability and detrusor hyperreflexia. Because the bladder is emptying frequently, bladder capacity is small; however, because not all contractions may be sufficiently strong to overcome outlet resistance, there is sometimes residual urine.

Detrusor instability is the single most common cause of incontinence in the elderly, accounting for 50 to 75 percent of incontinence in most series. It can be neurogenic in origin, occurring when central nervous system inhibition is diminished because of cortical damage associated with stroke, dementia, Parkinson's disease, or brain tumor. Alternatively, it can be of nonneurogenic or so-called vesicogenic origin. Bladder inflammation and irritation, both potent local factors, can override central nervous system suppression of micturition, especially in elderly patients with other impairments. Another vesicogenic cause of detrusor instability develops as the bladder initially responds to an obstructed outlet [7]. Finally, detrusor instability can be stress-induced, that is, precipitated by increasing intraabdominal pressure, a condition that complicates stress incontinence about 25 percent of the time [8]. In all of these conditions, bladder sensation is intact so that urge to void is sensed just prior to spontaneous micturition. If the patient is sufficiently alert and mobile, he may be able to predict when contractions

Table 24-1. Correlation of Pathophysiology with Clinical and Pathologic Classifications, Common Clinical Settings, and Implications for Therapy of Urinary Incontinence

Pathophysiology	Clinical Classification	Pathologic Classification	Common Clinical Settings	Treatment[a]
Contractile (detrusor) function				
Increased	Reflex	Reflex bladder (detrusor instability)	Herniated disk Spinal cord tumor	1. Antispasmodic 2. Anticholinergic 3. Alpha antagonist ⎱ if dyssynergia 4. Sphincterotomy ⎰ present 5. Intermittent catheter/condom drainage
	Urge	Uninhibited bladder (detrusor instability) Neurogenic	Cortical insult	1. Bladder training with incontinence chart 2. Behavior modification[b] 3. Psychotherapy[b] 4. Antispasmodic 5. Anticholinergic 6. Intermittent catheter/condom drainage
		Vesicogenic	Outlet obstruction Bladder irritation Stress-induced	1. Remove obstruction 2. Treat infection if present 3. Antispasmodic/anticholinergic

Decreased	Overflow	Detrusor insufficiency Atonic myogenic Atonic neurogenic Autonomous	Outlet obstruction Diabetes mellitus Sacral cord lesion	1. Remove obstruction if present 2. Credé maneuver and straining 3. Bethanechol 4. Alpha antagonist 5. Intermittent catheterization 6. Indwelling catheter
Outlet resistance Increased	Overflow Urge	Outlet obstruction Uninhibited bladder (detrusor instability)	BPH, fecal impaction BPH, ?fecal impaction	Remove obstruction
	Reflex	Detrusor-sphincter dyssynergia	Spinal cord metastasis	1. Alpha antagonist 2. Sphincterotomy if needed 3. Intermittent catheter/condom drainage
Decreased	Stress	Outlet incompetence	Pelvic floor relaxation[e] Postprostatectomy	1. Weight loss if obese 2. Pelvic exercises 3. Pessary if uterine prolapse 4. Estrogen vaginal cream 5. Anticholinergic/antispasmodic 6. Alpha agonist 7. Surgery if severe and refractory[d]

[a] Listed in suggested order to be tried (see text).
[b] If applicable [13,14].
[c] One-fourth have detrusor instability as well.
[d] [12]

will occur and get to the bathroom in time to remain continent. However, with clouding of the sensorium secondary to acute confusion, illness, medications, or progression of central nervous system disease, as well as with development of decreasing mobility, the predisposed patient with detrusor instability becomes incontinent.

Detrusor Insufficiency

Detrusor insufficiency (detrusor hyporeflexia) occurs when detrusor contractions are inadequate to overcome normal outlet resistance. The bladder becomes distended, thin-walled, and hypotonic or atonic. The cause is either neurogenic or myogenic. The neurogenic atonic bladder results from damage to sensory bladder afferents. The bladder's increasing distention is not sensed, overfilling occurs, and the detrusor decompensates. Examples include peripheral neuropathies from many causes, especially diabetes mellitus and tabes dorsalis, but also from herniated disks and subsequent to surgical damage of pelvic nerves.

The myogenic atonic bladder is usually secondary to chronic severe outlet obstruction. The bladder frequently becomes unstable and irritable initially but as obstruction becomes more complete, it enlarges and eventually decompensates. The distinction between neurogenic and myogenic causes is important in terms of diagnosis of etiologic and correctable factors, treatment, and prognosis.

Outlet Obstruction

Outlet obstruction can result from neurologic, functional, or anatomic causes. In neurologic entities, sphincter relaxation is not coordinated with detrusor contraction—a condition known as detrusor-sphintcer dyssynergia—and obstruction to outflow occurs. Functional or psychologic causes in which the patient does not relax the external sphincter appear to be uncommon in the elderly but no definite data exist. Anatomic causes of obstruction include prostatic hypertrophy, severe chronic fecal impaction, urethral stricture, and pelvic tumors. These are important causes of incontinence, not only because they can often be definitively treated, but also because recognition can prevent the development of chronic renal failure from hydronephrosis.

Outlet Incompetence

Outlet incompetence is usually ascribable to overstretching of pelvic musculature during childbirth or to previous prostate surgery that damages the sphincter mechanism. Because urethral mucosa contributes to outlet resistance and is maintained in women by estrogen, postmenopausal estrogen deficiency with atrophic urethritis and mucosal thinning can also cause or exacerbate outlet incompetence. Another, much less frequent cause of sphincter insufficiency is neurologic in nature, in which the sacral bladder reflex center is ablated by trauma, tumor, or herniated disk, a condition resulting in the so-called autonomous bladder (see the following section). In each of the entities causing outlet incompetence, except the autonomous bladder, the clinical presentation is stress incontinence. It should be recalled, however, that about 25 percent of these patients also have vesicogenic detrusor instability.

NEUROGENIC BLADDERS

Neurogenic bladders can present in a variety of ways and should be considered under their appropriate pathophysiologic category. The neurogenic uninhibited bladder occurs when frontal lobe inhibition of bladder contraction is impaired, as seen in Figure 24-1, lesion 1. Because afferent supply from the bladder to the parietal recognition center is intact, the patient senses an urge to void. The resultant bladder pathology is detrusor instability.

The neurogenic reflex bladder (Fig. 24-1, lesion 2) arises when a lesion in the spinal cord, such as a herniated disk or tumor, interrupts neural pathways above the sacral bladder reflex center. Since the sacral center is uninvolved, reflex filling and emptying of the bladder occur in uninhibited fashion and the pathology is again detrusor instability. The reflex bladder differs clinically from the neurogenic uninhibited bladder in two ways. First, afferent supply to the cortex is impaired and, thus, incontinence is not accompanied by an urge. Second, if the lesion involves many fibers ascending to the pontine micturition center, there is poor coordination of voiding and, thus, detrusor-sphincter dyssynergia may ensue.

The neurogenic atonic bladder (Fig. 24-1, lesion 3), as noted previously, overfills because the reflex arc is broken, and the consequent pathology is detrusor insufficiency. If the sacral bladder reflex center is affected, as in the neurogenic autonomous bladder (Fig. 24-1, lesion 4), the pathology is mixed. Because both detrusor and sphincter fibers are affected, detrusor insufficiency as well as sphincter insufficiency occur. The bladder is not as grossly distended as it is with the neurogenic atonic bladder because sphincter tone, and hence outflow resistance, is decreased and constant dribbling results.

When incontinence occurs because of nonneurogenic causes or from an uninhibited neurogenic bladder (Fig. 24-1, lesion 1), pathways to the parietal recognition center are intact; the patient should experience bladder distention, discomfort, and urgency. If these sensations are not appreciated, the patient most likely has one of the other neurogenic bladders: reflex, atonic, or autonomous (Fig. 24-1, lesions 2–4).

Although there are only four primary pathophysiologic mechanisms by which voiding can malfunction, especially in the elderly more than one mechanism may be operative. As alluded to previously, about a quarter of patients with stress incontinence also have detrusor instability. The patient with prostatic hypertrophy may initially develop detrusor instability, but, as obstruction worsens, the bladder may decompensate, giving rise to detrusor insufficiency and a myogenic atonic bladder. The patient may additionally have diabetes, so the atonic bladder may have a neurogenic component as well. These elements can frequently be dissected out by a thorough evaluation, however, and therapy can be directed at all or just the predominant pathophysiologic processes.

Evaluation

All elderly patients with urinary incontinence deserve a careful clinical evaluation and, if necessary, urodynamic study, including cystometry. Evaluation begins with a detailed history of the associated circumstances and duration and pattern of incontinence. Symptoms can be important clues. "Scalding" can result from atrophic vaginitis; dysuria may signify infection. The absence of either urge or sensation of bladder fullness implies a neurogenic cause for the incontinence (Fig. 24-1, lesions 2–4). The patient's symptoms alone, however, although valuable, may be misleading if taken out of the context of the full evaluation. For example, since the patient with an uninhibited neurogenic bladder will feel an urge and detrusor instability will lead to frequency, the bladder will usually contain only a small volume of urine. The stream thus will be small and mimic the symptoms of prostatic obstruction. This was documented by a recent study of patients aged 64 to 96 years old with "obstructive" symptoms. In only 15 percent was isolated obstruction discovered by urologic testing [9].

Many medications contribute to incontinence. Frequent offenders include psychoactive drugs such as hypnotics, tricyclic antidepressants, and neuroleptic agents, as well as potent diuretics that rapidly increase urine flow and produce incontinence in individuals with marginally compensated uninhibited bladders. Antihypertensives, which can induce orthostatic hypotension and thus limit the patient's mobility, are also commonly implicated. Anticholinergic agents, including medications for Parkinson's disease, as well as some cardiac medications (particularly disopyramide [Norpace]) inhibit detrusor contractions and may cause acute urinary retention with overflow incontinence.

A thorough physical examination is essential to seek signs of a distended bladder, stress incontinence, pelvic pathology, fecal impaction, prostatic hypertrophy, autonomic insufficiency, or other neurologic disorder. Testing perineal sensation and the anal wink (or bulbocavernosus reflex) can detect and differentiate neurogenic causes of incontinence, since these reflexes and perineal sensation share innervation with the bladder (Table 24-2). Postvoid residual volume should also be measured.

Laboratory investigation need not be extensive, but it should include a urinalysis, urine culture, and a metabolic survey. Urine cytology is warranted if sterile hematuria is present.

Table 24-2. Distinguishing Characteristics of Neurogenic Bladder Disorders

Clinical Finding	Type of Neurogenic Bladder[a]			
	Uninhibited	Reflex	Atonic	Autonomous
Urge	+	−	−	−
Distended bladder	−	−	++	±
Perineal sensation	+	−	−	−
Anal wink/bulbo-cavernosus reflex	+	+	−	−
Cystometry	Hyperreflexic	Hyper-reflexic	Hypo-reflexic	Hyporeflexic

[a] +, present; −, absent; ++, strongly present; ±, sometimes present.

CYSTOMETRY

If standard clinical evaluation is unrewarding, patients should be referred for urologic evaluation and, if available, urodynamics. Although we still do not know what the cystometric (CMG) appearance is in a normal elderly continent population, CMG can be important in identifying an underlying abnormality and in suggesting possible modes of therapy. The procedure is simple: the patient is catheterized, residual volume is measured, and the bladder is filled with either gas or fluid. The change in pressure is plotted as a function of the change in volume. In young subjects the residual volume is less than 25 ml, but it probably increases with age to less than 100 ml [10,11]. Normally, there is little or no increase in pressure during filling until bladder capacity is reached at 300 to 500 ml. Desire to void occurs at about 150 ml, but contractions are normally suppressed until voluntary voiding occurs at bladder capacity.

Other techniques used in the evaluation of the lower urinary tract are electromyography (EMG), uroflowmetry, and urethral profilometry. EMG, frequently performed with CMG, can detect denervation or dyssynergia of the sphincter. An anal probe or a needle is inserted in the periurethral sphincter. Normally, there is minimal sphincter activity when the bladder is empty, increasing activity as the bladder distends, and then electrical silence just before detrusor contraction. In cases of detrusor-sphincter dyssynergia, EMG will show simultaneous sphincter and detrusor activation. Uroflowmetry, in which the maximal velocity of urine flow is measured, can also be helpful if outflow obstruction is suspected, especially if it is used in conjunction with urethral profilometry.

Using these tests abnormal patterns can be divided into the same four pathophysiologic mechanisms outlined previously and can occur singly or in combination: (1) detrusor instability, with involuntary detrusor contraction at less than normal bladder capacity; (2) detrusor insufficiency with high volume, low pressures, and decreased or absent detrusor contractions; (3) increased or nonrelaxing sphincter tone or outlet obstruction; or (4) decreased sphincter tone. If cystometry is not available, the algorithm outlined in Figure 24-2, theoretically designed but as yet untested, may aid in determining the diagnosis.

Management

The importance of management should not be underestimated. Successful treatment of urinary incontinence may (1) permit removal of a chronic indwelling catheter; (2) reduce the risk of urinary tract infection with sepsis; (3) help prevent pressure sores and local infection; (4) eliminate the social stigma; and (5) allow many patients to remain at home who would otherwise be placed in long-term care facilities. Even amelioration of incontinence accomplishes many of these goals.

The first principle of management is to correct the precipitating event, if possible, by reducing enforced bed rest, treating the cause of the acute confusional state, disimpacting feces, prescribing estrogen for atrophic vaginitis or urethritis, administering antibiotics for acute urinary tract infection, changing the offending drug regimen, and correcting metabolic imbalances. More specific measures are guided by other etiologies discovered in the evaluation and are outlined in Table 24-1. In addition, general principles to be followed include fluid and alcohol limitation (especially after supper); formulation of a daily, frequent voiding routine; reduction of xanthine intake such as in coffee or tea; use of absorbent pads; and scrupulous attention to local hygiene and perineal skin care to avoid decubiti and local skin infection. Construction of a voiding chart with notation of when and how frequently the patient is incontinent is important in establishing a baseline that can direct and assess efficacy of therapy.

To maximize therapy for urinary incontinence it is often helpful to combine the four primary pathophysiologic categories into two broader groups: (1) difficulty with urinary storage, encompassing detrusor instability and outlet incompetence; and (2) difficulty with urine evacuation, including detrusor insufficiency and outlet obstruction. For instance, the patient with outlet incompetence suffers from impaired ability to store urine. The other component of storage is detrusor function. If therapy for outlet incompetence is inadequate to restore continence, adding treatment directed at reducing the frequency and force of detrusor contractions may correct the problem. Another patient may have predominantly an uninhibited bladder, but adding estrogen vaginal cream may increase outlet resistance sufficiently to reestablish continence. Conversely, a patient with prostatic hypertrophy and incontinence secondary to obstruction may undergo prostatic resection only to find his incontinence is exacerbated. Removing the obstruction unmasked the

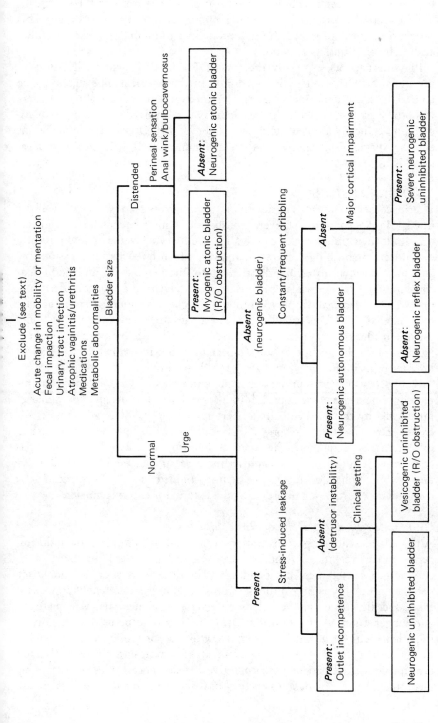

Figure 24-2. Algorithm for approach to diagnosis of urinary incontinence (if cystometry not available).

409

underlying detrusor instability, present in about one-third of these patients, and converted a problem of evacuation into one of urinary storage. This problem can be approached through modalities to inhibit detrusor instability and/or increase outlet resistance.

In some patients, especially those with advanced dementia, all efforts to restore continence meet with frustration. In these patients one may only be able to use a condom catheter in men or intermittent or indwelling catheters in both sexes to deal with the problem. Issues involved with long-term indwelling catheters are dealt with elsewhere [15,16]. Other paraphernalia, including diapers and special clothes, are summarized in another publication [17].

PHARMACOTHERAPY

Pharmacotherapy merits consideration, although its role is not yet well defined. Most agents are relatively nonspecific, with frequent adverse effects that limit their utility in the elderly. Their efficacy as well as safety critically depend on establishing a correct diagnosis, which often requires cystometry and may mean transferring the patient to another facility and additional consultation. Of the available clinical trials, few have included elderly patients and fewer have employed rational drug combinations despite the fact that such combinations usually represent an improvement in efficacy. Nonetheless, medications are frequently effective, and in a patient who has exhausted other therapeutic options, especially when incontinence will lead to long-term institutionalization, a drug trial is warranted.

Knowledge of lower urinary tract neuropharmacology is essential to employing a pharmacologic approach to incontinence. The detrusor is primarily innervated by the parasympathetic nervous system. Cholinergic agonists increase detrusor contractile force and frequency, while anticholinergic agents inhibit detrusor stability. The internal sphincter is primarily under alpha-adrenergic influence. Alpha agonists increase sphincter and urethral resistance while alpha-blocking agents reduce sphincter tone. No medication is consistently effective for disorders of the external urethral sphincter.

Uninhibited Bladder (Detrusor Instability)

Although anticholinergic medications can cause incontinence by inducing acute urinary retention, if the primary problem is detrusor instability, anticholinergics can be used therapeutically. The drug used most commonly for detrusor instability is propantheline (Pro-Banthine), an anticholinergic with more specific effects on the detrusor, fewer central nervous system effects, and longer duration of action than atropine. It should be used with caution in patients with glaucoma, coronary artery disease, or prostatism and avoided unless outlet obstruction has been excluded. However, in the frail, bedbound, multiply impaired patient with cognitive deficits, once causes of temporary incontinence and obvious obstruction have been ruled out, the most likely etiology of incontinence is detrusor instability. If conservative measures to control incontinence as outlined previously fail to work, an empiric trial of antispasmodics or anticholinergics, or both may be undertaken. The patient must be monitored carefully for urinary retention and catheterized promptly if this occurs.

Since detrusor instability can also be associated with irritative lesions in which neurovesical supply is unimpaired, a smooth muscle relaxant such as flavoxate (Urispas) might theoretically be preferable to anticholinergic therapy in these circumstances. Initial enthusiasm for flavoxate has waned recently, however [18,19], and its role is unclear at the present time. Oxybutynin, another smooth muscle relaxant, actually has modest anticholinergic effects as well but is probably no more efficacious than propantheline.

Outlet Incompetence

For sphincter insufficiency, alpha agonists causing an increase in sphincter tone have proved most effective; the two used most commonly are ephedrine and phenylpropanolamine (Propadrine). Phenylpropanolamine is favored by some investigators over ephedrine because it causes less central nervous system stimulation and is subject to less tachyphylaxis. Both drugs should be used cautiously in patients with hypertension or coronary artery disease. Imipramine, with more complex effects on the lower urinary tract, has also been used effectively. In addition to its primary alpha agonist effect, imipramine's milder anticholinergic properties also help to inhibit detrusor instability. In difficult cases in which features of both detrusor instability and sphincter incompetence are present, such as in a poor surgical candidate with severe stress incontinence, combined use of phenylpropanolamine and propantheline has been advocated [18,20].

Detrusor Insufficiency

The most effective drug for detrusor insufficiency, despite variable results, remains bethanechol (Urecholine). It has a narrower spectrum of action, less central nervous system effect, and a longer duration of action than acetylcholine. It is more useful for decompensated myotonic atonic bladders than it is for neurogenically induced atonic or autonomous bladders and should be reserved until mechanical obstruction has been excluded. Theoretical reasons for its frequent inefficacy have been outlined by Finkbeiner and Bissada [18]: first, it will not work well if increased detrusor contractility is opposed by asynchronous sphincter relaxation, which often accompanies the bladder condition for which bethanechol is employed; and second, bethanechol can occasionally induce this sphincter dyssynergia. Thus, if it fails to work adequately, combination with an alpha-adrenergic antagonist such as phenoxybenzamine may be beneficial. Bethanechol's adverse cholinergic side effects are primarily confined to the gastrointestinal system, but it is contraindicated in patients with asthma and should be used cautiously in patients with coronary artery disease and bradycardia.

Outlet Obstruction (Nonanatomic)
Increased outlet resistance due to detrusor–sphincter dyssynergia can occur secondary to neurogenic, functional, or drug-induced (bethanechol) causes. The most effective pharmacotherapy for this condition is an alpha antagonist to decrease sphincter tone, and phenoxybenzamine (Dibenzyline) is the most commonly used drug in this category. Its effectiveness can be predicted by response to parenteral phentolamine. As noted previously, it can be successfully combined with bethanechol. Side effects at low dose are uncommon but at high doses include orthostatic hypotension and reflex tachycardia. Elastic stockings may improve the former and the reflex increase in heart rate is frequently blunted in the elderly.

For a more extensive discussion of urologic pharmacotherapy, more detailed reviews should be consulted [18,20].

Summary
Urinary incontinence is a prevalent and particularly distressing symptom in the elderly that frequently leads to their placement in long-term care facilities and causes considerable morbidity. If it is approached optimistically, evaluated carefully, and treated rationally, it can often be reversed.

References
1. Hobson, W., and Pemberton, J. *The Health of the Elderly at Home.* London: Butterworth, 1955. Pp. 39–44.
2. Milne, J. S. Prevalence of Incontinence in the Elderly Age Group. In F. L. Willington (Ed.), *Incontinence in the Elderly.* New York: Academic Press, 1976.
3. Brocklehurst, J. C., et al. The prevalence and symptomatology of urinary infection in an aged population. *Gerontol. Clin.* 10:242, 1968.
4. Adams, G. F., and McIlwrath, P. M. *Geriatric Nursing.* Oxford, England: Oxford University Press, 1963.
5. DeGroat, W. C., and Booth, A. M. Physiology of the urinary bladder and urethra. *Ann. Intern. Med.* 92:312, 1980.
6. Bates, P., et al. The standardization of terminology of lower urinary tract function. *J. Urol.* 121:551, 1979.
7. Schoenberg, H. W., Gutrick, J. M., and Cote, R. Urodynamic studies in benign prostate hypertrophy. *Urology* 14:634, 1979.
8. McGuire, E. J., et al. The value of urodynamic testing in stress urinary incontinence. *J. Urol.* 124:256, 1980.
9. Eastwood, H. D. H. Urodynamic studies in the management of urinary incontinence in the elderly. *Age Ageing* 8:41, 1979.
10. Brocklehurst, J. C., and Dillane, J. B. Studies of the female bladder in old age. I. *Gerontol. Clin.* 8:285, 1966.

11. Thompson, J. Cystometry in the investigation of urinary incontinence. In W. F. Anderson and B. Isaacs (Eds.), *Current Achievements in Geriatrics.* London: Cassell, 1964.

12. Stamey, T. A. Endoscopic suspension of the vesical neck for urinary incontinence in females. Report on 203 consecutive patients. *Ann. Surg.* 192:465, 1980.

13. Frewen, W. K. An objective assessment of the unstable bladder of psychosomatic origin. *Br. J. Urol.* 50:246, 1978.

14. Jarvis, G. J., and Millar, D. R. Controlled trial of bladder drill for detrusor instability. *Br. Med. J.* 281:1322, 1980.

15. Stamm, W. E. Guidelines for prevention of catheter-associated urinary tract infections. *Ann. Intern. Med.* 82:386, 1975.

16. Warren, J. W., et al. Sequelae and management of urinary infection in the patient requiring chronic catheterization. *J. Urol.* 125:1, 1981.

17. Mandelstam, D. *Incontinence.* London: Disabled Living Foundation, 1977.

18. Finkbeiner, A. E., and Bissada, N. K. Drug therapy for lower urinary tract dysfunction. *Urol. Clin. North Am.* 7:3, 1980.

19. Briggs, R. S., Castleden, C. M., and Asher, M. J. The effect of flavoxate on uninhibited detrusor contractions and urinary incontinence in the elderly. *J. Urol.* 123:665, 1980.

20. Khanna, O. B. Disorders of micturition. Neuropharmacologic basis and results of drug therapy. *Urology* 8:316, 1976.

25. Anesthesia and Surgery

Kenneth L. Minaker
John W. Rowe

Although the elderly comprise only 11 percent of the population, they undergo between 20 and 40 percent of all surgical procedures and account for 50 percent of surgical emergencies [1] and three-quarters of postoperative deaths. Overall surgical mortality is four to eight times higher in patients over age 70 [2]. The percentage of elderly patients undergoing surgery will likely increase as more sophisticated and safe anesthetic and surgical techniques become available and aggressive postoperative care reduces postoperative morbidity. These geriatric patients will carry significant burdens of disability and disease, and correct management will involve consideration of the current risks and benefits of surgery in very old patients. This chapter will review the special preoperative assessment, operative management, and postoperative care of the elderly patient.

Multiple studies show a progressive gradual increase in surgical risk with age in adults until the eightieth year, after which the risk increases dramatically [3–5]. This is consistent with gerontologic observations that the process of aging exerts little impact on functional reserve until late old age. More important than chronologic age in determining the physiologic status and reserve of a surgical candidate is biologic age and a combination of disease, normal age-related physiologic changes, and unquantifiable variables such as the will to live. This underscores the crucial necessity for individualization of surgical risk and refusal to allow age alone to be a major criteria in determining whether a patient will undergo surgery.

Life Expectancy

One factor often underestimated is the life expectancy of the elderly. At age 65 American males can expect to live another 14 years and females 18.4 years. Even at advanced age, such as 85, mean life expectancy approaches six years and at age 90 approaches five years. This information has to be weighed against the natural history of the disease for which surgery is being considered.

It is often thought that surgery in the elderly is for palliation only and that cure is unreasonable. However, the relatively long life expectancy of our aged population and the slow natural history of some surgical diseases often result in surgery being a more attractive alternative, even in a relatively high-risk patient, than chronic morbidity.

The limitation of life expectancy at advanced age is due to the combination of the impact of aging and concomitant associated disease. The process of aging adds its own element of surgical risk and can basically be viewed as limiting the homeostatic reserve [6]. The prevalence of coronary artery, respiratory, and central nervous system disease all increase with age and can be expected to increase surgical risk.

Preoperative Assessment

Preoperative assessment aims to define the present functional status and quality of life of the patient, to identify special vulnerabilities for perioperative morbidity, and to develop a plan for proper preoperative preparation and postoperative management. It is often wise to be aware of the anticipated complications of specific types of surgery and to begin postoperative education and rehabilitation planning before the surgical procedure itself.

This is often a team effort. Starting with the physicians sensitive to geriatric problems, social service and nursing assessment add immeasurably to the preoperative and postoperative care of the patient, culminating in his or her safe discharge home. With this assessment in hand, the surgeon can decide whether to operate.

Specific care must be paid to the cardiopulmonary system and, depending on the urgency of the operation, improvement of the patient's condition before surgery may be approached on emergency or a more leisurely basis. It is crucial to correct hypovolemia, congestive heart failure, or electrolyte abnormalities prior to surgery. Careful attention to the nutritional state of the elderly patient may be justified in the more semielective types of surgery. Postponement of operations in an attempt to reverse long-standing but stable problems is misguided and allows the pathologic "surgical" process to continue.

The elderly surgical patient is likely to be taking numerous medications, and the question of continuing or discontinuing concurrent drug therapy is frequently raised. In general, individual assessment is necessary and continuation of concurrent drug therapy is being increasingly recommended. A general trend is to continue antihypertensive therapy, including beta blockade, up to the time of surgery [7]. Patients with parkinsonism who are receiving L-dopa should have the drug continued up to the time of surgery and resumed as soon as possible after operation [8]. Full digitalization preoperatively may alter the choice of anesthetics, but it is not standard policy to reverse the effects of digitalis or to wait for its effects to wear off before surgery.

Almost as important as the physical condition of the elderly patient is attention to his or her mental state. Sensory deprivation due to impaired vision and hearing must be recognized by all caring for the patient, and extra time should be spent in explaining each aspect of the operation so that anxiety is limited. Preoperative explanation by the anesthetist is not only a humanitarian necessity but has been demonstrated to improve the patient's postoperative course. If there is a past history of postoperative confusion or if any element of brain failure is present preoperatively, it is appropriate to anticipate deterioration in the postoperative period and have a planned and staged approach to management of the postoperative acute confusional state.

Pharmacokinetic and Pharmacodynamic Considerations

Aging influences drug handling in many ways important to anesthetic practice. The blunted respiratory response to hypercarbia or hypoxia is well known as is the gradual decrease in ventilation that occurs with advancing age. These result in a reduced reserve for response to surgical stress. The decrease in blood flow to important organs such as liver and kidney impacts on drug handling [9]. The progressive decline in serum albumin is important in the protein binding of drugs, and the increase in fat with advancing age alters distribution of inhaled lipid-soluble anesthetics. Increased vulnerability to decreases in core temperature during the course of anesthesia may further impair the biodegrading capacity of the aged surgical patient.

INHALED ANESTHETICS
Young and old patients differ in their handling of inhaled anesthetics. The rate of rise of alveolar halothane concentrations is slower in patients over the age of 40 than in younger adults, but arterial halothane concentrations are higher in the elderly, implying increase in anesthetic solubility in the blood of older patients. Venous halothane levels are lower in older patients, implying greater tissue uptake and higher metabolism of halothane in the elderly. After 15 minutes of anesthesia, older patients have been shown to take up 70 percent more halothane than those 40 to 60 years old. The influence of aging on pharmacokinetics of inhaled agents other than halothane has not been examined extensively, but it would appear that enflurane and methoxyflurane share similar characteristics to halothane. Older patients are more easily anesthetized, and the minimum alveolar anesthetic concentration that prevents response to surgical incision in 50 percent of patients decreases with advancing age [10].

INTRAVENOUS ANESTHETICS
The induction of elderly surgical patients with intravenous diazepam is accomplished with lower total doses than are required in young patients. Pentathol induction is more liable to be followed by delayed recovery of consciousness and causes a greater fall in blood pressure in the elderly. Both agents induce early anesthesia because of lipid solubility and altered metabolism. Increase in the volume of distribution results in slower drug clearance with advancing age and contributes to postoperative drowsiness, notably with diazepam. The benefits of the quick action of these agents must be weighed against the lengthy postoperative recovery and contrasted with the slower induction of inhaled anesthetics, which will be largely removed as the surgical procedure finishes.

MUSCLE RELAXANTS

Neuromuscular blockade seems more intense and prolonged, and antagonism to the induced neuromuscular block, that is, reversal of the paralysis, is more difficult with advancing age [11,12]. It has been suggested that the neuromuscular junction is increasingly sensitive to neuromuscular blocking by drugs and that clearance of these agents also is impaired in the elderly. Drugs useful in reversing neuromuscular blockade may also have impaired clearance. If this is confirmed, then short-acting reversing agents such as edrophonium chloride may have a longer, more pronounced effect in the elderly. Increased use of this drug with its known ability to decrease cardiac irritability relative to other reversing agents should improve anesthetic risk.

ANALGESICS

Analgesics perform several functions during anesthesia, including preoperative sedation and intraoperative and postoperative analgesia. Elderly patients have an increase in sensitivity to narcotic analgesics that may complicate anesthetic management [13]. It is uncertain whether enhanced sensitivity to narcotics results from pharmacokinetic changes or pharmacodynamic changes reflecting alterations in central nervous system sensitivity. The quantitation of analgesic effects of morphine in patients undergoing cancer surgery seems to indicate an approximate twofold increase in effectiveness in the elderly [14]. One must also consider that the placebo effect tends to be larger with advancing age. In the very scarce studies of pharmacokinetics of morphine with advancing age, it appears that the elimination half-life and volume of distribution is greater in elderly patients than in healthy young adults. The mechanisms for this might involve decreased hepatic metabolism. The observation that peak analgesia lags behind plasma morphine levels suggests that brain morphine levels are slower to decay than plasma levels. Pain intensity and relief as well as the effects of morphine on mental function require further correlation with pharmacokinetic factors.

Morbidity and Mortality

Anesthesia is becoming more safe in the elderly, with deaths during perioperative and postoperative periods showing a decline from 20 percent before 1960, to 10 percent in the early 1970s, to a 1979 report of 6.2 percent in patients over the age of 80 years [15]. The improved mortality figures reflect advances in surgical and anesthetic technique. In the early 1960s it was reported that perioperative and anesthetic deaths in 85 percent of cases were due to errors in management. Additionally, almost 28 errors in management occurred for each one that caused mortality and 17 percent of nonfatal errors were associated with more than transient morbidity [16]. Anesthetic deaths presently arise exclusively from the irreversibility of the underlying disease, with few of the deaths within 48 hours of operation apparently attributable to the effects of anesthesia or surgery per se [15].

The American Society of Anesthesiologists (ASA) physical status scale (Table 25-1) remains the best available predictor of noncardiac deaths and a fair predictor of cardiac deaths and should be understood by internists contributing to the perioperative care of elderly patients [17]. The largest lesson learned from recent studies is that in ASA classes II and III, the young and elderly have comparable risks from surgery, but that in classes IV and V there is still a disproportionate morbidity and mortality associated with elderly patients, with greater than 25 percent mortality in patients in these two classes.

Invasive preoperative monitoring of cardiopulmonary function using right-sided, balloon-flotation catheterization and arterial blood sampling provides a more detailed documentation of the relevant physiologic status. A recent study suggests that these methods are more predictive of surgical risk than bedside ASA III and IV classification in the elderly. Invasive methods can serve as ongoing monitors of preoperative physiologic "fine-tuning" and early detectors of decompensation during surgery [18]. These techniques represent the newest and most relevant methods of lowering perioperative risk in the elderly.

There is no qualitative change with advancing age in the causes of death in the perioperative period. Aspiration and sudden cardiac difficulty, including arrhythmias, myocardial infarction, and hypotension, are the major causes of death and morbidity. The method of anesthesia is relatively unimportant, and the duration of surgery is surprisingly not a major predictor of mortality.

Deaths occurring during the first 48 hours after surgery are distributed as follows: 10 percent occur during induction of anesthesia, 35 percent occur intraoperatively, and 55 percent occur in the remainder of the first 48 hours [19]. One-half of all deaths in the first 48 hours occur after the patients have returned to the ward and are therefore under the supervision of the surgeon and his or her team. The main types of postoperative morbidity remain the

Table 25-1. American Society of Anesthesiologists (ASA) Physical Status Scale

Class	Physical Status
Cl 1	Normally healthy individual
Cl 2	Patient with mild systemic disease
Cl 3	Patient with severe systemic disease that is not incapacitating
Cl 4	Patient with incapacitating systemic disease that is a constant threat to life
Cl 5	Moribund patient who is not expected to survive 24 hours with or without operation.
E	Added to any class patient undergoing emergency surgery

same with advancing age and reflect the age and disease-associated afflictions of the elderly.

CARDIAC MORBIDITY AND MORTALITY

The National Halothane Study has shown that the overall risk of 0.15 percent for myocardial infarction in the postoperative period is divided equally from the first to the fifth postoperative day. After the fifth day, the rate of infarction drops off dramatically [4]. Of postoperative geriatric deaths 50 percent are due to cardiac disease [2]. Cardiac problems leading to death are divided between arrhythmia, new myocardial infarction, acute pulmonary edema, and progressive congestive heart failure. Overall cardiac function appears to be the major predictor of morbid cardiac events, with congestive heart failure and the presence of a third heart sound carrying equal weight to previous evidence of myocardial infarction in predicting morbidity and mortality.

PULMONARY COMPLICATIONS

The sequence of hypoventilation, atelectasis, and pneumonia is estimated to occur in 20 to 40 percent of all postsurgical patients. The elderly are made particularly prone to this by associated debilitating disease, which prevents early mobilization and impairs mental function, thus interfering with adequate secretion removal. Postoperative mortality associated with pneumonia has been reported to be higher than 50 percent in the elderly age group [20].

Vigorous attempts at early mobilization are essential and require a full team approach, particularly when the patient is confused or disoriented. Careful attention to control of infection, adequate control of pain, and adequate hydration are important in maximizing the elderly patient's ability to cooperate with the required physical therapy.

A larger percentage of elderly patients undergoing thoracotomy will require greater than 24 hours of controlled constant volume ventilation postoperatively. In the over-80 age group, approximately one-quarter of the patients will require similar therapy after upper abdominal surgery [15]. Half of the nonfatal complications after thoracotomy in the elderly comprise atrial fibrillation, retained secretions, or persistent air leak [21]. Early detection and prompt attention are essential.

NONPULMONARY INFECTIONS

Peritonitis and gram-negative sepsis play dominant roles in postoperative morbidity in the elderly. In a 1979 series, gram-negative infection was the second leading cause of death in the postoperative period [15]. As most of this infection is nosocomial in origin, careful attention to handwashing, skin sterilization, and extensive bacteriologic monitoring of transmission routes is necessary. There is adequate evidence that attention to such detail can reduce the risk of this major complication.

POSTOPERATIVE DELIRIUM

Impaired ability to maintain attention and cognitive processes in the postoperative period is common in the elderly. The basic dysfunction in delirium is simultaneous diminution in the ability to think, perceive, and remember. The impact on compliance with the postoperative rehabilitation process is obvious. The common wide fluctuation in patient cooperation makes moment-to-moment individualization of supportive therapy difficult. Delirium with agitation manifests itself most often before the third postoperative day and commonly lasts for 1 to 2 days but may extend in some circumstances to as long as 15 days.

Postoperative delirium may be psychologically or biochemically derived [22]. Psychologically, the elderly can be expected to have a decreased ability to withstand stress. This vulnerability is increased in patients over 50. Additionally, patients with preoperative cognitive impairment may show a deterioration of psychologic functioning postoperatively without the customary lucid interval. Sensory deprivation and decreased ability to adjust to new surroundings, altered sleep patterns, unreasonable fears of surgery, and impaired coping mechanisms all make the elderly more prone to decompensation.

Constant involvement of family and familiar nursing and support staff in as quiet and familiar a surrounding as possible minimizes the stress associated with surgery in the elderly. The fact that eye operations are complicated by a high incidence of postoperative psychiatric states clearly underscores the contribution of sensory deprivation. The fact that cardiotomy induces a larger proportion of postoperative psychiatric complications than other surgical procedures suggests that preoperative anxiety levels about the heart and its function may contribute to greater postoperative stress.

Physiologic stress around the time of surgery plays a major part in inducing postoperative confusional states. Factors common in the elderly that may alter mental function postoperatively include hypothermia, hypoxia, enhanced catecholamine response to stress, and multiple drug therapy. This drug therapy may be related to anesthesia itself or due to concomitant psychoactive agents.

Surgical emergencies are disproportionately frequent in the elderly. With the intensive care required to manage such emergencies comes a greater disruption of both the psychologic and physiologic milieu of the patient. Subsequent sleep deprivation, fatigue, and pain obviously impair the ability of elderly patients to orient themselves in person, place, and time. The threat of death must be considered as a continuing stress.

Management of Postoperative Confusion

All physiologic variables should be corrected, including hypovolemia, electrolyte imbalance, and hypoxia. Appropriate analgesia should be administered. The patient should be oriented to his or her surroundings as much as possible and encouraged to participate in a convalescent routine. Not enough can be said for the continuing presence of a kind and considerate support staff.

Major tranquilizers are effective treatment for postoperative delirium. The hypotensive effects of phenothiazines in postoperative delirium may have been overemphasized. Newer agents such as acetophenazine and haloperidol carry much less hypotensive and cardioirritative action than chlorpromazine and thus represent safer therapy for postoperative delirium. Barbiturates should not be used since they often increase agitation. Restraints should be used only when absolutely necessary and then only when a staff member can be close at hand.

In summary, postoperative delirium or confusion is a crucial diagnostic and therapeutic challenge in the elderly. A checklist approach for environmental causes, infection, necrosis, metabolic causes, drugs, depression with agitation, and cerebral causes including hypoxia and new onset stroke must all be sought and corrected before additional medications are incorporated into any treatment regimen [23]. The common appearance of postoperative bladder problems should make it especially important that urinary retention be considered as a cause of postoperative confusion in the elderly.

Summary

The consensus is that age itself is no barrier to operation and that necessary surgery may be carried out quite safely, provided careful attention is given to preoperative assessment, the treatment of preexisting disease, careful anesthesia, expeditious surgery, and attentive postoperative observation, including treatment of complications and early mobilization. It is probable that in the future a greater number of elderly surgical candidates will derive benefit from more sophisticated perioperative monitoring and more efficient use of the anesthetic measures that are presently available.

References

1. Vowles, K. J. D. Surgery for the Aged. In K. J. D. Vowles (Ed.), *Surgical Problems in the Aged*. Bristol, England: John Wright and Sons, 1979.
2. Cole, W. Medical differences between the young and the aged. *J. Am. Gerontol. Soc.* 18:589, 1970.
3. Soper, K., and McPeek, B. Predicting Mortality for High Risk Surgery. In R. Hirsh, et al. (Eds.), *Health Care Delivery in Anesthesia*. Philadelphia: G. F. Stickley, 1980.
4. Banker, J., et al. (Eds.). The National Halothane Study: A Study of the Possible Association Between Halothane and Post-Operative Hepatic Necrosis. Bethesda, Md.: NIH, National Institute of General Medical Science, 1969.
5. Greenfield, L. *Surgery in the Aged*. Philadelphia, Saunders, 1975. Pp. 139–145.

6. Marx, G., Mateo, C., and Orkin, L. Computer analysis of post-anesthetic deaths. *Anesthesia* 39:54, 1973.
7. Prys-Roberts, C., Meloche, R., and Foex, P. Studies of cardiovascular responses of treated and untreated patients. *Br. J. Anaesth.* 43:122, 1971.
8. Ngai, S. Parkinsonism, levodopa, and anesthesia. *Anesthesia* 37:344, 1972.
9. Shock, N. W. The Physiology of Aging. In J. H. Powers (Ed.), *Surgery of the Aged and Debilitated Patient*. Philadelphia: Saunders, 1968.
10. Gregory, G., Eger, E., and Munson, E. The relationship between age and halothane requirement. *Anesthesia* 30:488, 1969.
11. Lippmann, M., and Rogoff, R. A clinical evaluation of pyridostigmine bromide in the reversal of pancuronium. *Anesth. Analg.* 53:20, 1974.
12. Baraka, A. Irreversible curarization. *Int. Care* 5:244, 1977.
13. Bellville, J., et al. Influence of age on pain relief from analgesics. *J.A.M.A.* 217:1835, 1971.
14. Kaiko, R. Age and morphine analgesia in career patients with postoperative pain. *Clin. Pharmacol. Ther.* 26:823, 1980.
15. Djokovic, J., and Hedley-Whyte, J. Prediction of outcome of surgery and anesthesia in patients over 80. *J.A.M.A.* 242:2301, 1979.
16. Dripps, R., Lamont, A., and Eckenhoff, J. The role of anesthesia in surgical mortality. *J.A.M.A.* 178:261, 1961.
17. Goldman, L. Letter. *N. Engl. J. Med.* 298:340, 1978.
18. Decuercio, L., and Cohn, J. Monitoring operative risk in the elderly. *J.A.M.A.* 243:1350, 1980.
19. Feigal, D., and Blaisdell, F. The estimation of surgical risk. *Med. Clin. North Am.* 163:1131, 1979.
20. Stahlgren, L. An analysis of factors which influence mortality following extensive abdominal operations upon geriatric patients. *Surg. Obstet. Gynecol.* 113:283, 1961.
21. Breyer, R. H., et al. Thoracotomy in patients over age seventy years. *J. Thorac. Cardiovasc. Surg.* 18:187, 1981.
22. Nadelson, T. The psychiatrist in the surgical intensive care unit. *Arch. Surg.* 111:113, 1976.
23. Robertson, J. Anesthesia and the Geriatric Patient. In T. C. Gray, J. F. Nunn, and J. Utting (Eds.), *General Anesthesia* (4th ed.). London: Butterworths, 1980.

26. Ethical Issues

Terrie T. Wetle
Richard W. Besdine

It is probable that no other domestic issue has caught the attention and conscience of the American public and federal system more than long-term care. Technological developments as well as changing social values and practices have led in recent years to dramatic changes in the delivery of long-term care to the aged chronically impaired. New health technology, including sanitation, prevention and treatment of infectious disease, and the development of life-support systems have led to an increased demand for long-term services for persons who, before these scientific advances, would not have survived to require services.

At the same time, the changing nature of families from large, extended multigenerational groups to smaller, nuclear units has begun to limit the potential for "informal," in-home care-giving. Family members are progressively less able or available to provide care, either because of the technological sophistication required or because the traditional care-givers (wives, daughters, and daughters-in-law) have entered the work force [1]. Finally, that group most likely to require long-term care services, the very old, is increasing proportionally faster (a 40 percent increase in those 85 years and older in the past decade) than any other age group in the population.

There is a general sense of suspicion and dissatisfaction regarding the delivery of long-term care. Circumstances of patient abuse, health hazards, and fraud are regularly reported for both institutionalized and noninstitutionalized persons. Increasingly, courts of law are called upon to determine the rights of patients to care, life, and sometimes death. These controversies, related to the delivery of long-term care, are in part a result of unrecognized or unresolved ethical dilemmas.

The care of chronically impaired persons carries the potential for ethical questions from many spheres of philosophy, law, and practice. No other group encompasses such a broad range of conditions, needs, and special problems. Any effort to address the ethical issues related to long-term care is quickly overwhelmed by the array of questions raised, ranging from issues of right to identification, diagnosis, and assessment, through issues related to the right to termination of treatment and "death with dignity." Between these anchor points are raised questions of access, equity, finance, decision-making responsibility, institutionalization, least restrictive alternatives, personal autonomy, normalization, deinstitutionalization, personal obligation, familial obligation, and societal responsibility.

Of the myriad of value dilemmas involved in the delivery of long-term care services, this chapter addresses three categories of questions. The first relates to issues of cost and equal access to service by examining collective versus individual responsibilities in paying for and providing care. The second category explores the individual autonomy of client/patients, and the third category questions the locus of decision-making, namely, who decides what for whom.

Cost and Equal Access: Individual versus Collective Responsibility

The total costs of providing long-term care are difficult to estimate. Speculations for the fiscal year 1980–1981 approximate $30 billion [2]. Every indication predicts both an increased demand for all long-term care services and increased costs per unit of service delivered. The first step in answering this question of cost and equal access is to address individual versus collective responsibility.

Under the concept of individual responsibility, each person is expected to provide for his or her own care through personal resources such as income, savings, and prepaid health and disability insurance. In an expansion of this philosophy, some would hold the families of client/patients responsible as well. Under the concept of collective responsibility, we as a society are considered responsible for the provision of certain types of care to some groups of persons. This may be accomplished through a variety of programs, including direct payment to the client/patient, vendor payments to service providers, or general support of agencies that provide care. Financing for these programs may be from local, state, federal, or philanthropic sources.

There is general agreement that some services are a matter of collective responsibility (for example, sanitation, law enforcement, or education). However, as we enter the realm of long-term care, there is substantial argument over public responsibility to provide service to the chronically impaired.

Happenstance development of laws and financing for long-term care have resulted in a variety of programs that reflect conflicting views of collective responsibility. In some instances, certain services are available to all persons who meet specific criteria: for example, part A of Medicare, for which any person over the age of 65 with the requisite number of quarters of participation in the social security program is eligible. Other services are available based on a physical illness of the patient, for example, Medicare reimbursement for hemodialysis, regardless of the patient's age or financial resources. Finally, some services are made available only to those who are unable to pay for them, exemplified by the Medicaid reimbursement for services to the medically indigent. Combinations of these views may be seen in programs with sliding fee scales or limited "spend-down" provisions.

The lack of clear policy related to collective responsibility leads to inequities in access to service, uneven levels and quality of care, and limited availability of a full range of services to the chronically impaired. For those areas in which collective responsibility *is* acknowledged (Medicaid and Medicare, for example) there is a strong bias toward institutional versus home-based care. Less than 3 percent of Medicare and about 1 percent of Medicaid reimburses home health care [3]. The implicit value statement appears to be that institutional care is a mattter of collective responsibility whereas community-based services are, for the most part, a matter of individual responsibility.

Changing social values have begun to alter this picture, however. As women (the traditional providers of care in the home setting) are less available to offer care to their husbands and parents, *and* as demand for formalized home health services increases, efforts to limit expenditures for institutional care have led to proposed legislation supporting home-based, community-based services. The controversy around these proposals provides clear evidence of conflicting views related to collective versus individual responsibility.

Autonomy of the Individual

A related set of questions is concerned with issues of individual autonomy or the right of the individual to be self-determining and independent. Language reflecting this value can be found in the Older Americans Act, the Federal Council on Aging's Bicentennial Charter for Older Americans, and the Nursing Home Patient's Bill of Rights.

From the Older Americans Act, older persons should be assured (among other rights) "freedom, independence, and the free exercise of individual initiative in planning and managing their own lives" [4]. The Federal Council on Aging's statement expands on this concept by adding ". . . this should encompass not only opportunities and resources for personal planning and managing one's life-style, but support systems for maximum growth and contributions . . ." [5]. The Nursing Home Patient's Bill of Rights declares that each patient should be ". . . fully informed . . . [and allowed] to participate in the planning of his medical treatment" and be ". . . treated with consideration, respect, and full recognition of his dignity and individuality." [6].

The ethical dilemma arises in the translation of these values into practice. What does it mean to assure the autonomy of the individual? Some would argue that this requires not only freedom to choose from an array of available services but also assurance that a *full* array of services is indeed available. This issue has entered into law through litigation on behalf of the developmentally disabled, in that Pennsylvania courts have held that clients should be provided care in the "least restrictive environment." Expanding the initial ruling, the Pennsylvania courts required certain areas to develop less restrictive alternatives appropriate to the needs of the client. A similar philosophy has led to the "normalization" or "mainstreaming" efforts for handicapped children in education.

In 1979 a class action suit, Linden versus King [7], was filed demanding that the Commonwealth of Massachusetts provide a full range of community alternatives for older persons who, without those alternatives, are or will be placed in nursing homes. It argues that the right of the individual to exercise autonomy requires that a full range of services be available. However, it has been documented that such a full range of services is not available in many communities [8,9]. What are the practical limits of this issue? Does society pay for community-based alternatives even when such services are more expensive than institutional care?

What should be done when the client/patient makes choices that will, in the long run, lead to increased suffering or societal expense? Who determines that the client/patient is competent to make care and life-style decisions and how is that determination made?

Locus of Decision-Making

The next question—who decides what for whom?—is at the heart of ethical concerns in long-term care and relates to all aspects of life for the chronically impaired person. Questions to be decided include:

Will a patient be placed in a nursing home or supported in his or her own home?
Will a cognitively impaired person be allowed to manage his or her affairs?
Will treatment be initiated for a seriously ill or severely impaired person?
Will treatment be terminated when the quality of life is severely reduced by pain or cognitive loss?

Not only are the answers to these specific questions in conflict, but there is great controversy regarding who should participate in these difficult decisions. On the one hand, some argue that the individual has the right to make *all* decisions regarding his or her life in even the most extreme circumstances [10,11]. Others believe that well-trained, experienced professionals are in a much better position to make care decisions than patients themselves. Still others believe that decisions should include all persons who have interest and involvement in the case. Obviously, no one format will fit all cases, but we would like to suggest some guidelines that may be useful.

1. Each client/patient has the right to a careful and complete assessment of health status, including functional and cognitive capabilities
2. Then, if the patient is cognitively intact, he or she should be informed of the resources and services that are available and relevant to his or her needs
3. Potential outcomes and risks of treatment or service should be carefully explained, and the client/patient then may choose to accept or refuse services and treatments offered

4. If service or treatment is refused, the decision stands; if treatment is
   sought, then the physician or program administrator decides in consultation with the patient and involved others whether the treatment or service
   is initiated

If there is cognitive loss, the process is more difficult. Robert Burt [12] in
his book *Taking Care of Strangers: The Rule of Law in Doctor-Patient Relations* reminds us that cognitive impairment, or "incompetence" as it is
referred to in the courts, is not an either-or issue but rather forms a continuum. A person who is competent to make some decisions may not be
competent to make others. For example, a woman in the earlier stages of
Alzheimer's disease may no longer be able to manage her own finances but
may understand the issues quite well enough to refuse or accept major surgery.

Physicians, families, and other providers of service have a responsibility to
include the client/patient in all appropriate decision-making. If errors are
to be made, they should be made on the side of autonomy rather than paternalism [13]. However, there *are* patients who are unable to take part in
decision-making, either because they are unconscious or severely emotionally
or cognitively impaired. In these circumstances, care decisions should involve
the collaboration of persons close to that client/patient through service responsibilities, familial, pastoral, or friendship ties.

The most commonly publicized cases under these circumstances involve
"death with dignity" or decisions to forego or terminate treatment, as evidenced by two recent State Supreme Court decisions. In the now famous
Karen Quinlan case [14], the New Jersey Supreme Court was asked to ap-
point Quinlan's father as guardian so that he could direct termination of
treatment for his unconscious daughter. In the Saikewicz case [15], the
Massachusetts Supreme Judicial Court ruled that a decision to withhold
painful treatment of incurable leukemia for an uncommunicative, profoundly retarded man should be made by a judge rather than an appointed
guardian. In both cases, however, the court relied heavily on the testimony
and opinions of "expert" witnesses and family members. It should be recognized that in the vast majority of such circumstances, decisions are made
without legal or judicial intervention, and there are virtually no recorded
criminal prosecutions against physicians for such actions or against family
members acting in collaboration with physicians [12,16].

The real issue, then, is to recognize that each of us will face the task of
making long-term care decisions. We will make these decisions as physicians
or social workers, as health planners or attorneys, as children or spouses, and
perhaps, someday for ourselves as patients. The quality of these decisions is
dependent, in large part, on our recognition and consideration of the ethical
components involved.

At every step of the identification, assessment, disposition, treatment, and finally death of the patient, ethical judgments are essential in the decision-making process. Failure to identify and evaluate the ethical aspects of any problem guarantees that service decisions will be fragmented, based on incomplete information, and inadequate over the long run. Little of our formal training as professionals prepares us for these difficult, often tragic choices. It is our responsibility as concerned researchers, educators, and practitioners to acknowledge, study, and discuss openly the ethical questions that impinge upon our work and the lives of our clients and, in this way, to improve the quality of life for those who are served and for those who serve them.

References

1. Smith, R. E. (Ed.). The subtle revolution: women at work. *The Urban Institute: Policy and Research Report.* Vol. 9, 1979. P. 1.
2. Congressional Budget Office. *Long Term Care for the Elderly and Disabled.* Washington, D.C.: U.S. Government Printing Office, 1977.
3. Butler, P. *Financing Non-Institutional Long-Term Care Services for the Elderly and Chronically Ill: Alternatives to Nursing Homes.* Washington, D.C.: Legal Services Corporation, 1978.
4. Older Americans Act, Public Law 89-73, July 14, 1965. See also Older Americans Act, as amended, Public Law 95-65, July 11, 1977.
5. Administration on Aging. *Federal Council on Aging Bicentennial Charter.* Washington, D.C.: Department of Health and Human Services, 1976.
6. Nursing Home Patient's Bill of Rights. See Code of Federal Regulations, 20 CFR 405.1121 (K) and 45 CFR 249.12(a)(1)b, 1974.
7. Linden vs. King. U.S. District Court of Massachusetts, 79-862-T, 1979.
8. O'Brien, J., and Wetle, T. *Analysis of Conflict in Coordination of Aging Services.* A Report to the Administration on Aging, Portland State University, Portland, Oregon, 1975.
9. Pearson, D., and Wetle, T. Long-Term Care. In S. Jonas (Ed.), *Health Care Delivery in the United States.* New York: Springer, 1980.
10. Szasz, T. *Law, Liberty and Psychiatry: An Inquiry into the Social Uses of Mental Health Practices.* New York: Macmillan, 1963.
11. Szasz, T. *Psychiatric Slavery.* New York: Free Press, 1976.
12. Burt, R. *Taking Care of Strangers: The Rule of Law in Doctor-Patient Relations.* New York: Macmillan, 1979.
13. Halper, T. The double edged sword: paternalism as a policy in the problems of aging. *Milbank Mem. Fund. Q.* 58:472, 1980.
14. In re Quinlan, 335 A.2nd. 647, 1976.
15. Superintendent of Belchertown State School vs. Saikewicz, 370 NE3d 417, 1977.
16. Veatch, R. *Death, Dying, and the Biological Revolution: Our Last Quest for Responsibility.* New Haven: Yale University Press, 1976.

27. Research in Gerontology

John W. Rowe

Advances in the care of the elderly ultimately depend on the development of increased understanding of the aging process. As interest in and support for gerontologic research increase, there is enhanced need for clear recognition of the methodologic obstacles inherent with this type of research. Experience has identified several perils and pitfalls that are characteristic of research in aging [1]. This chapter will review some of these special considerations with particular emphasis on clinical investigation.

Subject Selection

Several important considerations govern the conduct and evaluation of clinical gerontologic studies. The most important factor is subject selection. In the past, geriatric literature was often tainted by a lack of attention to the medical status of the subjects being studied. Not infrequently, medical students or hospital employees constituted the young group, while the old group was comprised of residents of long-term care facilities or, in some cases, patients in acute-care hospitals. Although these individuals were generally screened to exclude those with an abnormality of the particular organ system under study, they were often disabled or multiply impaired and were suboptimal for a study of the physiologic concomitants of normal aging. In such studies, differences between young and old individuals were a complex mixture of disease-related and age-related effects and failed to provide insight into the normal aging process.

During the past several years, a new phase in gerontologic research has emerged in which investigators carefully scrutinize study subjects in an effort to avoid, to whatever degree possible, contamination from disease processes. Careful attention to exclusion of diseased individuals and those taking medications, while it may be viewed as "cleaning up" the physiologic data, also entails risk. One must be aware that intensive screening of the population may result in a select group of elderly superperformers whose data do not reflect the influence of age-related changes. For instance, in attempting to exclude diabetics, one might adopt criteria by which individuals with a two-hour postprandial blood glucose greater than 140 mg/dl would be excluded. Since carbohydrate tolerance is well known to decline with age in non-diabetics, the application of this uniform criterion to all age groups would result in an increasingly stringent selection procedure with advancing age. The marked changes in carbohydrate tolerance with age would result in only a small fraction of individuals in the eighth or ninth decade of life qualifying for the study. Since systolic blood pressure increases with age, a similar selection effect would be introduced in studies excluding all individuals with systolic pressure over 130 mm Hg. In these examples, generally accepted age-adjusted criteria for normality are available and might be applied as a screening technique. However, such guidelines are lacking for most variables.

Investigators embarking on gerontologic studies should also be aware that differences in habits, such as alcohol or caffeine consumption or tobacco use, might introduce apparent age effects. A reasonable approach seems to be that of (1) avoiding the presence of overt clinical diseases or administration of medications and (2) carefully describing the study population and the selection criteria applied to all age groups.

An additional approach is inclusion of individuals from across the adult age range rather than just young and old adults. Such a strategy provides insight not only into the status of old individuals but also some view of the change in the variable during the life cycle. Since most age-related changes in physiologic variables have been found to be linear, the finding of a marked change in middle age or late middle age suggests the presence of an underlying disease process.

Clinical Relevance of Aging Changes

Once we define a normal change with age, it is important to understand that normality does not imply harmlessness. If healthy old individuals perform less well on glucose tolerance tests than young individuals, that does not imply that the carbohydrate intolerance of the elderly, which is "normal" for their age, is harmless. That conclusion would require a study of another dependent variable—for example, cardiovascular complications or death—since it may be that among the normal 80-year-olds, those with the worst carbohydrate tolerance are actually at greater risk for these complications. Although systolic blood pressure increases "normally" with age, that does not mean it is harmless. Advancing age is a risk factor for diseases and death. Just because we define some age-related changes as normative, let us not overlook their potential adverse effects.

On the other hand, it is important clinically to know which changes occur as a function of normal aging and which do not. Perhaps the most important change that occurs with age is no change. Too frequently physicians, because they lack a concept of normative aging, will ascribe a diagnosis to an individual with a normal age-related finding. Hematocrit, for instance, does not change with normal aging [2], and thus "anemia of old age" is not a meaningful diagnosis.

Cross-Sectional and Longitudinal Studies

Two general study designs are available to clinical gerontologists. In cross-sectional studies, groups of various ages are observed and age-related differences are sought. In longitudinal studies, serial prospective measurements are obtained in one group of subjects at specified intervals, and the slopes for these variables or the age-related changes are determined. Since the human life span is so long, most longitudinal studies follow subjects in several age cohorts throughout the adult age range concurrently; thus, slopes for different ages can be compared.

Cross-sectional studies must be interpreted with caution since there are several ways in which they may not reflect true age-related changes. One error in design is based on a common misconception of the human life cycle. It is often assumed that the growth-and-development phase ends before the age of 20 and is followed by a prolonged "plateau phase," during which the biologic or physiologic variable under study is stable, and then, at about the age of 60 years, by the onset of a fairly rapid decline. However, in terms of most of the variables that have been found to change with age, the growth-and-development phase ends near the age of 20 to 30 years and is followed by a gradual, often linear, decline. Misconceptions of the life cycle have also introduced error into animal studies in which the animals (particularly rats) used as the young adult group were still undergoing rapid growth and development and had not yet reached maturity.

Selective Mortality

In the interpretation of cross-sectional studies, it is important to remember that subjects over the age of 75 represent a sample of biologically superior survivors from a cohort that has experienced at least a 75 percent mortality. If the variable under study is related to survival, either because it is a risk factor or because it has a protective effect, a cross-sectional study will seem to show age-related differences that do not exist. This effect, called selective mortality, is shown in Figure 27-1. The figure concerns an imaginary study

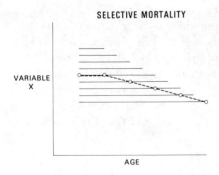

Figure 27-1. Influence of selective mortality on age trends in cross-sectional data. Horizontal lines indicate values for variable X, which does not change with age. Increasing levels of X are associated with increased risk of death (see text).

of the influence of age on the plasma concentration of "factor X," a risk factor that is found at widely varying levels in the population but does not change with age. Since X is related to survival, a group with a very high level will have a shortened life span, and, on the basis of this variable, a group with a low level will have a normal life span. In a cross-sectional study, values for the subjects 30 and 40 years old are similar in both means and variance. The 50-year-old cohort, however, has lost its members with the highest values, and the mean value is less, with a lower variance. This trend continues with advancing age, and the cross-sectional results wrongly suggest that factor X declines with age. This serious methodologic obstacle can be avoided with use of a prospective longitudinal study design, in which each subject is followed over time and the rate of change of each variable is calculated for each age group followed. As shown by the horizontal lines in Figure 27-1, no age effect is indicated if this method is applied to the study of factor X. An effect similar to that of selective mortality may be introduced in cross-sectional studies by any cause of variation in follow-up—including death, illness, and change in geographic location—that is related to the level of the variable under study.

Changes in Populations

Non–age-dependent differences between age groups of a population may introduce error into age trends based on cross-sectional observations. The origin of the differences between age groups might be quite diverse, including educational, nutritional, environmental, and other influences that would result in misleading data regarding the possible effects of age. This type of effect is shown in Figure 27-2, which contains cross-sectional and longitudinal data from the Framingham Study on the impact of age on weight [2]. Whereas the cross-sectional data, based on a single examination, indicate a decline in weight with age, the longitudinal data, based on five examinations over a period of 18 years, suggest a different trend. The 35-year-old subjects are increasing weight rapidly and approaching a weight, eight years after their initial examination, that is clearly higher than that initially recorded for the 43-year-old subjects. Since the analysis only includes subjects who survived for at least 18 years after the first examination, neither selective mortality nor another cause of variation in follow-up study is responsible for this effect. The longitudinal data, shown by the lines in Figure 27-2, indicate that weight is changing in the entire population and that the general tendency to gain weight decreases with age.

Drawbacks of Longitudinal Studies

Despite their advantages over cross-sectional studies, longitudinal studies may also have major drawbacks, including the need to observe a stable popu-

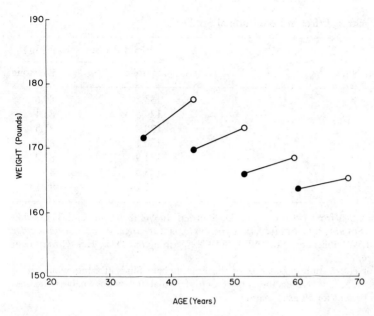

Figure 27-2. Influence of age on weight based on cross-sectional and longitudinal analyses. While the cross-sectional data (filled circles) suggest that weight declines with age, the longitudinal data (lines connecting filled and open circles) indicate that weight is actually increasing with age in all groups and that this effect becomes progressively less pronounced in the older age groups.

lation over a long period and a particular sensitivity to alterations in methods. Subtle changes in laboratory techniques over several years may introduce "laboratory drifts" that are difficult to separate from age-related changes. An example is the "aging" of a sphygmomanometer. In addition, when subjects return at regular intervals and become increasingly familiar with the testing environment, a "learning" or "stress" effect may introduce error into serial measurements.

An example of such an effect is depicted in Table 27-1 in which systolic and diastolic blood pressures at the first seven biannual examinations of the Framingham Study are depicted. The data were selected from a population who had completed all seven examinations, thus removing the possibility of selective mortality or differential follow-up. The researchers set out to determine the influence of age on blood pressure and the impact of high blood pressure on morbidity from heart disease. At the first visit, the averages were 133 systolic and 85 diastolic. Surprisingly, the second visit produced 129 systolic and 82 diastolic. At the third visit, blood pressure was 128 over 81 and still going down! Six years and many, many dollars later, they had found out that blood pressure declines with age—which was very unlikely! For the subsequent visits blood pressure rose, and the initial decrease is at-

Table 27-1. Stress Effect in Longitudinal Studies*

| Examination No. | Blood Pressure (mm Hg) | |
	Systolic	Diastolic
1	133.2	84.6
2	129.6	82.4
3	128.2	81.5
4	130.1	82.6
5	131.9	83.2
6	133.9	84.3
7	135.2	85.1

Source: Data taken from J. Gordon and D. Shurtleff. In W. B. Kannel and T. Gordon (Eds.), *The Framingham Study: An Epidemiologic Investigation of Cardiovascular Disease.* DHEW Publication No. (NIH) 74-478. Washington, D.C.: U.S. Government Printing Office, 1973.

* Data are for entire study population of the Framingham Study. Examinations are at two-year intervals. To exclude the impact of differential follow-up, analysis includes only subjects present for all examinations.

tributed to the "stress effect." Familiarity with the testing environment has a measurable effect. Four years passed before the first useful data for calculating slopes were collected. Perhaps one can make more frequent measures in the beginning to accustom participants to the testing environment rather than spend four years doing it. If one ignored the effect and calculated slopes using all the data, the slopes would be much less steep than those reflecting the actual effect of age.

Planning a Longitudinal Study

The major elements in a longitudinal study are the size of the samples, the frequency of measurements, and the duration of the study. Clearly, a variable that changes dramatically with age and is easily measured accurately need only be tested a few times before age-related changes are well defined. On the other hand, variables that change slowly with age and are difficult to measure accurately require frequent observations over a long period. Quantitation of the factors involved in the design of longitudinal studies has been made possible by the work of Schlesselman [3]. Appropriate strategies for each variable can now be estimated once reliable cross-sectional data or limited longitudinal data are available.

Recognition of these special considerations will improve the utility of the data for gerontologic studies and contribute to the necessary expansion of our understanding of the aging process as well as the interaction of aging-related and disease-related changes.

437

References

1. Rowe, J. W. Clinical research in aging: strategies and directions. *N. Engl. J. Med.* 297:1332, 1977.
2. Gordon, J., and Shurtleff, D. In W. B. Kannel and T. Gordon (Eds.), *The Framingham Study: An Epidemiologic Investigation of Cardiovascular Disease.* DHEW Publication No. (NIH) 74-478. Washington, D.C.: U.S. Government Printing Office, 1973.
3. Schlesselman, J. J. Planning a longitudinal study: I. Sample size determination. II. Frequency of measurement and study duration. *J. Chronic Dis.* 26: 553, 561, 1973.

Index

senile, 246
  compared to osteoporosis, 247
  and trauma in falls, 394
Osteoporosis, 148, 246–254
  causes of, 247–249
  complications of, 250–254
  circumscripta, 259
  diagnosis of, 249
  management of, 247, 249–250
  in menopause, 160, 161, 243, 244,
    247, 249, 250
Oxazepam, 51, 128, 129, 130
Oxybutynin, in detrusor instability, 411
Oxygen
  arterial tension of, 371, 372
  basal consumption of, 323–324
  cerebral consumption of, 56
  maximum rate of consumption of,
    189
  therapy at home, 378
Oxytocin, side effects of, 176

Pacemaker, cardiac
  age-related changes of, 192
  artificial, 204
Pacemaker theory of aging, 23
Paget's disease of bone, 254–263
  local manifestations of, 257–260
  systemic manifestations of, 261
  treatment of, 261–263
Pain
  abdominal, acute, 314
  cognitive impairment in, 105
  drug therapy for, 42, 45–46
    analgesic agents in, 42, 45–46, 277,
      418
    anesthetic agents in, 415–423
  in legs, 230–233
    in intermittent claudication, 227–
      228, 230, 233
  in osteoarthritis, 274, 275
    management of, 277, 278
  in osteoporotic compression fractures,
    251, 252
  in Paget's disease, 255, 257, 258, 261,
    262
  in peripheral vascular disease, 230,
    231

at rest, 230
Palsy, progressive supranuclear, 73
Pancreas, 308–309
  in normal aging, 308
  pathologic conditions of, 218, 308–
    309, 314
Pancreatitis, 308
  acute, 314
  management of, 308–309
Pantothenic acid, 330
Paranoid thinking and behavior, 91, 93,
  115
Parasympathetic function in aging, 151
Parathyroid gland, 147–149
  age-related changes in, 147–148
  adenomas of, 149
  in hyperparathyroidism, 148–149,
    248, 280
  in pseudogout, 280
  surgery of, 149
Parathyroid hormone levels
  age-related changes in, 147–148
  in hyperparathyroidism, 148–149
  in osteoporosis, 248
Parkinsonism, 71–73, 111
  dementia associated with, 111
  differential diagnosis of, 81
  drug-induced, 48, 49, 119
  drug therapy for, 48, 72–73, 365
  orthostatic hypotension in, 218
Parotid gland
  in normal aging, 298
  in Sjögren's syndrome, 286
Pathologic conditions in elderly
  multiple, 8–9, 10, 39
  social pathology as cause of, 29–32
Pelvic examinations, 10
Pelvic tumors, urinary incontinence in,
  404
Pelvis, Paget's disease of, 259, 261
Pemphigus vulgaris, 389
Penicillamine, 284
Penicillin, 363, 364
  in pneumonia, 353
Pentothal, 417
Peptic ulceration of stomach and duodenum, 301–303
  management of, 52, 303–304